FOURTH EDITION

Project Planning, Implementation, and Evaluation

A GUIDE FOR NURSES AND INTERPROFESSIONAL TEAMS

James L. Harris, PhD, APRN-BC, MBA, CNL, FAAN

Linda A. Roussel, PhD, RN, NEA-BC, CNL, FAAN

Catherine Dearman, RN, PhD

Patricia L. Thomas, PhD, RN, NEA-BC, ACNS-BC, CNL, FAAN, FNAP, FACHE

JONES & BARTLETT
LEARNING

World Headquarters
Jones & Bartlett Learning
25 Mall Road
Burlington, MA 01803
978-443-5000
info@jblearning.com
www.jblearning.com

Jones & Bartlett Learning books and products are available through most bookstores and online booksellers. To contact Jones & Bartlett Learning directly, call 800-832-0034, fax 978-443-8000, or visit our website, www.jblearning.com.

Production Credits
Vice President, Product Management: Marisa R. Urbano
Vice President, Product Operations: Christine Emerton
Director, Content Management: Donna Gridley
Director, Project Management and Content Services:
  Karen Scott
Director, Product Management: Matthew Kane
Product Manager: Tina Chen
Content Strategist: Paula-Yuan Gregory
Project Manager: Jessica deMartin
Project Specialist: Lori Weidert
Senior Digital Project Specialist: Angela Dooley
Digital Project Specialist: Rachel DiMaggio
Senior Marketing Manager: Jennifer Scherzay

Content Services Manager: Colleen Lamy
VP, Manufacturing and Inventory Control: Therese Connell
Product Fulfillment Manager: Wendy Kilborn
Composition: S4Carlisle Publishing Services
Project Management: S4Carlisle Publishing Services
Cover Design: Michael O'Donnell
Text Design: Michael O'Donnell
Senior Media Development Editor: Troy Liston
Rights & Permissions Manager: John Rusk
Rights Specialist: Benjamin Roy
Cover Image (Title Page, Part Opener, Chapter Opener):
  © Yavdat/Shutterstock.
Printing and Binding: McNaughton and Gunn

24834-0

Library of Congress Cataloging-in-Publication Data
Names: Harris, James L. (James Leonard), 1956- editor. | Roussel, Linda,
  editor. | Dearman, Catherine, editor. | Thomas, Patricia L., 1961-
  editor.
Title: Project planning, implementation, and evaluation : a guide for
  nurses and interprofessional teams / edited by James L. Harris, Linda
  Roussel, Catherine Dearman, Patricia L. Thomas.
Other titles: Project planning and management (Harris)
Description: Fourth edition. | Burlington, MA : Jones & Bartlett Learning,
  [2023] | Preceded by Project planning and management : a guide for
  nurses and interprofessional teams / edited by James L. Harris, Linda
  Roussel, Catherine Dearman, Patricia L. Thomas . Third edition. [2020].
  | Includes bibliographical references and index.
Identifiers: LCCN 2021044277 | ISBN 9781284248340 (paperback)
Subjects: MESH: Nursing Administration Research--methods | Quality
  Improvement | Program Evaluation | Program Development--methods |
  Planning Techniques | Interprofessional Relations
Classification: LCC RT89 | NLM WY 105 | DDC 362.17/3068--dc23
LC record available at https://lccn.loc.gov/2021044277

Printed in the United States of America
27 26 25 24 23   10 9 8 7 6 5 4 3 2 1

Contents

CHAPTER 6 Using Findings from Organizational Analysis and Clinical Needs Assessment to Frame Improvement Projects and Implementation 127

CHAPTER 7 Synthesizing, Leveling, and Assessing the Fidelity of Evidence in Support of Project Implementation and Proposed Interventions 149

Preface

Textbooks are references for students, faculty, interprofessional teams, and consumers of care. As healthcare organizations are challenged to maintain a competitive edge and relative advantage, multiple strategies are required. What one views as a crisis situation in one healthcare organization may provide an opportunity for creativity and innovation in another. This situation offers transformative, transformational, and challenging opportunities. As a result, meaningful interprofessional quality improvement projects add quantum value and contribute to new evidence.

The authors' dedication as educators, administrators, clinicians, and nurse researchers led to them updating this fourth edition of the text in an attempt to meet the constant healthcare changes, as well as reflect updates in the recent release of the *Future of Nursing Report 2020–2030,* the revised *Essentials of Nursing,* and the myriad of challenges within any organization. As healthcare environments continue to require up-to-date information, the acknowledgment of interpretive design, biotechnologies, computational technologies, interprofessional project team assignments, and learning, they form collaborative improvement teams. The collective talents and insights of teams and their engagement are necessary if the challenges of providing quality, safe, and efficient care are to be met. As interprofessional teams work together, new behaviors develop and an understanding that embraces the contributions from other disciplines emerges.

The authors contend that the content in the *Fourth Edition* is not all-inclusive, but rather a snapshot for designing, updating, and evaluating interprofessional quality improvement projects that transcend a global care continuum. This edition's content provides an introspective foundation for successful project planning and management, interprofessional team management, appreciative inquiry, implementation science, team synergy, use of a needs assessment, and metrics to shape sustainable project outcomes. Based on comments from students, faculty, external reviewers, biomedical librarians, and institutional review boards, this text features essential information related to influences and determinants of projects. Based on additional comments, this edition also incorporates information on team science, big data, literature synthesis, evidence fidelity, and organizational alignment to projects.

The authors have provided information in the *Fourth Edition* that will challenge interprofessional teams to become innovative forces dedicated to developing projects that improve healthcare delivery, innovation, and discovery. These skills enhance a team's vision, which serves as a compass to guide meaningful projects and spread evidence, add value, and engender a culture of sustainable change.

James L. Harris
Linda Roussel
Catherine Dearman
Patricia L. Thomas

Acknowledgments

The authors acknowledge each of the contributors of this text, mentors who have guided our visionary careers, and the review comments from diverse individuals and disciplines represented. In an era of constant change imposed by a pandemic and need to join forces toward normalization, the call for action by transformational leaders who support and encourage interprofessional quality improvement team activities is paramount. Projects create pathways for patient-centered care, as well as opportunities for synergy, evidence-based knowledge creation, and directions for the future to meet the demands of a global society facing any future healthcare crises.

To our families, colleagues, and external reviewers who supported this edition, we offer our gratitude for the encouragement and guidance. To the staff at Jones & Bartlett Learning, your consistent support and unwavering direction are equally appreciated.

James L. Harris
Linda Roussel
Catherine Dearman
Patricia L. Thomas

Contributors

Michael Bleich, PhD, RN, NEA-BC, FNAP, FAAN
President and CEO
NursDynamics, LLC
Senior Professor and Director,
VCUSON Langston Center for
Innovation in Quality and Safety
Ballwin, MO

Lolita Chappel-Aiken, PhD, RN
Chair of Graduate Programs
Division of Nursing
School of Health Sciences
Winston-Salem State University
Winston-Salem, NC

Clista Clanton, MSLS
Biomedical Library
University of South Alabama
Mobile, AL

Catherine Dearman, PhD, RN
Adjunct Faculty
University of West Florida
Pensacola, FL

Todd Harlan, DNP, RN
Associate Professor of Nursing
Chair, Community Mental Health
Nursing
University of South Alabama
Mobile, AL

James L. Harris, PhD, MBA, APRN-BC, CNL, FAAN
Professor of Nursing
University of South Alabama
Mobile, AL

Carolyn Thomas Jones, DNP, MSPH, RN
Lead Instructor, Master of Applied
Clinical and Preclinical Research
Assistant Professor of Nursing, College
of Nursing
The Ohio State University
Columbus, OH

Shea Polancich, PhD, RN
Assistant Professor of Nursing
University of Alabama, Birmingham
Birmingham, AL

Bettina Riley, PhD, RN
Associate Professor Nursing
University of South Alabama
Mobile, AL

Dionne Roberts, PhD, FNP-C, CNE
Associate Professor & FNP/DNP
Program Director
FNP (MSN and DNP) Director
Winston-Salem State University
Winston-Salem, NC

Linda Roussel, PhD, RN, NEA-BC, CNL, FAAN
Professor of Nursing
Cizik School of Nursing
The University of Texas Health Science
Center at Houston
Houston, TX

Patricia L. Thomas, PhD, RN, NEA-BC, ACNS-BC, CNL, FACHE, FNAP, FAAN
Associate Dean Nursing Faculty Affairs
and Associate Professor
Cohn College of Nursing
Wayne State University
Detroit, MI

Kathryn M. Ward-Presson, DNP, RN, NEA-BC
Jonas Scholar in Veterans
Healthcare Alumni
Raleigh, NC

Lonnie K. Williams, MSN, RN
Educational Consultant
Washington, DC

Janet E. Winter, DNP, MPA, RN, FNAP
Associate Dean of Undergraduate
Programs in Nursing
Cook DeVos Health Science Center
Kirkhof College of Nursing
Grand Valley State University
Grand Rapids, MI

Case Exemplar Contributors

Jennifer Anne Blalock, RN
Former Graduate Student
University of South Alabama
Mobile, AL

Amy Campbell, DNP, MSN, RN
Assistant Professor
University of South Alabama
Mobile, AL

Catherine Dearman, PhD, RN
Adjunct Faculty
University of West Florida
Pensacola, FL

Wes Garrison, DNP, RN, MBA
Associate Chief Nursing Officer
Northeast Georgia Medical Center
Gainesville, GA

Kimberly Goins, MSN, RN
Ardmore, AL

Todd Harlan, DNP, RN
Associate Professor of Nursing
Chair, Community Mental Health
Nursing
University of South Alabama
Mobile, AL

James L. Harris, PhD, APRN-BC, MBA, CNL, FAAN
Professor of Nursing
University of South Alabama
Mobile, AL

Carolyn Thomas Jones, DNP, MSPH, RN
Lead Instructor, Master of Applied
Clinical and Preclinical Research
Assistant Professor of Nursing, College
of Nursing
The Ohio State University
Columbus, OH

Theodora Ledford, MSN, RN, CNL
Clinical Nurse Leader
Charles George VA Medical Center
Asheville, NC

Jacqueline M. Lollar, DNP, RN
Assistant Professor of Nursing
University of South Alabama
Mobile, AL

K. Michele Lyons, MN, RN
Southeastern Louisiana University
Hammond, LA

Margaret Mitchell, DNP, MN, FNP
Former Graduate Student
University of South Alabama
Mobile, AL

Terri Poe, DNP, RN, NE-BC
Chief Nursing Officer
University of Alabama Hospitals
Birmingham, AL

Bettina Riley, PhD, RN
Associate Professor
University of South Alabama
Mobile, AL

Linda Roussel, PhD, RN, NEA-BC, CNL, FAAN
Professor of Nursing
Cizik School of Nursing
The University of Texas Health Science
  Center at Houston
Houston, TX

Heather Surcouf, DNP, MSN, BSN, FNP
Methodist Health Systems Foundation
Slidell, LA

Patricia L. Thomas, PhD, RN, NEA-BC, ACNS-BC, CNL, FACHE, FNAP, FAAN
Associate Dean Nursing Faculty Affairs
  and Associate Professor
Cohn College of Nursing
Wayne State University
Detroit, MI

Kathryn M. Ward-Presson, DNP, RN, NEA-BC
Jonas Scholar in Veterans Healthcare
  Alumni
Raleigh, NC

Lonnie K. Williams
Educational Consultant
Washington, DC

Swapna Thomas, DNP, APRN, FNP-BC
Primary Care Practice
Houston TX

Key Foundations of Successful Quality Project Planning, Implementation, Evaluation, and Management: An Overview

James L. Harris
Bettina Riley

CHAPTER OBJECTIVES

1. Differentiate between a quality improvement project, project plan, and project management for deliverable outcomes.
2. Discern the differences between the scope of quality improvement projects and research.
3. Discuss the importance of legislation, health policy, and economic conditions when designing quality improvement projects.
4. Identify historical influences, determinants, and unintended consequences/ risks related to a well-defined quality improvement project in a culturally diverse healthcare environment.
5. Identify requisite skills and techniques of the project leader and designated team members whether on-site or virtual when designing value-based quality improvement projects from inception to completion, including dissemination of outcomes.

KEY TERMS

Continuous quality improvement
Design
Diversity
Economics
Environment
Evidence-based
Health disparities
Health policy
History
Influences and determinants
Just culture
Legislation
Management
Organizational culture
Outcomes

Political environment
Project budget
Project life cycle
Project management
Project plan
Quality improvement
Regulations
Research
Social factors
Stakeholders
Sustainability
Teams
Unintended consequences
Value
Virtual environment

ROLES

Analyzer
Communicator
Designer

Educator
Leader
Manager

PROFESSIONAL VALUES

Civility
Ethics
Inclusivity
Integrity

Norms
Patient- and customer-centeredness
Quality
Values

CORE COMPETENCIES

Analysis
Appreciative inquiry
Assessment
Communication
Critical thinking
Emotional intelligence
Evidence-based practice

Health policy knowledge
Innovation
Regulatory knowledge
Risk anticipation and mitigation of
    unintended consequences
Systems thinking
Understanding of civility and diversity

Introduction

Vision coupled with transformational change is central to the future success of efficient healthcare delivery in an evolving global economy. What was once merely pondered by many in the healthcare arena has now evolved into sustainable project plans and value-based programs that are driven by the basic instinct of survival. With release of the 2020–2030 Future of Nursing report (National Academies of

Sciences, Engineering, and Medicine, 2021), new vistas of appreciative inquiry await a mindful revolution of individuals, teams, and global leaders dedicated to seamless integration and coordination of improvement (Stratton-Berkessel, 2016). New paths of improvement will be charted that are dedicated to a culture of health, reduced health disparities, and improved health and well-being of society. Appreciative inquiry will guide each improvement, highlighting current industry trends, and act as a catalyst for organizational change.

As individuals and teams consider the daunting task of establishing a culture of health, reducing health disparities, and improving the health and well-being of society, they must recognize that having a project idea and implementing it are two different actions. Understanding the scope of a project, the dynamics associated with stakeholder and partnership involvement, culture, information technology, team dynamics, economics, and the political environment can easily result in a state of project paralysis. In the current healthcare industry, the path to an innovative project must include micro-, meso-, and macro-level input linked to global considerations for substantive change and influence that evidence ongoing opportunities.

Successful planning and implementation of any project are supported by the notion that for an effective system to be strengthened, it requires systems thinking and attention to how the parts work together to create a seamless whole (Crisp, 2010). As knowledge is gained from project outcomes, knowledge transfer becomes an imperative. Evidence is spread and systems of care are strengthened and sustained. This is relevant in the current environment, where the focus of work is on obtaining the right outcomes, as opposed to past decades, where performing the right processes was emphasized (Porter-O'Grady & Malloch, 2015, 2017). Likewise, the relevance is increasingly predominant in a global market driven by value-based versus volume-based care delivery and reimbursement (Frist, 2016; Simatupang et al., 2017).

This chapter focuses on differences between a quality improvement project, project plan, project management, and research related to deliverable outcomes. The importance of legislation, health policy, and economic conditions when designing projects will also be addressed. The importance in identifying historical influences, determinants, and unintended consequences or risks in culturally diverse settings is examined. In addition, the skills and tools of an improvement team leader and identified members for a sustainable project are described as work environments become increasingly virtual.

Quality Improvement Projects, Project Plans, and Project Management: Necessary Distinctions for Deliverable Outcomes

The genesis of any quality improvement project is planning, but ongoing management of the project is essential as well. All projects have a beginning, duration, and an end, which collectively constitute the project's life cycle. Project outcomes may, for example, be adopted in the form of evidence-based guidelines or viewed as opportunities for conducting additional inquiry and validation studies before incorporating them in practice. It is critical, however, not to immediately adopt findings from a small project, as they may not be generalizable to a broader context. According to Peters (1999), approximately 50% of the work completed in organizations may be considered as projects. Many staff working on projects as de facto members or managers may not possess the critical path and earned value analysis skills, which are key to orchestrating and managing a project from inception to completion (Lewis, 2011).

What is a quality improvement project? Projects are temporary endeavors that focus on producing a unique operational entity such as a product, service, or result differing from that obtained in prior projects (Project Management Institute, 2013). Through a systematic process, outcomes are produced that improve system efficiency and patient experiences. Regardless of the project, it should be based on the idea of accomplishing a goal for systems, stakeholders, and/or customers.

When does the project begin? A series of iterative processes, activities, and actions precedes the initiation of a project. One fundamental consideration is readying the project environment by identifying and validating the need for the project, developing the plan, and obtaining system buy-in and/or approval from stakeholders. Identifying and engaging stakeholders early and throughout the improvement project is pivotal to success. The value of stakeholder involvement cannot be underestimated in any project as new partnerships are formed, their interests are represented, ownership is reinforced, and support becomes center stage (Ives, 2019).

A project plan encompasses several components that collectively culminate in a realistic and well-planned sequence of actions and processes. The project plan goes beyond a general project scope and includes the details necessary to make a meaningful and value-based addition that reduces or eliminates variation in a work unit or an entire system. As the project proceeds and causative factors are eliminated, productivity and measureable quality outcomes are evident.

According to Tuthill (2014), the project plan includes a project budget, a work and activity breakdown and schedule, an overall project schedule, and any supporting documents. Haughey (2014) identifies other related parts of the project plan, including project goals, deliverables, schedule, and supporting documents (human resources, communications, and risk management plans). Additionally, other project plan considerations were outlined by Billows (2014), whose project plan template provides for scope definition, major deliverables, risk identification, team resource requirements, and decomposing individual tasks. A variety of project-planning programs are available commercially and often used by larger, more complex projects within systems.

Thinking and rethinking what one needs or desires in relation to the project plan are key aspects of complex ecosystem planning to extend beyond the workplace view (Merrifield, 2009). This author identified three important "rethinking questions" for any student or project planning team:

1. Does the project exactly correlate with any of the organization's key business goals?
2. Does the project have a strong connection to the organization's brand or corporate identity?
3. Does the effort required for the project result in increased organizational performance and change the value of the project to achieve organizational effectiveness?

What is project management? The *Project Management Body of Knowledge (PMBOK) Guide* defines project management as "application of knowledge, skills, tools, and techniques to project activities to meet project requirements. Project management is accomplished through the application and integration of the project management processes of initiating, planning, executing, monitoring and controlling, and closing" (Project Management Institute, 2013, p. 6). Of interest, the *PMBOK Guide* has, as its primary objective, the explanation of how each of the processes may be accomplished in practice.

Although consistent management of activities is essential for project completion, project management extends beyond managing and scheduling activities. Project management entails a combination of tools, people, and systems (Lewis, 2011). Tools may include computers, software applications and platforms that include electronic management systems, and daily planners. People include organizations and project teams who engage in processes geared toward goal accomplishment within systems. Management of people may present as a challenge in this endeavor, and leaders and communicators must use multiple skills to coach and mentor individuals toward achieving the common goal. The manager's emotional intelligence may be tested along the way, as will be examined further in this chapter.

Regardless of the depth or breadth of the project, plan, and management, the various stages of the project life cycle must not be neglected. Tuthill (2014) identified this cycle as having four phases:

1. Initiating the project (including identifying customer-driven factors and obtaining leadership approval and support)
2. Planning (including human and physical resources)
3. Executing (monitors, control, and cycle of efforts)
4. Project closing (training, operations, and support)

Project planning across the life cycle should additionally consider the project's feasibility, value, key drivers for success, skills and tools needed, and processes whereby project teams may be managed in virtual environments. Virtual work environments have gained popularity in the last decade as more employees work from distant locations, especially when operating in a contingency or crisis situation as demonstrated during the COVID-19 pandemic. Likewise, virtual work environments proved advantageous as organizations remained responsive to customers and stakeholders with fewer expenditures dedicated to office space, supplies, and indirect costs (Bloch, 2017).

Differentiation of Quality Improvement Projects and Research

Creating an environment receptive to change and evidence-based practice requires a series of purposeful actions and partnerships. Actions include various quality improvement projects that are led by interprofessional team members that culminate in sustainable practice change and outcomes. As project teams form, partnerships emerge and a common goal is established. Including researchers as equal partners on the quality improvement project team is an asset, thus avoiding a waste of valuable resources. This creates opportunities for the design and methodology, allowing teams to disseminate relevant information to the larger community. This opportunity informs decisions with reliable and evidence-based data (Marjanovic et al., 2017).

Often, individuals use language indiscriminately. Differentiating between quality improvement and research is essential to avoid barriers that lead to misunderstandings by quality improvement team members. For purposes of this chapter, the following definitions of *quality improvement* and *research* apply.

Quality improvement focuses on systems, processes, and functions associated with clinical quality, satisfaction, and cost outcomes. Meaningful quality improvement projects contribute to a better understanding of care processes through the application of knowledge. Research involves a process of systematic inquiry, whereby knowledge is developed, refined, and/or expanded. Research answers questions to develop knowledge grounded in a scientific method (Melnyk & Fineout-Overholt, 2005, 2019). Although there are connections between quality improvement and research, differences also exist. These differences include intent, design, setting benefits, generalizability of findings, oversight, subject and risk consent, ethical justification, and dissemination. Research can focus on quality improvement initiatives, but a quality improvement project is not always considered research (Gregory, 2015). Further consideration of the differences is discussed in Chapter 2.

Importance of Legislation, Health Policy, Economic Conditions, Culture, Social and Environmental Factors, Values, and Norms When Designing Quality Improvement Projects

Demonstrating effectiveness in healthcare operations is required for sustainability in today's market. Doing more with less has resulted in organizations charging teams to design quality improvement projects that strengthen efficiency and accountability while achieving sustainable outcomes. Cost, quality, safety, and access provide a basis for innovative improvement teams. Innovation is a critical value of alignment between the multiple forces affecting health care and decisions that follow (Porter-O'Grady & Malloch, 2015). To appreciate the impact of innovation in health care, sharing the project outcomes that used identified dissemination plans must become the lifeblood of a 21st-century organization and be linked to new ideologies of business and a data-rich environment (Porter-O'Grady & Malloch, 2017). The shift from volume-based to value-based care has required innovative leaders to shift previous mental models of care to those that ensure advancement of the health of a nation (Centers for Medicare and Medicaid Services, 2013; U.S. Department of Health and Human Services, 2011). Likewise, quality improvement project design must balance innovation with value if a return on investment is realized. Using a cost–benefit model, project teams can create opportunities for practice change, whereby evaluation of outcomes is based on implementation with their fidelity to the original project design. This necessitates for project designs to reflect all work processes and activities subject to ongoing inquiry and reassessment (Porter-O'Grady & Malloch, 2015, 2017). Incentives that balance innovation with value also have sizable implications for survival in the current healthcare arena. Incentives should be developed based on evidence-based economies, fairness, and equitability that have an intuitive appeal that benefits patient outcomes and system efficiency. Economics will continue to shape the landscape of health care and the design of quality improvement projects as reimbursement processes are reformed.

As a quality improvement team begins to design a project, examining the impact of legislation and health policy provides insight into the demand to demonstrate effectiveness. Legislation, regulations, and health policy are grounded in evidence, inform budgets and management decisions, and strengthen accountability (Pew-MacArthur Foundation, 2015). The exponential number of federal regulations affecting the healthcare industry increasingly requires multiple resources to manage and meet mandates. According to the American Hospital Association (AHA, 2017), 629 regulations are mandated by four agencies (Centers for Medicare and Medicaid, the Office of Civil Rights, the Office of Inspector General, and the Office of the National Coordinator of Information Technology) that promulgate the requirements with additional directives forthcoming.

Laws and public policies do not exist in a vacuum. Action taken in one domain may have unintended consequences in another domain while having synergistic, positive effects in yet another (Senterfitt et al., 2013). If quality improvement teams dismiss this reality, a disconnect will prevail, and the efficacy of project improvement project design, implementation, and outcomes will be jeopardized.

There is no question that the culture of an organization, social and environmental factors, and values and norms also affect the design, implementation, and adoption of quality improvement project outcomes. Universally, change in health care is driven by projects that result from errors, inefficiency, and survival instincts. Getting to the root cause of an issue becomes the foundation for a well-designed and executed quality improvement project. Innovation of key stakeholders is a key to integrating organizational culture for sustainability of quality improvements.

Projects are advanced as leaders acknowledge the importance of context and culture. Assessing organizational culture is pivotal to planned change and adoption of improvements. Organizations that value quality improvement project team activities and their outcomes create windows of opportunity. As a result, the full potential of employees is realized, and care access, delivery, and efficiency are advanced. This requires moving from an organizational culture that blames others to adoption of a just culture (Khatri et al., 2009).

A just culture is an environment where an atmosphere of trusting, encouraging, and rewarding others for providing essential safety-related information occurs (Reason, 2008). A just culture addresses two areas: (1) the role of punitive sanction in the safety of the healthcare system and (2) the effects of a punitive sanction as a remedy for human error as a help or hindrance to safety efforts (Marx, 2001). With adoption of a just culture based on consideration of human limitations, numerous advances in healthcare practices and operations have been achieved, yet advances are needed in cultural transformation (Kennedy, 2016).

Social and environmental factors are important to consider for any quality improvement project team. These factors are the largest predictor of health outcomes and are influential in changing practices (Senterfitt et al., 2013). Health and health-related problems result from multiple factors. For example, factors such as educational level, employment, environment where individuals live and work, and support are primary determinants of health outcomes. As quality improvement teams design projects, remaining aware of these factors is essential if outcomes are realized (Mosadeghrad, 2014). Consider the current debate surrounding requirements for immunizing infants and preschoolers. Addressing the social and environmental factors related to immunizations requires others to interpret evidence, advocate for adherence, and align messages that are supportive of universal practices. Similarly, the adoption of quality improvement project findings can be impacted by social group acceptance and the environment targeted for change. Advocacy for change becomes paramount in these circumstances.

One's values and norms in society also influence quality improvement projects. If individuals or organizations have conflicting values associated with a project, the likelihood of the development or success is endangered. Societal norms also affect acceptance of a project and its outcomes. If the norm is to only adopt changes from one specific group, new projects and ideas are destined for disapproval or failure. An environment of constant evaluation and adaptation is essential.

The convergence of team efforts and consideration of the aforementioned factors form a collective network of knowledge and facts as improvement projects are developed, implemented, and evaluated. Ruland (2010) concluded that reliable data increase decision quality, diminish errors, and strengthen the adoption of projects and outcomes. Regardless of the system, whether local, national, or international, data guides legislation, policy formulation, and decisions. However, this will require individuals to question if existing policy and practices are achieving the balance between potential risks and benefits (Heitmueller et al., 2014).

Some of the most prominent healthcare organizations arise from the accumulation of knowledge. When a healthcare organization improves services, others adopt what works and benefit from its knowledge. The spread of this knowledge and its universal adoption result in situations that influence the economic outlook, sustainability, quality of services, and satisfied consumers.

Quality improvement project design must balance innovation with value if a return on investment is realized. Using a cost–benefit model, project teams can create opportunities for practice change, whereby evaluation of outcomes is based on implementation with their fidelity to the original project design. This calls for project designs to reflect all work processes and activities subject to ongoing inquiry and reassessment (Porter-O'Grady & Malloch, 2015). Incentives that balance innovation with value also have sizable implications for survival in the current healthcare arena.

Historical Influences, Determinants, and Unintended Consequences/Risks Associated with Quality Improvement Projects

The current healthcare system is driven by the need to respond to a rapidly changing environment and delivery of quality care. Healthcare quality is a universal marker that systems use to measure if care and desired outcomes are achieved (Batalden & Davidoff, 2007). The status quo is no longer acceptable. Current assumptions and processes must be challenged and replaced with robust improvements driven by measurable quality, safety, and value-based outcomes. Influences, determinants, and any unintended consequences or risks must be considered if improvements are valuable and sustainable within organizations. This requires positive engagement and actions by the entire healthcare team if systems of care are changed. Change must be based on clear expectations relevant to the situation that foster relevant learning (Nelson et al., 2007). This is not a linear process, but a series of explorations resulting in meaningful outcomes (Moran, 2014).

History guides individual and group actions (Fairman & D'Antonio, 2013). This includes preparation and dissemination of policies, funding allocations, system improvements, and the design of quality improvement projects. Making sense and understanding the value of history when designing a quality project are invaluable. Historical data provide a lens to assess prior improvement attempts, processes, and variations in outcomes. History offers evidence that guides the work of quality improvement project teams and provides direction when choices are vague and lack basis.

Gaining insight into an organization's quality improvement project attempts and determinants of success is made easier when one considers three domains: process, structure, and outcomes (Donabedian, 1985). Process provides the context necessary to understand approaches that guide quality improvement project development and engagement of team members. Structure includes the specific elements that are most likely to have relevance and attain desired outcomes. Outcomes provide pathways for documenting the efficacy and impacts of the project. Outcomes are further evident as project data are analyzed and communicated, and changes are adopted across the healthcare system.

Beyond the value of history and determinants of quality improvement project success are unintended consequences and project risks. Anticipating and managing the unintended consequences and potential risks can be difficult even for a skillful leader. Unintended consequences extend beyond clinical effectiveness and include dismissal of evidence, social factors, financial impacts, and stakeholder partisanship. Evidence may be dismissed in geographical regions, cultures, and groups. Evidence may be jeopardized when controversy and differing opinions exist, limiting the development of a meaningful quality improvement project. Thus, environments may not be conducive to change based on the current evidence. Evidence is desirable to ensure interventions are optimized, negative outcomes are minimized, and resources are used effectively. Realizing an immediate financial gain or incurring upfront costs may be viewed as a risk and limit the full impact of a quality improvement project or its adoption. Partisanship among and between stakeholders may also affect buy-in of a quality improvement project, thus preventing or curtailing the design and initiation of projects that solidify quality, safety, and value-added outcomes.

Addressing and remaining cognizant of unintended consequences and potential risks require the actions of all quality improvement team members. Advocating for the use of current evidence, interpreting the need for an evidence-based quality improvement project, and using available tools and resources are essential determinants of success.

Requisite Skills and Techniques of an Improvement Team Leader and Members for Sustainable Projects in Healthcare Systems

In the fast-paced, ever-changing healthcare landscape, a plethora of project leader and team member skills and techniques are needed throughout the life cycle of a project, especially quality improvement ones. The basic nature of individuals to learn and use new techniques creates a positive sense of competition and often uncertainty that can benefit project activities and outcomes (Khan, 2012). The idea that evidence-based quality improvement project outcomes transform practice and advance quality is a strategic differentiator tool for sustaining a competitive edge (Mosadeghrad, 2014). Achieving equilibrium between practice and quality offers a strategic regimen that ensures all evidence is available as quality improvement projects are envisioned, developed, and completed. However, this does not occur in a singular process, but requires use of various tools and techniques that support meaningful projects. Envisioning a future state where the path forward can readily be recognized and followed by others is a deliberate action that leads to meaningful projects and supports their sustained management. The ability to manage the delicate maneuvers of leading, engaging, and inspiring others toward greatness is among the many skills needed by a project leader. Investment in skill development and core competencies for project planning and management is central to shaping business outcomes in all industries, especially in health care.

Applying human factors engineering in health care allows one to gain the knowledge needed to examine human behavior and interaction with others or with their surroundings and apply information for greater efficacy (Carayon & Wood, 2010; Gosbee & Anderson, 2003; Weinger & Gaba, 2014). Human factors engineering can further assist both the novice and expert project planner and manager in gaining insight into processes quickly and being able to initiate actions for course correction, as indicated. The patient's journey through the multifaceted and complex systems should be a consideration of the process (Carayon et al., 2020).

The skills and techniques needed for success with a project include an array of critical approaches. Although there is no singular set of skills and techniques that guarantees success, some options are mutually beneficial to teams, individuals, and organizations. The process for instilling these skills and techniques into practice requires first understanding each of them and then linking it to goals and measurable, sustainable outcomes. The skills and techniques will be examined in this text, keeping in mind no particular skill or technique is necessarily better than—or a replacement for—another.

Throughout an improvement project, keeping activities focused on the customer is important, especially when the organization depends on those customers for revenue and most of its market share. When the customer is satisfied, loyalty is preserved and repeat business occurs. For example, if a manager requests the development of a quality improvement project that will increase customer satisfaction, it is important to first understand customer needs and expectations and then to communicate those needs and expectations throughout the organization, while measuring value and reporting results. The understanding is gleaned through an organizational analysis and assessment tools, which are explored in Chapters 5 and 6.

Every project requires a designated leader to establish the project's direction and goal. Although there may be informal leaders, the project leader should possess the skills needed to create and maintain the environment where others engage in meeting the project's goal. Creating opportunities to encourage others and involve them in both the current project and future projects is a mark of transformational leaders, who continually inspire and recognize others' contributions.

Being an effective communicator who possesses emotional intelligence will engage others and provide the leverage necessary to initiate and complete projects in an expeditious fashion (Galli, 2020; Goleman, 2005). However, this outcome will not occur without the ability, awareness, and cultural sensitivity to address cultural and diverse differences in today's workforce. All individuals process information differently because of their diverse backgrounds and cultural beliefs. Being aware and sensitive can facilitate progress on projects (Saxena, 2014; Seibert et al., 2002; Young & Guo, 2016).

Planning and organizational skills, such that one can assimilate information from various assessment processes and break down information into discrete parts, can set the stage for effective ongoing management of the project. Individual creativity may flourish when these skills are applied to organize outcomes for dissemination.

Managing Projects and Teams in a Virtual Environment

One of the great rewards of technology is the opportunity to have global project team members contribute remotely. Project managers can leverage the strengths and talents of multiple individuals that match the project plan, strategy, and desired outcomes. As Porter-O'Grady and Malloch (2015) explain, teams are small systems and often mirror the complexity in other levels of the larger system. The effectiveness and performance of a project team, whether virtual or not, are contingent upon a combination of attributes and skill sets. These personal assets include, but are not limited to, individual competence, interpersonal skills, flexibility, accommodation, creativity, strong work ethic, and a focus on outcomes, to name a few. If the team has no identified purpose or end point, there is no meaning to the work to be accomplished. Projects may fail or yield limited outcomes that are not sustainable, and future virtual teams may be considered suspect.

As the moral compass for the virtual team, the leader should bring diplomacy to bear in the discourse with staff, managers, stakeholders, and/or distractors. In particular, it is the virtual team leader's responsibility to defend the project and virtual team by shielding the overarching goal from distractors (Sturmberg & Martin, 2012). Adaptability becomes pivotal to success and is often more important than anticipation in such an environment.

Managing a team, whether onsite or virtual, can be rewarding as well as challenging. Virtual Hires (2014) identified nine guidelines that apply when selecting and managing individuals and teams in virtual environments, which are easily applicable to on-site teams:

1. Perform a project evaluation. Project leaders must be knowledgeable about goals, tactics, and deliverables if they are to communicate effectively with prospective team members.
2. Determine the skill sets needed by team members. Match the skills of team members to the delegated tasks and mutually reach consensus on assignments. Leveraging individual strengths promotes measurable outcomes.
3. Identify and anticipate obstacles. Knowing what has been attempted previously to resolve a problem or opportunity can only benefit the present outcomes. Conversely, disregarding this information can mean a loss for the plan, as the strategy may actually require only a minor redesign or assignment of a team member with matching skills and competencies.
4. Constantly engage members and encourage bidirectional communication. Contact with virtual team members often is employed to verify needs for

supervision and encouragement. Likewise, the team member can communicate successes and challenges encountered that require intervention.

5. Establish a timeline and milestones. Identify expectations and the schedule needed to move the project toward completion. Monitor progress at designated intervals. Share accomplishments with all virtual members and stakeholders.

6. Ensure individual team member accountability. Recognizing the importance of each individual member's investment in achieving the critical priorities of a specific project and their buy-in to the larger institutional performance is a critical success factor.

7. Be cognizant of cultural differences. Being aware and sensitive to the diversity of virtual team members is important to avoid conflicts and delays in completing assigned tasks.

8. Manage conflict and difficult team members. Avoiding a conflict will only perpetuate the issue and result in inefficiency of the individual and team function. Although crucial conversations may be difficult on a personal level, they are valuable for resolution of identified issues that may create project paralysis.

9. Provide education and training. Just-in-time or accelerated learning techniques may be required to assure all team members are on the same page with respect to the project goal and strategies. Using practical application examples and techniques matched with evidence, flexibility, and innovative teaching strategies can strengthen project outcomes and create synergy among virtual team members.

Effective governance and ownership of any project is critical to its success. A poorly articulated and organized management structure, overlapping roles and decision-making authority, and mismatched roles and team members can prevent a project from achieving any momentum or producing valuable outcomes. The designated leader is the guardian of a finite project, who is charged with creating the structure and practices needed to guide the plan forward and strategically align it with the enterprise's overall direction.

The expansive use of virtual teams provides a substantial trend in the healthcare arena, where changing reimbursement models and movement toward greater industry transparency have placed substantial pressure on organizations to deliver stronger performance and improved value. In the long term, this trend is expected to continue. In turn, current improvements and projects focused on cost and quality performance will impel healthcare organizations toward higher standards requiring visionary leaders and dedicated project teams positioned to meet the challenges facing the healthcare industry.

Summary

- Planning successful projects requires a series of deliberate and purposeful activities and a well-developed budget that result in an attainable goal.
- Projects may be limited to the microsystem or may extend to the meso- and macrosystem level(s) within an organization or industry.
- Projects are finite in scope, whereas program management extends across a system or industry.

- Leadership is central to successful projects and their sustainability.
- Projects benefit systems, stakeholders, and various customers.
- Envisioning a futuristic state opens avenues for changes in behavior and value-based project outcomes.
- Technology affords opportunities for global project team membership where talents are leveraged toward an achievable goal.
- The status quo in health care is no longer acceptable. Current assumptions and processes must be challenged and replaced with robust quality improvement projects driven by measurable quality, safety, and value-based outcomes.
- Influences and determinants must be considered if improvements are valuable and sustainable within organizations. This requires positive engagement and actions by the entire care team if systems of care are changed and sustainable.
- Quality improvement focuses on systems, processes, and functions associated with clinical quality, satisfaction, and cost outcomes.
- Research involves a process of systematic inquiry, whereby knowledge is developed, refined, and/or expanded.
- History guides individual and group actions. Making sense of, and understanding the value of, history when designing a quality improvement project is invaluable. Historical data provide a lens to assess prior improvement attempts, processes, and variations in outcomes.
- Process provides the context necessary to understand approaches that guide quality improvement project development and engagement of team members. Content includes the specific elements that are most likely to have relevance and attain desired outcomes. Outcomes provide pathways for documenting the efficacy and impacts of the project.
- Cost, quality, and access provide a basis for innovative improvement teams.
- Current legislation, regulations, and health policy are grounded in evidence that informs budgets, guides management decisions, and strengthens accountability.
- The spread of this knowledge and its universal adoption result in situations that influence the economic outlook, sustainability, quality of services, and satisfied stakeholders and consumers.
- The culture of an organization, social and environmental factors, and diverse values and norms affect the design, implementation, and adoption of quality improvement project outcomes.
- A just culture is an environment where an atmosphere of trusting, encouraging, and rewarding others for providing essential safety-related information occurs.
- Social and environmental factors are the largest predictors of health outcomes and are influential in changing practices.
- Values and norms in society influence the outcomes of quality improvement projects.
- Evidence-based quality improvement projects transform practice and advance quality. Such projects are a strategic differentiator tool for sustaining a competitive edge.
- Achieving equilibrium between practice and quality offers a regimen to ensure all evidence is available as quality improvement projects are developed and completed.
- Multiple tools and techniques exist that offer quality improvement project teams to identify latent or hidden failures in a system.

Reflection Questions and Learning Activities

1. Reflect on your current work environment and identify how leaders and stakeholders within the organization impact project successes, sustained practice change, and spread of evidence.
2. Identify and discuss a technological advance that may assist you in developing a capstone or improvement project.
3. What attributes contribute to a virtual project team's success? How can you ensure positive changes and outcomes as the project leader?
4. You are tasked with developing a quality improvement project. What are the primary components to include in the project plan?
5. When developing a quality improvement project or proposal, what are the primary considerations to ensure success and practice change outcomes are sustained?
6. Select a quality improvement project. What are the tools and techniques that will assist you throughout the process?
7. How would you differentiate between structure, process, and outcome indicators? How may each be incorporated in a quality improvement proposal?
8. How would you evaluate the quality improvement project's outcomes?

References

American Hospital Association. (2017). *Regulatory overload report. Assessing the regulatory burden on health systems, hospitals, and post-acute care providers.* https://www.aha.org/guideposts/2017-11-03-regulatory-overload-report

Batalden, P. B., & Davidoff, F. (2017). What is "quality improvement" and how can it transform healthcare? *Quality Safe Health Care, 16*(1), 2–3. https://doi.org/10.1136/qshc.2006.022046

Billows, D. (2014). *Project plan template: How to create a project plan.* http://4pm.com/project-plan-template

Bloch, R. (2017). Advantages and disadvantages of a virtual workforce. *The Hartford.* https://www.thehartford.com/business-playbook/in-depth/virtual-workplace-advantages-disadvantages

Carayon, P., & Wood, K. E. (2010). Patient safety: The role of human factors and systems engineering. *Studies in Health Teaching and Informatics, 153,* 23–46.

Carayon, P., Woolridge, A., Hoonakker, P., Hundt, A. S., & Kelly. M. M. M. (2020). SEIPDS 3.0: Human-centered design of the patient journey for patient safety. *Applied Egonomics, 84,* 103033. https://doi.org/10.1016/j.apergo.2019.103033

Centers for Medicare and Medicaid Services. (2013). *Bundled payments for care improvement (BPCI) initiative: General information.* http://innovation.cms.gov/initiatives/bundled-payments

Crisp, N. (2010). *Turning the world upside down: The search for global health in the 21st century.* RSM Press.

Donabedian, A. (1985). The quality of care: How can it be assessed? *JAMA, 260*(12), 1743–1748.

Fairman, J., & D'Antonio, P. (2013). History counts: How history can shape our understanding of health policy. *Nursing Outlook, 61*(5), 346–352. https://doi.org/10.1016/j.outlook.2013.07.001

Frist, B. (2016). From volume to value: Achieving bold change in our healthcare payment systems. *Forbes.* https://www.forbes.com/sites/billfrist/2016/06/30/from-volume-to-value-achieving-bold-change-in-our-healthcare-payment-systems/#349507349c82

Galli, B. J. (2020). Effective strategies for communication management in a project management environment. *International Journal of Applied Logistics, 10*(2), 1–7. https://doi.org/10.4018/IJAL.2020070105

Goleman, D. (2005). *Emotional intelligence.* Bantam Books.

Gosbee, J., & Anderson, T. (2003). Human factors engineering design demonstrations can enlighten your RCA team. *Quality Safe Healthcare, 12,* 119–121. https://doi.org/10.1136/qhc.12.2.119

Gregory, K. (2015). Differentiating between research and quality improvement. *Journal of Perinatal and Neonatal Nursing, 29*(2), 100–102. https://doi.org/10.1097/jpn.0000000000000107

Haughey, D. (2014). *Project planning a step by step guide.* http://www.projectsmart.com/articles/project-planning-a-step-by-step-guide.php

Heitmueller, A., Henderson, S., Warbuton, W., Elmajarid, A., Pentland, A., & Darzi, A. (2014). Developing public policy to advance the use of big data in health care. *Health Affairs, 33*(9), 1523–1530. https://doi.org/10.1377/hlthaff.2014.0771

Ives, S. (2019). *Quality improvement in healthcare for 2020.* https://pliohub.com/what-is-quality-improvement-healthcare-definition/

Kennedy, B. (2016). Toward a just culture. *Nursing Management, 46*(6), 13–15.

Khan, M. E. (2012). *Relationship between project attributes, project performance, and project governance dimensions—building the theoretical framework.* Paper presented at PMI Global Congress 2012—EMEA, Marsailles, France. Project Management Institute.

Khatri, N., Brown, G. D., & Hicks, L. L. (2009). From a blame culture to a just culture in health care. *Health Care Management Review, 34*(4), 312–322. https://doi.org/10.1097/hmr.0b013e3181a3b709

Lewis, J. P. (2011). *Project planning, scheduling and control: The ultimate hands-on guide to bringing projects in on time and on budget* (5th ed.). McGraw-Hill.

Marjanovic, S., Ghiga, I., Yang, M., & Knack, A. (2017). *Understanding value in health data ecosystems.* Rand Corporation.

Marx, D. (2001). *Patient safety and the "just culture": A primer for health care executives.* Columbia University.

Melnyk, B. M., & Fineout-Overholt, E. (2005). *Evidence-based practice in nursing and healthcare.* Lippincott Williams & Wilkins.

Melnyk, B. M., & Fineout-Overholt, E. (2019). *Evidence-based practice in nursing and healthcare* (4th ed.). Wolters Kluwer.

Merrifield, R. (2009). *Re-think.* Pearson FT Press.

Moran, K. (2014). Setting the state for the doctor of nursing practice scholarly project. In K. Moran, R. Burson, & D. Conrad (Eds.), *The doctor of nursing practice scholarly project. A framework for success* (pp. 3–14). Jones & Bartlett Learning.

Mosadeghrad, A. M. (2014). Factors influencing healthcare service delivery. *International Journal of Health Policy Management, 3*(2), 77–89.

National Academies of Sciences, Engineering, and Medicine. (2021). *The future of nursing 2020–2030: Charting a path to achieve health equity.* The National Academies Press. https://doi.org/10.17226/25982

Nelson, E. C., Batalden, P. B., Homa, K., Godfrey, M. M., Campbell, C., Headrik, L. A., & Wasson, J. H. (2007). Creating a rich information environment. In E. C. Nelson, P. B. Batalden, & M. M. Godfrey (Eds.), *Quality by design. A clinical microsystems approach* (pp. 178–196). John Wiley & Sons, Inc.

Peters, T. (1999). *The wow project.* Fast Company. http://www.fastcompany.com/36831/wow-project

Pew-MacArthur Foundation. (2015). *Legislating evidence-based policymaking. A look at state laws that support data-driven decision-making.* http://www.pewtrusts.org/en/research-and-analysis/issue-briefs/2015/03/legislating-evidence-based-policymaking

Porter-O'Grady, T., & Malloch, K. (2015). *Quantum leadership: Building better partnerships for sustainable health.* Jones & Bartlett Learning.

Porter-O'Grady, T., & Malloch, K. (2017). *Quantum leadership: Building better partnerships for sustainable health* (2nd ed.). Jones & Bartlett Learning.

Project Management Institute. (2013). *A guide to project management body of knowledge (PMBOK guide)* (5th ed.). Project Management Institute.

Reason, J. (2008). *The human contribution: Unsafe acts, accidents, and heroic recoveries.* Ashgate Publishing.

Ruland, C. (2010). Translating evidence into practice. In W. L. Holzmer (Ed.), *Improving health through nursing research,* 238–246. Wiley-Blackwell.

Saxena, A. (2014). Workforce diversity: A key to improve productivity. *Procedia Economics and Finance, 11*, 76–85. https://doi.org/10.1016/S2212-5671(14)00178-6

Seibert, P. S., Trejo, L. S., & Zimmerman, C. G. (2002). A checklist to facilitate cultural awareness and sensitivity. *Journal of Medical Ethics, 28*, 143–146.

Senterfitt, J. W., Long, A., Shih, M., & Teutsch, S. M. (2013). How social and economic factors affect health. *Social Determinants of Health, 1*, 1–22.

Simatupang, T. M., Piboonrungroj, P., & Williams, S. (2017). The emergence of value chain think-ing. *International Journal of Value Chain Management*, 8(1), 1–19.

Stratton-Berkessel, R. (2016). *Appreciative inquiry for collaborative solutions: 21 strength-based work-shops*. Pfeiffer.

Sturmberg, J. P., & Martin, C. M. (2012). Leadership and transitions: Maintaining the science in complexity and complex systems. *Journal of Evaluation in Clinical Practice*, 18(1), 186–189.

Tuthill, J. M. (2014). *Practical project management for informatics! How to manage a project without losing your mind*. Presentation at API Annual Conference.

U.S. Department of Health and Human Services. (2011). *Hospital value-based purchasing pro-gram*. http://www.cms.gov/Outrearch-and-Education/Medicare-Learning-NetworkMLN/MLN Products/downloads/Hospital_VBPurchasing_Fact_Sheet_ICN907664.pdf

Virtual Hires. (2014). *15 tips for effectively mapping your virtual employee*. http://www.virtualhires .com/resources.cgi?file=15-tips-to-effectively-managing- your-virtual-employee

Weinger, M. B., & Gaba, D. M. (2014). Human factors engineering in patient safety. *Anesthesiology*, 120(4), 801–806. https://doi.org/10.1097/ALN.0000000000000144

Young, S., & Guo, K. L. (2016). The necessity of cultural competence for health care providers in nursing practice. *The Health Care Manager*, 35(2), 94–102.

Case Exemplars

Guidepost for Students Selecting a Meaningful Capstone Project Topic

Jacqueline M. Lollar

As a former labor and delivery nurse in a teaching hospital and a current nurse educator, Sandy had always wanted to remain in the teaching and learning role. She began to recognize she had an excellent opportunity to advance her education. Sandy had a great desire to earn a doctorate of nursing practice (DNP) degree and began discussing her options with mentors and colleagues. The university in which she was teaching had started a simulation program, which Sandy had been involved in from its inception. She knew she wanted to incorporate human patient simulation and education into her capstone project.

When conducting literature searches related to simulation and nursing education, Sandy found that medication errors were a recurring theme. The first idea she considered for her proposed capstone project was to implement simulated scenarios into the various nursing courses to decrease medication errors by student nurses and newly graduating novice nurses. That way, the students would be able to use their knowledge and skills in medication administration without causing harm to live patients. If an error occurred, the students would be able to see the immediate reaction to a medication error.

After having numerous meetings with her faculty advisor and discussing the process for a needs assessment, Sandy completed a needs assessment at the institution. Upon its completion, it was evident that the institution's faculty were already integrating medication administration in each simulated scenario. Thus, Sandy's idea was abandoned because medication administration was already a current practice at the College of Nursing. Additionally, with the guidance of her advisor, Sandy realized the project should have a more inclusive systems-change approach that would be better suited to a hospital setting. A change that could be incorporated into one unit in a hospital had the potential to change the entire culture of education throughout each department within a hospital.

After more meetings with her faculty advisor, Sandy began to explore the practices of area hospitals to determine the use of human patient simulation for educational purposes. One area hospital's labor and delivery unit shared a birthing simulator, Noelle, with another area hospital's labor and delivery unit. Each hospital had Noelle to use for a 6-month period of time. The labor and delivery nurse educator desperately wanted to utilize the simulator for educational purposes but had no expertise in its application. The nurse educator began explaining that the unit had numerous novice nurses and wanted them to participate in simulated scenarios focused on high-risk, low-volume obstetric patients. Additionally, she commented that The Joint Commission would be evaluating the hospital soon and the nursing staff was very weak in knowledge related to the National Patient Safety Goals (NPSGs). A shared belief between Sandy and the nurse educator working with the project was that competence in the discipline of nursing is paramount. Maintaining a level of competence is imperative for nursing staff to provide quality and safe patient care. However, competency is challenging to measure because of its many different components. The proposal of annual competencies, including NPSGs, was discussed at length with the nurse manager and nurse educator. At this time, buy-in for Sandy's capstone project was obtained.

Further conversations and meetings followed with the unit educator to determine the specific obstetric emergencies and NPSGs to be included in the annual competencies. The obstetric emergencies finally selected included fetal distress, amniotic fluid embolism, placental abruption, and postpartum hemorrhage. At the time, 10 NPSGs were in existence. Four NPSGs were selected for inclusion in the simulated scenarios based on common errors and staff needs: improve the accuracy of patient identification, improve the effectiveness of communication among caregivers, improve the safety of using medications, and accurately and completely reconcile medications across the continuum of care (The Joint Commission, 2008).

Sandy then began working closely with her faculty advisor to make the project both meaningful and sustainable. Her advisor questioned, "What theory would be the driving force for the project?" After conducting numerous literature searches and conversations with the faculty advisor, Sandy identified Dr. Patricia Benner's theory, from novice to expert, as the foundation for the project.

At this point, the DNP project had a theoretical basis and needed a model for change. The ACE Star Model of Knowledge Transformation, the model used for the quality improvement project, enabled the discovery of knowledge to be implemented and transformed into practice. The ACE model consisted of five cyclical phases: discovery, summary, translation, integration, and evaluation (Bonis et al., 2007). While planning and implementing the project of using human patient simulation for annual competency validation for labor and delivery nurses, each phase of the ACE model was encountered.

Many variables were significant in planning for the implementation of each phase of the project. First, the institutional review board (IRB) had to approve the project to maintain protection for those subjects participating in the project. Although the project was one of quality improvement, protection of the participating subjects was an important aspect of the project, including future publication options. IRB approval was required before any steps in the implementation phases could begin at the institution. The information provided in the IRB application explained the purpose of the systems change project, as well as the risks and benefits to the participants. The faculty advisor played a major role in assisting and advising Sandy throughout the IRB approval process.

Information throughout the IRB application described the process of implementing the use of human patient simulation for annual competency validation. Although there were no anticipated risks associated with the quality improvement project, there was a minimal risk that staff might experience the normal anxiety typically associated with performance during the annual competency validations. Job security would not be compromised as a result of poor performance during the annual competencies. If a nurse did not perform at a level to meet the goal of 100% compliance, the staff nurse would be provided with review information and given more opportunities to repeat the simulated experience until the desired performance was achieved. However, the projected positive outcome would be an increase in the nursing staff's confidence in their management of obstetric emergencies, especially with high-risk, low-volume patients.

All labor and delivery nurses were required to participate in the annual competencies. Data collected for competency validation were kept confidential. The results of the successful completion of the annual competencies were stored in the nurse's personnel folder to maintain confidentiality. However, some level of privacy and confidentiality was lost because of group participation, evaluation, and debriefing.

Approximately 60 labor and delivery nurses participated in the annual competency validation. The anticipated outcomes of the annual competency validations were positive. The goal of 100% compliance was met with each labor and delivery nurse. Human patient simulation provided an excellent learning opportunity for the labor and delivery nurses.

Continuous quality improvement was evident throughout the entire systems change process. The project provided benefits to both the hospital staff and their obstetric patients. Because the purpose of the project was one of quality improvement, the Institute of Medicine (IOM) aims were an important factor in the project, although each aim was not distinctly defined in this case. In general, the IOM aims included patient-centeredness, safety, effectiveness, efficiency, timeliness, and equity (Institute for Healthcare Improvement, 2009). Each aim was addressed in Sandy's quality improvement project, but the aim of safety was clearly a focal point throughout the implementation of the project. The project also incorporated evidence supporting human patient simulation as an effective learning tool for staff nurses. Experience is imperative for nurses to develop critical thinking skills and achieve competence. Once critical thinking skills and proficiency of psychomotor skills have been established, patient safety can be ensured.

The component was in place from the initial meeting with the nurse manager and nurse educator. Many inquiries were made during the project regarding different strategies for future simulated experiences for annual competencies. At the completion of the project, educational information and modules for the educator, as well as the staff nurses, were given to the unit educator for future use of the simulator. Information included in the modules dealt with pathophysiology, incidence, assessments, interventions, evidence-based practice articles, and case studies related to each of the obstetrical emergencies. Additionally, general information regarding The Joint Commission, accreditation, NPSGs, and elements of performance were included in the nurse's educational module.

Additional training and information were provided for educating the unit educator to maintain the sustainability of the project. Hands-on training, ranging from assembly of the simulator to moulaging to running scenarios, was provided to enable the unit educator to become proficient in using the simulator. A user manual was also developed for the unit educator, which included written and pictorial guides for future use.

Finally, several evaluation tools were developed and used for various aspects of the project and given to the nurse educator. One evaluation tool was developed to evaluate competence for each nurse with the obstetric emergencies as well as the chosen NPSG to be completed by the unit educator. Upon completion of the simulated scenarios, the staff nurses were given another evaluation tool to evaluate the experience during the scenarios.

Because it was well received by the institution and all of those involved, Sandy's project had great potential for sustainability. The labor and delivery unit educator planned to continue to use human patient simulation for annual competency validations. Also, other departments in the hospital were interested in using human patient simulation for various educational needs. One very exciting possibility was interprofessional use of human patient simulation, which was under discussion by the departments. The dissemination of findings, a very important factor, was also guided and supported by the faculty advisor. The project was presented at various conferences and introduced to surrounding hospitals.

The guidance by Sandy's advisor throughout the entire process of the quality improvement project and systems change was critical to the project's success. Without the direction and education provided by the advisor related to evidence, the project's theoretical basis, the project plan, the IRB process, analysis of data, and dissemination of the results, the project would not have had a solid foundation or the ability to maintain sustainability. Incorporating the use of human patient simulation for annual competency validation in a labor and delivery unit was a process that encompassed multiple strategic methods and various models. Obstetric emergencies are rare occurrences, but the nursing staff must be competent and maintain the ability to respond to them quickly and appropriately. The advisor, Sandy, the nurse educator, and the nurse manager firmly supported the use of human patient simulation for annual competency validation. The simulated scenarios assisted in bridging the gap between real patients and the learning opportunities for the labor and delivery nursing staff. Additionally, the incorporation of the NPSGs into the simulated experiences assisted the organizations in maintaining compliance with The Joint Commission standards.

Reflection Questions

1. What are the benefits of completing a needs assessment before developing a clinical project? Consider which parts of a needs assessment may benefit you later as you engage in a clinical project.
2. How might a faculty advisor guide students throughout the clinical project?
3. How does completing the IRB process benefit the clinical project and its sustainability?

References

Bonis, S., Taft, L., & Wender, C. (2007). Strategies to promote success on the NCLEX-RN: An evidence-based approach using the ACE Star Model of Knowledge Transformation [Electronic version]. *Nursing Education Perspectives, 2*, 82–87.

Institute for Healthcare Improvement. (2009). *Science of improvement: Setting aims.* http://www.ihi .org/resources/Pages/HowtoImprove/ScienceofImprovementSettingAims.aspx

The Joint Commission. (2008). *National Patient Safety Goals.* http://www.joint commission.org

Praxis: The Benefit to the Chief Nursing Officer as Projects Are Planned and Implemented

Wes Garrison

In any professional discipline, the overarching question of what guides practice is essential to understanding the framework within which practice occurs (Cody, 2013). Many factors influence the integration of theories and experiences that form the practice choices of an individual, and understanding the interrelation of those factors allows the individual to pursue knowledge, articulate practice, and communicate ideas more effectively. The process of integrating those theories and experiences is the underlying concept of praxis. As explained by Rolfe (1993), praxis is an ongoing, circular process of reflection in action whereby theory and practice continually inform, modify, and guide each other. Understanding the integration of informal theory and practice, a nurse executive can advance the profession and improve practice through a continual, circular process of reflection and action as projects are planned, implemented, and evaluated.

As the healthcare industry is evolving into a more technology-driven and resource-limited business model, the role of the nurse executive is becoming more business-focused. Certainly, clinical knowledge and skill are required for effective leadership of a nursing workforce, but a nurse executive also must understand how to direct quality care efficiently and communicate and collaborate effectively. Nurse executives must lead quality improvement initiatives to ensure cost-effective delivery of quality care (Carlson & Staffileno, 2013). Using relevant influences to form a nursing praxis to guide leadership allows for a structured, intentional approach to practice. By intentionally operating within the framework of a personal praxis, a nurse executive will continually improve leadership and advance the profession as projects evolve.

Ideological, Theoretical, and Ethical Influences

For a chief nursing officer (CNO), embracing an analytic approach as the primary philosophical viewpoint for practice allows for quantifying and measuring a variety of operational metrics. Based on empiricism, an analytic approach involves quantifiable data and definable results (Monti & Tingen, 1999). Empirical data allow a CNO to analyze relationships between quality improvement measures and cost-savings strategies. However, incorporating the continental approach to understand qualitative factors also is important for addressing less quantifiable aspects of nursing care and leadership (Monti & Tingen, 1999). Integrating both the analytic and continental approaches into leadership practice provides for a greater understanding of the nursing meta-paradigm and other relevant theoretical influences that guide projects throughout all phases.

From the broader framework of Fawcett's (1984) nursing meta-paradigm, Orem's (1991) Self-Care Deficit Nursing Theory (SCDNT) acts as an instructive guide for teaching organizational goals for improving patient health and decreasing readmissions. McMahon and Christopher's (2011) middle-range theory for teaching the aesthetic skill of nursing presence is also an excellent guide for the continued education of nurses. In addition to nursing theories, the field of complexity science offers important guidance for practice in the explanation and understanding of complex adaptive systems. CNOs must recognize the potential butterfly effect when even a small project or practice change is implemented (Florczak et al., 2012).

Operating within an ethical framework is also imperative to effective and professional nursing practice. The theory of virtue ethics offers an appropriate context for professional practice. Focusing on the qualities of compassion, discernment, trustworthiness, integrity, and conscientiousness, virtue ethics provides a guideline for developing the qualities necessary for professionalism and for integrating those qualities into practice (Chism, 2013). In any leadership activity, a CNO must recognize the importance of instilling in nurses the ethical standards required for practice. By integrating the virtue ethics framework with the hospital-specific code of ethics, a nurse executive can communicate effectively to the nursing workforce the ethical expectations for practice. Keeping in mind the relevance of an ethics framework and its transparency is also pivotal as any project transpires.

Utilization of Framework: A Case Study

Understanding the benefit of a nursing praxis can be demonstrated by analyzing a CNO's personal praxis (**Figure 1-1**) in the context of the phenomenon of interest of nurse residency programs (NRPs) for new graduate registered nurses (RNs). Analyzing empirical data related to a high level of RN vacancies across the hospital, the CNO quantified the operational impact of the vacancies. Hospital volume was increasing, but the size of the RN workforce remained stagnant. Hospital policy required any RN being hired to have at least 2 years of RN experience. Available qualitative information revealed engagement and organizational loyalty within the existing RN workforce were decreasing because of the work demands caused by the vacancies.

Understanding the ethical obligation to provide quality care and the stewardship responsibilities for leading nursing practice, the CNO discerned the need to change the policy on hiring only experienced RNs. This change required implementing an NRP to address the needs of RNs transitioning to professional practice. In designing the NRP, the CNO stressed the importance of communicating the SCDNT for health promotion and the use of nursing presence theory to guide training simulations. Understanding the complex, adaptive nature of the hospital, the CNO anticipated a positive butterfly effect as the NRP eliminated vacancies, increased RN engagement, and improved the quality of care. As the NRP proceeded, the CNO planned to collect data on the effects of the NRP and determine which data will influence the CNO's praxis (Figure 1-1) for future guidance.

Figure 1-1 Chief Nursing Officer Framework for Praxis

Reflection Questions

1. What are two benefits of praxis to nurses assigned to clinical and administrative roles?
2. How can you use the benefits of praxis to enhance your nursing knowledge and practice?

References

Carlson, E. A., & Staffileno, B. A. (2013). Establishing and sustaining an evidence-based practice environment. In M. A. Mateo & M. D. Foreman (Eds.), *Research for advanced practice nurses, from evidence to practice* (2nd ed., pp. 69–86). Springer.

Chism, L. A. (2013). The DNP graduate as ethical consultant. In L. A. Chism (Ed.), *The doctor of nursing practice* (2nd ed., pp. 179–212). Jones & Bartlett Learning.

Cody, W. K. (2013). Values-based practice and evidence-based care: Pursing fundamental questions in nursing philosophy and theory. In W. K. Cody (Ed.), *Philosophical and theoretical perspectives for advanced nursing practice* (5th ed., pp. 5–13). Jones & Bartlett Learning.

Fawcett, J. (1984). The meta-paradigm of nursing: Current status and future refinements. *Journal of Nursing Scholarship, 16*, 84–87. http://www.nursingsociety.org/Publication

Florczak, K., Poradzisz, M., & Hampson, S. (2012). Nursing in a complex world: A case for grand theory. *Nursing Science Quarterly, 25*, 307–312. https://doi.org/10.1177/0894318412457069

McMahon, M. A., & Christopher, K. A. (2011). Toward a mid-range theory of nursing presence. *Nursing Forum, 46*, 72–82. https://doi.org/10.1111/j.1744-6198.2011.00215.x

Monti, E. J., & Tingen, M. S. (1999). Multiple paradigms of nursing science. *Advances in Nursing Science, 21*, 64–80. http://journals.lww.com/advancesinnursingscience/pages/default.aspx

Orem, D. E. (1991). *Nursing: Concepts of practice* (4th ed.). Mosby.

Rolfe, G. (1993). Closing the theory-practice gap: A model of nursing praxis. *Journal of Clinical Nursing, 2*, 173–177. https://doi.org/10.1111/j.1365-2702.1993.tb00157.x

Effective Virtual Teams

James L. Harris

To nurture innovation, creativity, and measurable outcomes, cultures are required that are supportive of virtual teams. Virtual teams offer opportunities for collaboration and generation of knowledge from different individual, organizational, and geographical perspectives. The Department of Veterans Affairs Office of Nursing Services is an excellent example of how virtual project teams are formed, work collaboratively to standardize standards of practice, spread innovation, and generate evidence (Thorne-Odem et al., 2015).

Virtual Field Advisory Committees (FACs), composed of clinical experts and staff from 152 Veterans Affairs Medical Centers, were formed, and a program coordinator provided national oversight. Each FAC identified key priority areas within the specialty area (gap analysis) and developed projects that focused on improving veteran care and providing tools and resources for staff in order to meet care needs. Outcome metrics were identified in order to track team effectiveness and outcomes that were aligned with national performance measures. FACs collaborated with multiple internal and external stakeholders, quality indicators, and competency-based assessment processes.

As indicated in this brief example, virtual teams provide value to organizations and patient care, and they engender staff engagement. Although this was only one example, numerous healthcare organizations form virtual teams daily and collectively engage interprofessional teams to meet benchmarks and improve care.

Reflection Questions

1. How can you effectively contribute to a virtual team?
2. What are the key determinants of an effective virtual improvement team?

Reference

Thorne-Odem, S., Engstrom, C., Sommers, E., & Daly, A. (2015). Creating innovative models of nursing care. In C. Rick & P. B. Kritek (Eds.), *Realizing the future of nursing: VA nurses tell their story* (pp. 531–544). U.S. Department of Veterans Affairs Veterans Health Administration.

Increasing Therapeutic Communication Skills Using Behavioral Simulation

Bettina Riley

Based on an identified need to improve therapeutic communication skills in an undergraduate nursing course, behavioral simulation was used. This was based on one component of a team-based learning (TBL) strategy, the use of active learning versus passive learning techniques to increase knowledge (Michaelsen et al., 2008). Parmelee (2010) purports that TBL improves knowledge and critical thinking among nursing students.

The behavioral simulation session focused on a specific patient safety goal (i.e., depression with suicide risk) and was linked to suicide risk assessment, which was cited as a major patient safety goal by The Joint Commission (2017). The behavioral scenario emphasized the importance of suicide risk assessment, building on the establishment of a trusting, therapeutic nurse–patient relationship. The simulation experience utilized standardized patients trained in a prepared scenario before the event. Training emphasized depression criteria with suicidal ideations. The participants included 96 undergraduate nursing students who were involved in a pre-simulation educational TBL activity on suicide and suicide risk assessment. Next, individual students interviewed a standardized patient for purposes of completing a psychiatric assessment focused on suicide risk. Students were rotated through eight simulation rooms, and students and peers videotaped the assessment for future review. Debriefing sessions, led by psychiatric mental health faculty, followed each behavioral simulation. The purpose of debriefing was expression of feelings and exploration of benefits for clinical application. Student and faculty evaluations of the TBL, simulation, and debriefing experiences have been very positive. Positive evaluations by students centered on the ability to have a safe practice zone for acquiring assessment skills, particularly in sensitive-topic areas—over 93% of nursing students expressed more confidence in the ability to assess suicide risk, and over 90% of the students found that the standardized patient scenario, combined with the TBL, was helpful and effective. Anecdotal findings from faculty included comments suggesting that when students went to community and inpatient clinical sites after the behavioral simulation, they exhibited greater confidence and knowledge in clinical assessment of suicide risk and therapeutic communication skills.

Reflection Questions

1. What are other components of TBL that can be developed to enhance learning and competency development in baccalaureate nursing students?
2. In what ways can TBL activities be evaluated?

References

Michaelson, L. K., Parmelee, D. X., McMahon, K. K., & Levine, R. E. (2008). *Team-based learning for health professions education. A guide to using small groups for improving learning.* Stylus Publishing, LLC.

Parmelee, D. X. (2010). Team-based learning: Moving forward in curriculum innovation: A commentary. *Medical Teacher, 32*(2), 105–107.

The Joint Commission. (2017). National Patient Safety Goals effective January 2017. Behavioral health care accreditation program—Goal 15. *Behavioral Health Care: National Patient Safety Goals,* 1–4. https://www.jointcommission.org/assets/1/6/NPSG_Chapter_BHC_Jan2017.pdf

Increasing Access to Mental Health Treatment Using the Internet: A Quality Improvement Project Proposal

Jennifer Anne Blalock

Background

Although the Affordable Care Act (ACA) continues to face challenges, it nevertheless has presented an opportunity to improve mental health treatment. Underfunded and underutilized mental health treatment is desperately in need of change. The age of technology and widespread use of the internet present a new avenue for access and mental healthcare delivery. Rural populations will be able to receive more efficient and timely care.

Han et al. (2015) report that in 2012, approximately 9.6 million Americans older than the age of 17 were diagnosed with a serious mental illness (SMI). Depression alone affects 35 million Americans older than 65 years of age (Golden &Vail, 2014). Richards et al. (2015) acknowledge that depression is among the leading causes of disability worldwide, creating a significant economic burden, and the gap in treatment for depression is estimated to be 56.3%. Several contributing reasons are identified, including stigma associated with mental health treatment, physical and financial access to care, and availability of services. Costs of treatment for patients with an SMI are significant. However, the cost of preventive care, such as therapy and medication management, is considerably less than the cost of inpatient care or criminalization of those left untreated. According to Stensland, Watson, and Grazier (2012), the average hospital's cost of care delivery was highest for patients with Medicare and lowest for those who were uninsured. To use two common diagnoses, treatment for depression ranged from $6,990 for 8.4 days to $3,616 for 4.4 days, and alcohol use disorder treatment ranged from an average of $5,908 for 6.2 days to $4,147 for 3.8 days. Hoban (2013) compared the cost of mental health treatment, including medication management and outpatient services, for those on Medicaid to the cost of arrest and involvement in the criminal justice system; those arrested cost the government an average of $95,000 during the study period compared with $68,000 for those not arrested and channeled into mental health treatment. Although treating mental illness is expensive, the cost of NOT treating mental illness is more so. With this and similar studies in mind, a proposal to increase outreach and provide new access to care is presented.

Addressing the Treatment Gap

As healthcare providers in the United States struggle to meet the needs of mental health consumers, the use of the internet, or eMental Health, has become an attractive option. Batterman et al. (2015) reviewed four models of eHealth implementation in the community and found that all four were effective in the treatment of depression. ePrograms demonstrated several advantages to patients, particularly in the availability of services and increased access. By providing a common point of access, patients were able to locate both free and paid services in the community, allowing for self-referral without initial contact with a primary care physician (PCP). Handley et al. (2014) provide further support for internet-based mental health treatment, noting that such services make treatment options available to rural communities that would otherwise lack access to a mental health provider. Their results indicate that eHealth is as effective in treating mental health disorders as face-to-face contact and reduces the anxiety some patients experience in these interactions. Not only do web-based programs increase care access, but they also improve the timeliness of treatment, as there is no wait time and adherence to normal business hours is not necessary.

Proposed Project Implementation

Psychiatric providers will have the option of utilizing web-based services in several ways: continuation of already established, ongoing therapy; as a component of aftercare treatment upon completion of intensive services; and provision of a 24-hour crisis line to direct new patients to web-based services as determined appropriate by telephone triage. More patients can be treated, including those without access to transportation or those hesitant to seek face-to-face treatment. Use of eServices will be established on a sliding scale and fee-for-service copays based on insurance providers, providing additional revenue. Free services can also be included, funded by endowments or special purpose funds.

A business model with three layers will be developed, creating an eMental Health program: the patient layer (patients or payers that use the service), the operational service layer (operations, equipment, management, training, legal, billing, reimbursement), and the infrastructure layer (the telecommunication itself, including internet and wireless services). Implementation of eMental Health services can be integrated as part of the already-existing services as part of a behavioral health program, which encompasses two residential facilities as well as outpatient care.

For successful delivery of this relatively new concept, a development team will be necessary. This team will incorporate a variety of practitioners, including psychiatrists, medical physicians, nurses, and social workers, as well as a clinic manager, hospital administrator, and information technology (IT) development and support staff. Practice guidelines will be developed (hours of operation, policies specific to web interactions, etc.). Although these can run parallel to and include those already in place for existing psychiatric care facilities, attention to internet-related confidentiality must be considered. A new policy will be written. IT staff are critical in the development of web-based program components, with input from direct-care users, and in identifying costs and limitations. Design of the program will be done within the existing computer programs, thus reducing the cost of new software and licenses. Training time for staff already familiar with the platform will be reduced. Having an electronic medical record operational will strengthen the success of the eMental Health program. Once fully operational, with outcome measures that support continued use of an eMental Health program, additional delivery methods can be considered and employed, such as smartphone applications. Nicholas et al. (2017) found, in a study of individuals diagnosed with bipolar disorder, that the mobility of smartphone apps further increased accessibility, was cost effective, and allowed more client anonymity.

Evaluation

The structure of this proposal includes the use of computers and Wi-Fi, both public, such as those available in libraries, and those located within the patient's home. Staff involved in the program will utilize technology provided in on-site facilities. However, some home access may be granted as determined by the program director. Additional staffing will be needed to address the increased referrals anticipated from the implementation of eServices. The numbers required will likely increase over time as use of the program broadens. Use will be monitored to determine how many new staff are required. Initially, patient interactions will be managed with current staff plus one new psychiatrist, two family psychiatric nurse practitioners (FPNPs), and two additional psychiatric RNs. Web-based client interactions will be a portion of total patient contacts, the majority of which will remain face-to-face. Web visits will be billed at a lower cost than face-to-face visits, with some patients receiving pro bono services.

Process measures of the eHealth program will include tracking referrals and comparing data collected at three points: before program initiation, during the implementation phase, and later, during the sustainability phase. It is important to know not only if the number of referrals increased but also the number of patient contacts within the website. User-friendliness is a critical measure for web-based interactions and should be assessed regularly to ensure ease of use by patients and staff. The use of patient-satisfaction surveys will be critical in determining this aspect of the program. These can be mailed for completion or "attached" at the end of an internet session. Staff surveys will be utilized to determine areas that work well and those that require modification.

More important than use alone, the program needs to be effective and increase access to mental health services. The outcome of the program will be determined by comparing the number of patient psychiatric contacts before initiation of web-based services to those after implementation. This should be calculated at 6-month intervals for the first 18 months. The number of crisis inpatient admissions must also be compared to determine if web-based services produced a reduction in admissions by providing more access to psychiatric care by 50%. Pre- and postevaluations by patients will be conducted to gain an understanding of what patients found helpful and what needs to be improved. In addition, pre- and postsymptom assessment will be completed to determine effectiveness.

The return on investment for eMental Health services should not be anticipated as a black-and-white, financially based result. Initial investment costs could take several years to demonstrate cost savings related to decreased inpatient admissions or revenue created by increased patient contacts. Rather, the main purpose of the investment is enhancement of care quality. Swensen et al. (2013) note four instances of poor care quality that can be improved with this program: overuse care, defective care, inefficient care, and underuse care. By broadening effective psychiatric services, all of these can be addressed among individuals with mental health diagnoses. Overuse of inpatient psychiatric crisis admissions can be reduced, more effective and efficient care can be provided, and access to care can be increased. Although these changes, over time, have the potential to reduce costs to Medicare, Medicaid, and private insurance, the reason to adopt the program is not financial gain. This initiative is recommended to improve quality of care, not produce a financial return. By investing more in patients, genuine care and concern for patients' health outcomes will be evident, contributing to an improved reputation in the community and, ultimately, gaining increased credibility and potentially more patient flow and revenue as a result.

Conclusion

Web-based services provide a new opportunity for growth in the initial and ongoing treatment of patients with mental health diagnoses. Although use of this form of treatment remains in the introductory phase, the capacity to further the development of this approach is promising. Providing mental health care to a larger portion of the population by significantly increasing access, particularly for patients hesitant to engage face-to-face, those in rural communities, or those simply lacking transportation, is a valid rationale for the proposal. The timeline may vary, but it is anticipated to take approximately 18 months from the first team meeting to a full live rollout. Financially, the return on investment cannot yet be clearly defined, although in time reduced cost for services and increased revenue are anticipated. Mental health is a global issue and one that remains underfunded and underrecognized. With the inception of web-based services, the chance to become an innovator and a leader in the rapidly changing world of health care is possible. More importantly, many more patients can benefit from mental health treatment that was previously out of reach.

Reflection Questions

1. Consider that the mental health clinic where you are employed has experienced a 40% face-to-face missed-appointment rate. What options would you propose to the program director and why?
2. Reflect on a change in an organization. What are key considerations that resulted in the success or failure associated with the change, and why? What would you propose to improve the change?

References

Batterman, P. J., Sunderland, M., Calear, A. L., Davey, C. G., Christensen, H., Teesson, M., & Krouskos, D. (2015). Developing a roadmap for the translation of e-Mental Health services for depression. *Australian & New Zealand Journal of Psychiatry, 49*, 776–784. https://doi.org/10.1177/0004867415582054

Golden, R. L., & Vail, M. R. (2014). The implications of the Affordable Care Act for mental health care. *Journal of American Society on Aging, 38*, 96–103. www.asaging.org/generations-journal-american-society-aging

Han, B., Gfroerer, J., Kuramoto, J., Ali, M., Woodward, A., & Teich, J. (2015). Medicaid expansion under the Affordable Care Act: Potential changes in receipt of mental health treatment among low-income nonelderly adults with serious mental illness. *American Journal of Public Health, 105*, 1982–1989. https://www.apha.org/publications-and-periodicals/american-journal-of-public-health

Handley, T. W., Kay-Lambkin, F. J., Inder, K. J., Attia, J. R., Lewin, T. J., & Kelly, B. J. (2014). Feasibility of internet-delivered mental health treatments for rural populations. *Social Psychiatry and Psychiatric Epidemiology, 49*, 275–282. https://doi.org/10.1007/s00127-013-0708-9

Hoban, R. (2013, July 1). NC state study shows why it costs less to treat mentally ill than incarcerate them. *North Carolina Health News.* http://www.northcarolinahealthnews.org/2013

Nicholas, J., Fogarty, A. S., Boydell, K., & Christensen, H. (2017). The reviews are in: A qualitative content analysis of consumer perspectives on apps for bipolar disorder. *The Journal of Medical Internet Research, 19,* 1–18. https://doi.org/10.2196/jmir.7273

Richards, D., Timulak, L., O'Brien, E., Hayes, C., Sharry, J., & Doherty, G. (2015). A randomized controlled trial of an internet-delivery treatment: Its potential as a low-intensity community intervention for adults with symptoms of depression. *Behaviour Research and Therapy, 75,* 20–31. https://doi.org/10.1016/j.brat.2015.10.005

Stensland, M., Watson, P. R., & Grazier, K. L. (2012). An examination of costs, charges, and payments for inpatient psychiatric treatment in community hospitals. *Psychiatric Services, 63,* 666–671. https://doi.org/10.1176/appi.ps.201100402

Swensen, S. J., Dilling, J. A., McCarty, P. M., Bolton, J. W., & Harper, C. M. (2013). The business case for health-care quality improvement. *Journal of Patient Safety, 9,* 44–52. www.journalpatientsafety.com

Quality Improvement Projects and Quality Improvement Research: Advancing Translational Science

Linda Roussel

CHAPTER OBJECTIVES

1. Identify similarities and differences between quality improvement projects and quality improvement research.
2. Describe ethical considerations in quality improvement work.
3. Define quality improvement and its primary elements.
4. Describe improvement science and its role in examining the methods and factors that best facilitate quality improvement.
5. List considerations related to implementation science, translational science, and dissemination of both quality improvement projects and quality improvement research.

KEY TERMS

Improvement science
Innovation
Project planning

Quality improvement
Value

ROLES

Advocate
Leader

PROFESSIONAL VALUES

Evidence-based practice   Quality
Patient-centered care

CORE COMPETENCIES

Assessment   Leadership
Coordination   Management
Design   Risk mitigation

Introduction

Differentiating between a quality improvement project and research study can be challenging, because both involve defining a problem, planning and implementing an intervention or change to tackle the problem, then analyzing and evaluating the effect of the change on the problem (Gregory, 2015). Quality improvement activities are data-driven and involve human participants; therefore, it is not surprising that quality improvement and research can overlap with research methodologies common to human subjects' research. In situations where overlap exists between quality improvement and research methodologies, the federal regulations that protect human research participants may apply. When there is ambiguity about the type of work being conducted, team leaders are required to reflect on the intent, design, setting, benefit, and generalizability of the project findings. In addition, the oversight required, risk to participants, and ethical justification for the project need to be considered as part of determining which type of project the team is conducting.

The Institute of Medicine (IOM, 2001) describes six aims for quality care: it should be safe, timely, efficient, effective, equitable, and patient-centered. These aims provide key issues and concerns that guide quality improvement projects and research. According to a Hastings Center Report (2007), quality improvement is essential to the ongoing management of the healthcare system for delivering safe, quality clinical care and not an independent, knowledge-seeking enterprise. When there is uncertainty about the type of scholarly activity (quality improvement/research) being conducted, it is incumbent on systems' leaders to be mindful of the intent, design, setting, benefit, and generalizability of the project findings. (Additional considerations include the coaching required to complete the work, ethical concerns, and risks to participants. This is essential to better understanding the type of scholarly activity being conducted and the determination of quality improvement versus research (Jennings et al., 2007)).

Dubler et al., (2007) describe aspects of quality improvement and research that provide insights into distinguishing characteristics that guide best practices in considering both methods of improvement for patients and healthcare systems. For example, the aspect of level of subject knowledge and participation in quality improvement projects is general awareness as compared with research requiring individual informed consent. Quality improvement is an essential aspect of evidence-based health care; it is necessary as well as acceptable to consent to receive health care, which also includes consent to a reasonable level of cooperation with quality improvement activities. The degree of necessity for healthcare operations is considered nonexistent in research although it is implicit in quality improvement work. Assignment of interventions in research may be random, whereas quality improvement projects are often piloted for small tests of change. The nature of intervention in quality improvement projects may not be clear related to effectiveness, whereas research may demonstrate unclear efficacy. These aspects are essential to decision-making in overall operational goals of advancing innovation and improved delivery systems.

The Health Resources and Services Administration (HRSA, 2011) defines quality improvement as a systematic and continuous process that leads to measurable improvement in healthcare services and the health status of a targeted patient population. As a process for improving quality outcomes, strategies are employed in an intentional way to assure that there is flow from the gaps (needs assessment) to the planning, implementing, and evaluation phases. The IOM (2001) defines quality in health care as a direct relationship between the level of improved health services and the expected health outcomes of individuals and populations. Quality improvement strategies are integral to projects that focus on safety, improvement, and innovation. Studying improvement interventions and possible research study types informs quality improvement research. Understanding the basic principles of quality improvement and quality improvement research is the cornerstone of projects that are impactful and add value.

This chapter seeks to define quality improvement and identify the primary elements in the quality improvement cycle. Ways in which quality improvement projects and quality improvement research are differentiated are described as well. In addition, this chapter considers related improvement sciences, such as translational and implementation science.

Quality Improvement

Quality improvement requires thoughtful leadership in nursing as a major driver in advancing positive healthcare outcomes. Shewhart (1931) first studied quality from an industrial perspective, which led him to introduce concepts such as customer needs, reduction in variations in process, and elimination of the need for frequent inspections. Intrigued by Shewhart's work, Deming (1982) was able to determine that quality was a major driver for positive outcomes in industry; in turn, he introduced quality methodology to post–World War II Japanese engineers and executives. Deming's methods were strategically applied by the Japanese automobile industry, which enabled members of this industry—and other Japanese industries—to gain worldwide recognition for the quality of their products and services (Deming, 1982). Shewhart's and Deming's work on quality control has since informed the work of the Institute for Healthcare Improvement (IHI) and the Model for Improvement (MFI). The MFI is considered foundational to many of the quality models, such as Six Sigma, Lean Toyota, and the define–measure–analyze–improve–control (DMAIC) process (IHI, 2015c).

From the IOM's perspective, quality is considered within an organization's current system and is defined as how work gets done. Healthcare performance, however, is defined based on the organization's efficiency, care outcomes, and patient satisfaction levels. Quality is directly aligned with an organization's service delivery approach or underlying systems of care. Innovation is necessary to achieve a different level of performance and improve quality. From a project planning and management perspective to improve quality, it is important to understand the principles underpinning quality initiatives. The IOM purports that, although a quality project may be unique to the organization, all successful quality initiatives integrate four key principles:

1. Quality improvement work as systems and processes
2. Focus on patients
3. Focus on being part of the team
4. Focus on use of the data

Quality Improvement as Systems and Processes

If an organization is to make improvements, then understanding its own delivery system and key processes is critical to beginning this work. Quality improvement approaches recognize available resources (inputs) and tasks carried out (processes), which collectively determine quality of care (outputs/outcomes). For example, inputs may include people, infrastructure, materials, information, and technology. Consideration is given to the professionals and providers within the system, as well as to the supplies and equipment needed to carry out the project. According to Portela et al., (2015), quality improvement projects tend to be applied and, in some cases, self-evaluating. Although not directed at generating new knowledge, quality improvement projects may add considerable understanding of evidence-based uptake if the work is well conducted and cautious in their inferences (Portela et al., 2015).

Processes involve activities focusing on what is to be done and how the project will be carried out. Consequently, process-flow maps and concept maps are useful tools in illustrating the steps in carrying out the work. The process map, which comes to health care from engineering, provides a visual diagram that chronicles events or steps culminating in outcomes. The visualization of those steps provides a concrete look at how the work (process) is carried out, as well as who is accountable for that work and how efficiently the work flows, and can illuminate areas for improvement. Knowledge of how work flows may indicate the need for redesign, and the proposed plan can be compared to previous processes that are not working. In a blog post, IHI faculty members Little and Barbati (2015) describe five steps for creating value through process mapping and observations. The *first step*, identifying a care segment that has opportunities for improvement, involves looking at care segments with high consumption of resources, such as labor, supplies, time, and space. Opportunities for improvement could also include eliminating nonvalue-added clinical and administrative tasks. Interviewing experts (people involved in the process) and developing a first draft of a care segment process map is the *second important step* of process improvement. Preparing a list of frequently asked questions can be useful in optimizing the interviewee's time and talents. *Third,* it is best to start with Post-It notes, later converting to an electronic process map. This step allows for recognizing missing steps and illuminating misunderstandings, and it facilitates the ability to refer to the framework for improvement opportunities. A *fourth step* involves observing the care segment twice to validate the process map. Repeating the process twice allows for "catching" variations and provides a perspective on the general flow of expectations that can be validated from the team's practice experiences. A *fifth step* includes connecting the dots (closing the loop) with practice experts after the observation experience. This involves sharing findings with subject-matter experts and managers to further validate opportunities for improvement. This step also allows for identifying nonvalue-added processes, which may be barriers, leading to these processes only occurring 20% to 40% of the time. Tools and improvement strategies can be found at the IHI's website (Little & Barbati, 2015).

Gaps in the process can lead to further explorations, such as a thorough failure mode and effects analysis (FMEA). FMEA is a tool used for risk mitigation, which is essential to achieving safe, quality outcomes (IHI, 2015a). This type of analysis requires that each step (or process) be assessed for severity and frequency, with a hazard score being constructed to summarize these results. High hazard scores (8 or greater) alert the improvement team that emergent action is needed, particularly when the processes involve more than a single point, have few or no controls, and are not detectable (IHI, 2015b).

Outputs or outcomes may consider results or patterns such as health services delivered, changes in health behaviors and health status, and patient satisfaction. Health service delivery systems may be small, simple, and straightforward, such as a well-baby clinic, or multilayered and complex, such as a large corporate proprietary system. The efficiency and efficacy of the system depend on the services being individualized and attending to specific needs within the system. When the system considers the resources, activities, and results that exist and that are desired, quality improvement projects and programs can be customized to address unmet needs.

Focus on Patients

Patient-centered care is not a new concept; indeed, it has been reinforced as a competency for educating healthcare professionals in the 21st century (IOM, 2001). Patient-centered care evolved with the resurgence of the holistic roots of health care and initially had limited appeal given the complexity of the present healthcare system. Defined as engaging patients in a true partnership, patient-centered care involves personalizing care to include patients' normal routines and values. Such aims were considered daunting objectives when first introduced, and unrealistic at best. With increased technology and patient involvement, however, the creation of a healing physical environment, including one in which spiritual and emotional needs are met, has become mainstream practice.

So important is patient-centered care that the Hospital Consumer Assessment of Healthcare Providers and Systems (HCAHPS) created a survey that affords patients the opportunity to share information about their experiences with the healthcare system. In other words, this standardized tool assesses the way care is provided from the patients' perspective. Considering care from the patients' perspective considers more than just clinical treatment, medications, and technology. Although core measures provide data that evaluate hospitals' care quality, at a minimum from a standard-of-care perspective, the patient experience is not necessarily taken into consideration when evaluating overall care delivery. HCAHPS considers aspects of the healthcare experience that patients report is important to them on a personal level, such as communication with nurses and physicians, cleanliness and noise

levels, pain control, and quality of discharge instructions and medication information. Publicly reported scores of individual hospital systems have health systems on
high alert, given that patients can now compare the way care is delivered by various
systems and decide which is the best fit for them as individuals. With the advent
of value-based purchasing, HCAHPS data have become increasingly important as
a basis for reimbursement, further informing and advancing patient-centered care.
Responding to these demands by delivering patient-centered care has also become
an important business imperative.

The healthcare system's focus on patients is an important measure of quality
that considers the patients' needs and expectations. When a focus on patients is
present, services are created and designed by paying attention to the following factors: systems that affect patient access; care provision that is evidence-based; patient
safety; support for patient engagement; coordination of care with other parts of the
larger healthcare system; and cultural competence, including assessing the health
literacy of patients, patient-centered communication, and linguistically appropriate
care (HRSA, 2011).

Focus on Being Part of the Team

Quality improvement is a "team sport." Quality improvement as a team process denotes the importance of the team coming together to take advantage of the knowledge, skills, experience, and perspectives of individual providers and professionals
within the team to make sustainable improvements and produce innovations. Team
effectiveness can happen when the following elements are in play: considering the
process or system as complex; acknowledging that no one person in an organization
knows all the dimensions of an issue; recognizing that the process involves more
than one discipline or work area; advocating for solutions that require creativity;
and realizing that staff commitment and buy-in are needed.

Vickberg and Christfort (2017) describe four styles that give leaders and teams
a common language for understanding how people work and focus on improving
collaboration and interprofessional competency. According to the authors, the styles
bring useful perspectives and unique approaches to making decisions, generating
ideas, and addressing problems. Being able to identify styles provides a common
nomenclature, allowing for team structures that can maximize diversity and inclusion. The four styles are *Pioneers*, *Guardians*, *Drivers*, and *Integrators*. The *Pioneers*
are bold thinkers, creative, value risk, and trust their gut. They are imaginative,
ignite energy, and focus on the big picture. *Guardians*, in contrast, appreciate order,
rigor, and organizational stability. They are data-driven and want facts, figures, and
research-driven evidence to support their decisions. They are pragmatic and are
reluctant to take on risks, always weighing all sides of an argument before taking a
thoughtful position. Valuing challenges, generating momentum, and getting results
are characteristics of *Drivers*. That is, "drivers tend to view issues as black-and-white
and tackle problems head on, armed with logic and data" (Vickberg & Christfort,
2017, p. 52). The fourth style, *Integrators*, brings teams together and making connections. Integrators are diplomatic, focused on gaining consensus, and believe that
most issues are relative. They appreciate that relationships and responsibility to the
team are of the utmost importance. Intuitively bringing these styles together in teams
could be beneficial for cognitive diversity, increasing creativity and innovation, and

improving decision-making. In the authors' research, most top leaders are Pioneers or Drivers and report concern for groupthink because of their vocal styles. Guardians and Integrators were noted as being more stressed-out than any other styles; thus, looking for ways to maximize their strengths and easing their stress by making them feel psychologically safe are essential strategies for maximizing team effectiveness (Vickberg & Christfort, 2017).

Vickberg and Christfort (2017) provide strategies for managing the styles, specifically, pulling opposites closer, elevating the "tokens" on the team, and paying close attention to sensitive introverts (p. 54). Pulling opposites closer together can be accomplished by starting on small projects, then taking on bigger ones as the team opposites create complementary partnerships on the team. By generating productive friction and appreciating the differences, leaders can facilitate powerful collaborations. Elevating minority styles can enhance team functioning. For example, if you are trying to elicit Guardians' perspectives, it is best to give them time and the details they need to prepare for a discussion or a decision, allowing them to contribute in ways that are comfortable for them, for example, in writing. This allows them the opportunity to have their "voice heard" without having to compete for the floor because they likely will not push to speak. Pioneers' ideas are often expansive, so providing whiteboards and encouraging others to use the markers available for interacting through sharing ideas would be important to increasing contributions and collaboration. Planning timed discussions ahead of the meetings will allow Guardians, who prefer structure, the opportunity to relax into the free-flowing exercise. Vickberg and Christfort recommend that the team leader ask members to brainstorm ahead of the scheduled meeting so that the roundtable discussions may be conducted in a way that allows the team leader to give the floor to members who may be reticent to offer their ideas. A useful strategy if there are few members of a particular style is to ask team members to "think like" that style and doing so early in the meeting so that the majority viewpoint does not dominate the discussion (p. 55). Paying close attention to sensitive introverts involves encouraging anyone in the minority to share their "voice" early on before dominant styles forge ahead. Guardians and quiet integrators often are risk averse and so will see no reason to render their opinion to challenge prevailing wisdom. Team leaders who fail to recognize the various styles (particularly the quiet Integrators and Guardians) may miss the benefits of these styles. For example, these styles tend to be conscientious, thorough, and good at spotting errors and potential risks as they can focus intensely for long periods of time. Because they are good listeners, these styles often highlight others' great ideas and often take on and excel at the detail-oriented work that Pioneers and Drivers may prefer to pass on. Although it may seem labor intensive to "draw out" these quieter styles by slowing the pace, reducing information overload, providing quieter and more private work environments, or running interference so that they can focus with minimal distractions, the benefits outweigh the costs.

All quality improvement projects engage individuals as part of a team and implement quality improvement as a team process. Projects such as improving time to referring providers, increasing patient engagement, reducing wait time, and ensuring providers' use of evidence-based guidelines are team efforts that can go far toward achieving sustainable improvements. Active involvement of team members is critical, as each individual skill set and contribution leads to a synthesis and cooperation of ideas and solutions that would not have the same impact if they were implemented in isolation.

Another key component of a well-organized and functioning quality improvement team is an effective infrastructure, such as leadership and policies or procedures that design and facilitate the work of the team. A strong infrastructure provides the team with tools, resources, clarity of expectations, and a medium for communication (HRSA, 2011).

Focus on the Use of Data

A centerpiece of quality improvement is the use of data. Data can be used to determine how effectively current systems are working and what occurs when changes are applied, as well as to document successful performance. By using data, the team can accomplish several tasks. First, the quality improvement team members can separate what they believe is happening from what is actually happening within the system. A baseline can then be established to determine which, if any, changes made would be an improvement. It is likely that baseline scores will be low (this is acceptable), so the aim is to improve the rates and scores (e.g., patient satisfaction, falls, pressure ulcers, wait times, restraint use). By tracking data and comparing the baseline to the postintervention data, the team can determine the efficacy of solutions; likewise, by monitoring procedural changes, it can evaluate whether improvements are sustained over time. In this way, data serve as powerful sources by which to determine whether the changes made led to improvements, and they allow for comparisons of performance across sites.

Quantitative and qualitative methods of collecting data are essential to quality improvement projects. The use of numbers (rates, scores) and frequencies represents a quantitative research method that results in measurable data. Statistical process control, for instance, provides a wealth of information that can measure efficiency in care delivery. Examples include calculating how frequently patients access the emergency department and receive adequate health screenings. Run charts are useful in tracking improvement as they provide several benefits. For example, they help improvement teams develop goals by illustrating how well (or poorly) a small test of change is performing. Additionally, they can assist in deciding when changes are true improvements by showing a pattern of data that can be observed as changes are made. Run charts also give direction in real time on improvement and information about the value of specific changes (IHI, n.d.).

Although numbers, rates, and frequency provide excellent ways to measure improvement efforts, the use of qualitative methods sheds light on the depth and breadth of the experience of care delivery. Data that are qualitative in nature are observable (not measurable), consider patterns and relationships between systems, and are contextual in nature. Qualitative methods may include patient and staff satisfaction surveys, focus groups, interviews, and participant-observation experiences. Analyzing the data (transcripts) by identifying domains and themes through thematic analysis provides the story and voice of the participants (Caulfield, 2019).

Healthcare organizations can obtain data from several sources, including health records, patient and staff satisfaction surveys, external evaluations from accrediting and regulatory agencies, and community assessments. Using data sources in a methodical way within the infrastructure of an organizational system illuminates opportunities for improvement and allows for ongoing monitoring. Standardized performance measures focus on specific data for quality improvement programs.

Healthcare organizations are encouraged to collect data on performance measures that are impactful and add value to both the patient experience and the overall operation of the healthcare system. Such outcomes should guide the organization's decisions regarding which data are collected and measured.

Ethical Considerations for Protection of Human Participants in Quality Improvement Activities

There are several ethical elements to be concerned with when engaging in quality improvement work. These elements may include social and scientific value, scientific validity, fair subject selection, favorable risk/benefit ratio, and respect for participants (Jennings et al., 2007). Social and scientific value purports that, when considering gains from the quality improvement work, the team's ability to justify the resources expended and the risks to participants must be considered. From a scientific validity perspective, one should question if the quality improvement activity is methodologically sound and rigorously structured to accomplish its goals. Fair subject selection is concerned with determining a fair distribution of the burdens and benefits of quality improvement. When considering a favorable risk/benefit ratio, the team focuses on the design of the quality improvement activity that minimizes risks and maximizes potential benefits. It is also important to determine that the risk to an individual participant is in proportion to the benefit of the person and to society. Respect for participants in quality improvement activities needs to be designed to protect the privacy of participants through confidentiality. While maintaining confidentiality, quality improvement findings should be readily shared with team members in the healthcare system. That is, participants should expect to be informed about findings from the quality improvement activity that are clinically relevant for their own care. Along with this premise, patients and healthcare providers also should expect to receive basic information about the program of quality improvement activities within their healthcare system. Jennings et al. (2007) purport that low-risk quality improvement should generally have the same review and standards as routine healthcare delivery, whereas higher-risk quality improvement requires routine and orderly review within the standards of practice arrangements for clinical supervision or through an advisory group.

Quality Improvement Programs and Quality Improvement Research

With a quality improvement program, the quality improvement team considers the systematic activities that are designed and implemented to monitor, assess, and improve the organization's quality of health care for the population it serves. Higher levels of performance are reflected upon when reviewing the cyclical activities that are implemented to optimize resources and services for the patients served. There is a creative tension between innovation, sustained improvement, and ongoing delivery of evidence-based standards of care. Organizational quality improvement programs incorporate all quality improvement activities within the healthcare system.

The Donabedian model of structure, process, and outcomes provides a theoretical framework for integrating quality improvement strategies within the system (Donabedian, 1988). Leadership and interdisciplinary teams are essential to sustained quality improvement programs. Likewise, knowledge of the infrastructure and the principles of quality improvement is foundational to a successful quality improvement program. Leaders ask the question of how quality improvement processes work to support the success of the quality improvement program. A few benefits can be achieved from implementing a quality improvement program, including improved patient (clinical) outcomes that focus on process outcomes (screenings) and health outcomes (blood glucose and blood pressure readings within normal parameters). Other benefits of quality improvement programs are improved efficiency of managerial and clinical processes, such as reducing waste and maintaining financial viability.

According to HRSA, by improving processes and outcomes that reflect high-priority health needs, a system can reduce costs associated with system failures and redundancy. Quality improvement processes are typically budget-neutral, meaning that the costs incurred to make the changes are offset by the savings obtained through those efforts. Quality improvement programs put proactive processes in place and solve problems before they occur, making sure that systems of care are consistent, reliable, and predictable. These actions can go far in creating a culture of improvement, because they ensure that errors are tracked, reported, and addressed. Critical issues are often resolved because greater attention is paid to monitoring improvement initiatives and variations in standards of care.

Portela et al. (2015) offer ways to study improvement interventions using a variety of study types. The authors' literature search included reviewing several institutional sites, including the Health Foundation, IHI, and Improvement Science Research Network. Principles, strengths, weaknesses, and opportunities for study designs for improvement interventions are described. For example, considering quality improvement projects, the authors found that quality improvement projects should incorporate a theoretical base and qualitative methods in a more systematic way to allow for predicting and explaining the mechanisms for change involved. The authors note that more scientific rigor is needed in the application and reporting of Plan-Do-Study-Act (PDSA) cycles and other methods/techniques applied. Effectiveness studies, including randomized controlled trials (RCTs), quasi-experimental designs, observational (longitudinal) studies, and systematic reviews, are described. Specifically, strengths of systematic reviews are their ability to generate more powerful evidence, whereas weaknesses include uncritical incorporation and interpretation of studies, leading to inadequate conclusions. Low use of meta-analyses was also noted. The authors go on to report that because of the growth of systematic reviews on the effectiveness of quality improvement interventions, there is a need for more critical appraisal of the studies, including more meta-analyses, and to deal with complex interventions in diverse contexts.

With a culture of improvement in place, communication is enhanced both within the system and among community organizations. Improved communication focused on quality may result in stronger clinical partnerships and open funding opportunities. An effective quality improvement program can result in a balance of quality, efficiency, and profitability in its achievement of organizational goals (HRSA, 2011).

Quality Improvement Research

Quality improvement projects may come under the federal definition of research and may require institutional review board (IRB) review and approval if they involve human participants or individually identifiable data. Quality improvement programs and quality improvement research should not pose any risk to individuals, infringe on individual privacy, or breach individual confidentiality. Research in this context is defined as follows: 45 CFR 46.102(d) of the federal regulations defines research as a systematic investigation, including research development, testing, and evaluation designed to develop or contribute to generalizable knowledge. (Reproduced from the *Institutional Review Board Guidebook* [U.S. Department of Health and Human Service, 1993]. http://www.hhs.gov/ohrp/archive/irb/irb_chapter1.htm. Accessed February 8, 2015.)

One characteristic that distinguishes a quality improvement program from quality improvement research is whether the activities are intended or created to develop or contribute to generalizable knowledge. Results or research findings, when they are generalizable knowledge, can be applied to populations or situations beyond those being immediately studied. When quality improvement initiatives are not intended to yield generalizable knowledge, IRB review is not mandatory.

In contrast, quality improvement research that is planned to go beyond the scope of the unit, department, or services would require IRB approval. For example, the quality improvement team may want the results from its analysis and the interpretation of its quality initiative to be disseminated across a larger scope and to a broader community of scholars. In other cases, quality improvement research may be intended for application beyond the current quality control efforts or improvements, as when new procedures or processes are shared with a larger audience (outside of one system).

If at least one of these descriptions of quality improvement research applies to the team's quality improvement plan, the next consideration would be whether the proposed activities and strategies are a systematic investigation. When applying the concept of systematic investigation, the team would determine whether information beyond what is routine for patient care will be collected. For example, adding surveys or more data collection through qualitative means, which is typically not part of routine care delivery, would go beyond a quality improvement program. Another consideration with a systematic investigation would be to determine if the team will be assessing the effectiveness of processes or procedures and comparing two or more treatments, interventions, or processes. When such comparison is contemplated, and manipulation is done to determine if one practice is better, the effort would qualify as quality improvement research. When quality improvement activities entail a systematic investigation that will develop or contribute to generalizable knowledge, per 45 CFR 46.102(d), IRB review is mandatory (HHS, n.d.).

Quality improvement research may be required for writing implementation research grants. Proctor et al. (2012) provide 10 key ingredients, possibly best practices, for writing implementation research grant proposals. These ingredients include key questions to ask as well as review criteria. The 10 ingredients are as follows:

1. The care gap or quality gap
2. The evidence-based treatment to be implemented

3. Conceptual model and theoretical justification
4. Stakeholder priorities, engagement in change
5. Settings' readiness to adopt new services/treatments/programs
6. Implementation strategies/process
7. Team experience with the setting, treatment, and implementation process
8. Feasibility of proposed research design and methods
9. Measurement and analysis section
10. Policy/funding environments, leverage, or support for sustaining change (p. 3)

Considering the 10 key ingredients can strengthen your grant proposal. Review criteria are also offered and include significance impact, significance innovation, approach innovation, impact innovation, and environment. Knowing and responding to key questions and review criteria can best prepare the implementation science researcher in developing a strong, comprehensive grant proposal.

Specifically, when considering the implementation strategy/process ingredient, the researchers ask, "Are the strategies to implement the intervention clearly defined and justified conceptually?" The review criteria would include significant impact and innovation. Considering the ingredient of measurement and analysis section, the researcher would pose the following questions:

1. Does the proposal clarify the key constructs to be measured, corresponding to the overarching conceptual model or theory?
2. Is a measurement plan clear for each construct?
3. Does the analysis section demonstrate how relationships between constructs will be tested?

The review criteria to consider when focused on the measurement and analysis section considers the approach investigator team and provides key ways to address how the researchers will tackle this critical ingredient (Proctor et al., 2012).

At the outset, many quality improvement projects have only local (organizational) assurance/improvement intentions; during the process of data collection or analysis; however, it may become clear that the findings could be generalizable or benefit others. In such a case, IRB review should occur—that is, IRB review is necessary whenever there is an intention to make findings generalizable.

Translational Science: Quality Improvement and Research Implications

Translational science investigates implementation strategies that work to promote use of evidence-based practices (EBPs) for whom, in what types of settings, and identifies the methods by which they work. Advancing translation science can expedite integration of evidence in practice to improve population health, care delivery, and health outcomes (Henly et al., 2015). Translational science includes quality improvement and research perspectives.

Although nurses are the largest subgroup in the healthcare system, they lack representation on decision-making bodies. Quality improvement activities can increase nurses' influence and involvement in decision-making at the policy level. A Gallup survey conducted by the Robert Wood Johnson Foundation, titled "Nursing

Leadership from the Bedside to the Boardroom: Opinion Leaders' Perception" (Gallup/Robert Wood Johnson Foundation, 2010), reported that the persons surveyed considered government executives (75%) and health insurance executives (56%) as being able to exert more influence on health reform than nurses, whom they ranked as having only 14% influence (Khoury et al., 2011). These numbers demonstrate that nurses, especially those in positions of authority, need to encourage the development of leaders within the profession and advocate for interprofessional quality improvement team activity. Quality improvement programs provide an excellent opportunity for nurses to become involved in sustainable changes and policy development.

Beyond quality improvement's immediate impact and results, consideration should be given to dissemination of both quality improvement projects and quality improvement research. Translational science, including improvement and implementation sciences, is also important to developing quality improvement science.

Healthcare providers and consumers of health care are becoming more aware that research results that may have broad application do not always readily translate into improved health outcomes. The implementation and dissemination of research and science rely on a multidisciplinary set of theories and methods aimed at improving this process of translation from research evidence to pragmatic health-related practices. Implementation research investigates how interventions can best be integrated into diverse practice settings and underscores direct engagement with the institutions and communities where health interventions are introduced. Team science and organizational and cultural perspectives are also integrated into translational science, as the gold standard of research (RCTs) often does not consider the details necessary for application of findings.

Disseminating quality improvement projects and research can take many forms, such as local stakeholder engagement; poster and podium presentations at regional, national, and international venues; and publication of manuscripts that share findings obtained, barriers overcome, and lessons learned. An excellent resource for dissemination of results is the Agency for Healthcare Research and Quality's (AHRQ) Health Care Innovations Exchange (AHRQ, n.d.). The Innovation Exchange is a web-based resource created to assist healthcare professionals in sharing and adopting innovations that improve healthcare quality. The website includes a clearinghouse of innovative ideas and opportunities to learn and share ideas with others.

Using research evidence to develop EBP guidelines is also important in the application and translation process of quality improvement projects and research. The National Guidelines Clearinghouse (NGC), another initiative of the AHRQ, was originally created by the AHRQ in partnership with the American Medical Association and the American Association of Health Plans (now America's Health Insurance Plans [AHIP]). The mission of the NGC is "to provide health professionals, healthcare providers, health plans, integrated delivery systems, purchasers, and others with a readily usable mechanism for accessing objective, detailed information on clinical practice guidelines and to further their dissemination, implementation, and use" (NGC, 2017).

Quality improvement projects and research can also be disseminated through manuscript submissions. A useful tool in writing up quality improvement projects is the Standards for Quality Improvement Reporting Excellence (SQUIRE) guidelines. According to its sponsoring organization, the SQUIRE guidelines assist authors in writing up excellent, usable articles about quality improvement in health care. The guidelines serve to report findings that may be easily discovered and widely disseminated. The SQUIRE website notes that high-quality writing about improvement, lists of available resources, and discussions about the writing process can enhance dissemination and adoption of best practices. Sponsors of the SQUIRE guidelines include the Dartmouth Institute for Health Policy and Clinical Practice, the Robert Wood Johnson Foundation, Quality and Safety in Healthcare, and the IHI (SQUIRE, 2017).

Quality improvement projects and research can also be shared through the Honor Society of Nursing, Sigma Theta Tau International. Its e-Repository hosts communities and collections that can be accessed and applied in practice, as well as a method of disseminating quality projects and research. According to the website, the Henderson Repository, a resource of Sigma Theta Tau International, offers the following benefits:

- *Online dissemination.* This global digital service collects, preserves, and shares nursing research and EBP materials.
- *Free open access.* There is no charge to submitting nurse authors and no access fee for online patrons.
- *Peer review.* Submissions to collections under the Independent Submissions community are peer reviewed (Sigma Theta Tau International, n.d.).

Dissemination of evidence and information takes many forms, and methods for quality improvement and quality improvement research can be shared with many colleagues through these means. Evidence-based journal clubs and clinical scholars' programs are other ways to raise the level of conversation, create a spirit of inquiry, and enhance the culture of improvement in health care.

Summary

- Quality improvement projects and quality improvement research share common aims for making healthcare systems safe and quality driven.
- It is important to consider the ethical and regulatory issues for quality improvement projects and research.
- Leading a quality team that is focused on patient-centered care and using data to inform the process are essential to the work of clinical nurse leaders, executive leadership students, doctors of nursing practice (DNP), and highly functioning interprofessional project teams.
- The foundational work for the development of quality improvement projects and research is key to sustaining success over the long term.

Reflection Questions

1. Describe quality improvement projects you are currently involved in as part of your practice immersion experience.
2. Identify the types of data (quantitative, qualitative) that you plan to collect, and create a data analysis and management plan for your quality improvement project or research study.

3. Using the styles described by Vickberg and Christfort (2017), identify the styles in your team meeting, outlining strategies in place to increase team members' contributions and collaboration.

4. Outline potential ethical and regulatory issues that may impact your quality improvement project or quality improvement research study.

References

Agency for Healthcare for Research and Quality. (n.d.). *Innovation exchange*. https://innovations.ahrq.gov

Caulfield, J. (2019). *How to do thematic analysis*. https://www.scribbr.com/methodology/thematic-analysis/

Deming, E. W. (1982). *Out of crisis*. MIT Center for Advanced Engineering Study.

Donabedian, A. (1988). The quality of care: How can it be assessed? *Journal of the American Medical Association, 260*(12), 1743–1748. https://doi.org/10.1001/jama.1988.03410120089033

Dubler, N., Blustein, J., Bhalia, R., & Bernard, D. (2007). Informed participation: An alternative ethical process for including patients in quality improvement projects. In B. Jenning, M. Baily, M. Bottrell, & J. Lynn (2007), *Health care improvement: Ethical and regulatory issues* (pp. 74–93). Hasting Center.

Gallup/Robert Wood Johnson Foundation. (2010). *Nursing leadership from bedside to boardroom: Opinion leaders' perceptions*. https://www.rwjf.org/en/library/research/2010/01/nursing-leadership-from-bedside-to-boardroom.html

Gregory, K. (2015). Differentiating between research and quality improvement. *The Journal of Perinatal and Neonatal Nursing, 29*(2), 100–102. https://doi.org/10.1097/jpn.0000000000000107

Health and Human Services. (n.d.). *Office of Human Research Protections. Federal policy for the protection of human subjects* ("common rule"). https://www.hhs.gov/ohrp /regulations-and-policy /regulations/common-rule/index.html

Health Resources and Services Administration. (2011). *Quality improvement*. https://www.hrsa.gov /sites/default/files/quality/toolbox/508pdfs/qualityimprovement.pdf

Henly, S., McCarthy, D., Wyman, J., Heitkemper, M., Redeker, N., Titler, M. G., McCarthy, A., Stone, P., Moore, S., Alt-White, A., Conley, Y., & Dunbar-Jacob, J. (2015). Emerging areas of science: Recommendations for nursing science education from the Council for the Advancement of Nursing Science Idea Festival. *Nursing Outlook, 63*(4), 398–407. https://doi.org/10.1016/j .outlook.2015.04.007

Institute for Healthcare Improvement. (2015a). *Failure mode effect analysis tool*. http://www.ihi.org /resources/Pages/Tools/FailureModesandEffectsAnalysisTool.aspx

Institute for Healthcare Improvement. (2015b). *How to improve*. http://www.ihi.org/resources /Pages/HowtoImprove/default.aspx

Institute for Healthcare Improvement. (2015c). *The breakthrough series: IHI's collaborative model for achieving breakthrough improvement*. http://www.ihi.org/resources/Pages/IHIWhitePapers /TheBreakthroughSeriesIHIsCollaborativeModelforAchievingBreakthroughImprovement.aspx

Institute for Healthcare Improvement. (n.d.). *Run chart tool*. http://www.ihi.org/resources/Pages /Tools/RunChart.aspx

Institute of Medicine. Committee on Quality Health Care in America. (2001). *Crossing the quality chasm: A new health system for the 21st century*. National Academy Press. http://www.iom.edu /About IOM.aspx

Jennings, B., Baily, M. A., Bottrell, M., & Lynn, J. (2007). Health care quality improvement: Ethical and regulatory issues. *The Hastings Center*. https://www.thehastingscenter.org/wp-content /uploads/Health-Care-Quality-Improvement.pdf

Khoury, C. M., Blizzard, R., Moore, L. W., & Hassmiller, S. (2011). Nursing leadership from bedside to boardroom: A Gallup national survey of opinion leaders. *Journal of Nursing Administration, 41*(7/8), 299–305. https://doi.org/10.1097/nna.0b013e3182250a0d

Little, K., & Barbati, M. (2015). 5 steps for creating value through process mapping and observations. *Institute of Healthcare Improvement [Blog post]*. http://www.ihi.org/communities /blogs /5-steps-for-creating-value-through-process-mapping-and-observation

National Guideline Clearinghouse. (2017). *Help & about*. https://www.guideline.gov/

Portela, M. C., Pronovost, P. J., Woodcock, T., Carter, P., & Dixon-Woods, M. (2015). How to study improvement interventions: A brief overview of possible study types. *BMJ Quality & Safety, 24*, 325–336. https://doi.org/10.1136/bmjqs-2014-003620

Proctor, E. K., Powell, B. J., Baumann, A. A., Hamilton, A. M., & Santens, R. L. (2012). Writing implementation research grant proposals: Ten key ingredients. *Implementation Science, 7*(96), 1–13. http://www.implementationscience.com/content/7/1/96

Shewhart, W. A. (1931). *Economic control of quality of manufactured product*. D. Van Nostrand.

Sigma Theta Tau International. (n.d.). *Virginia Henderson Global Nursing e-Repository*. http://www.nursinglibrary.org/vhl

Standards for Quality Improvement Reporting Excellence. (2017). *Revised Standards for Quality Improvement Reporting Excellence SQUIRE 2.0*. http://squire-statement.org

U.S. Department of Health and Human Services. (1993). *Institutional review board guidebook*. https://www.hhs.gov/ohrp/education-and-outreach/archived-materials/index.html

Vickberg, S. M. J., & Christfort, K. (2017). Pioneers, drivers, integrators, and guardians. *Harvard Business Review, 95*(2), 50–57. https://search.ebscohost.com/login.aspx? direct=true&AuthType=ip,uid&db=bth&AN=121396241&site=ehost-live

Case Exemplars

Quality Teams Approach to Discharge Planning

Terri Poe

A team of DNP students engaged their quality team at their practice site to improve discharge planning by reducing nonvalue-added activities. The students, working together as a team of acute care nurse practitioners (ACNPs), noted a pattern of increasingly long waits for patients to be transferred to another level of care. To confirm that the pattern they experienced was a "true gap," they engaged their team members, the quality committee, and the chief nurse executive (CNE) to share their concerns. To obtain data to examine the outcomes, they were required to submit a question and begin a search of the external evidence. Through their translational courses, the students were able to step through the quality improvement process, beginning with obtaining internal data through a microsystems analysis and a FMEA, identifying a gap, searching for external evidence (synthesizing the research), and working with the MFI to begin a small test of change. As they progressed in their quality improvement work, they were able to bring team members along by charting a team, examining the process (through a process flow map), and using PDSA as a methodological framework for their scholarly project.

Reflection Questions

1. How can faculty best assure that doctoral students and interprofessional teams consistently go through a quality improvement process in which they will be able to engage their local stakeholders?
2. After completing the first iteration of the PDSA method, what would you suggest is the best way for doctoral students and teams to disseminate their results from the first cycle?

Action Plans as an Effective Asthma Management Tool: A Proposed Quality Improvement Project

Heather Surcouf

Asthma affects more than 22 million Americans. Asthma exacerbations lead to missed school, low quality of life, missed days on the job, hospitalizations, and emergency department visits. Multiple studies support asthma action plans (AAPs) as effective tools for asthma management.

At one school-based health center in Louisiana, the AAP completion rates declined markedly after adoption of an electronic health record (EHR). A project utilizing EHR reminders to prompt providers to complete AAPs was proposed. These reminders were set up to "pop up" in the EHR when an AAP is due. The provider recorded which action was taken (e.g., AAP completed, rescheduled, canceled) to move beyond the pop-up. These reminders automatically did the reset to appear on a yearly basis. The project relied on the Donabedian Model of Quality Care for theoretical structure. The Deming cycle and PDSA method of quality monitoring were used to assure continued quality improvements.

Specific project goals included the following: (1) increased provider AAP completion rates, (2) continued Office of Public Health clinic funding secondary to AAP benchmark satisfaction, and (3) reduced asthma exacerbation-related clinic visits. Congruent with the guidelines of the American Association of Colleges of Nursing (AACN) and advanced nursing practice (DNP Essentials), this project evaluated provider use of information systems and technology to support and improve patient care using the AAP (AACN, 2006, p. 12).

Records of patients with asthma (ages 14–21) were audited both before and after project implementation for the presence of a completed, up-to-date AAP. Preimplementation data and postimplementation data for two separate 9-month periods were compiled through a retrospective review of the electronic records of patients seen in the clinic for a 9-month period before the study and for a 9-month period after the study's implementation, based on their diagnosis of asthma. Records included for review were determined through the electronic record's reporting program. Results were tabulated using a frequency table (i.e., the number of patients with asthma with a completed AAP and the number of patients with asthma without a completed AAP). A second frequency table was used to tally the number of asthma-related visits for the same study periods using identical ICD-9 codes. Lastly, providers were given an anonymous survey before and after the intervention to gauge their familiarity with EHR reminders as well as their opinion regarding their effectiveness.

Reflection Questions

1. What is the value of an action plan in managing clinical symptoms?
2. How can medical record reminders promote patient-centered care delivery?
3. Identify tools that are useful in implementing quality improvement projects. Which of the tools are most useful when developing and implementing projects?

Reference

American Association of Colleges of Nursing. (2006). *Doctor of nursing practice (DNP) essentials.* http://www.aacnnursing.org/Education-Resources/AACN-Essentials

Bibliography

Bell, L. M., Grundmeier, R., Localio, R., Zorc, J., Fiks, A. G., Zhang, X., Stephens, T. B., Swietlik, M., & Guevara, J. P. (2010). Electronic health record-based decision supports to improve asthma care: A cluster-randomized trial. *Pediatrics, 125*(4), e770–e774. https://doi.org/10.1542/peds .2009-1385

Centers for Disease Control and Prevention. (2007, May 4). *CDC vital signs: Asthma in the U.S.* http:// www.cdc.gov/vitalsigns/asthma

Ducharme, F. M., & Bhogal, S. K. (2008). The role of written action plans in childhood asthma. *Current Opinion in Allergy and Clinical Immunology, 8*(2), 177–188. http://www.ncbi.nlm.nih .gov/pmc/articles/PMC3522127

Halterman, J. S., Fisher, S., Conn, K. S., Fagnano, M., Lynch, K., Marky, A., & Szilagyi, P. G. (2006). Improved preventive care for asthma: A randomized trial of clinician prompting in pediatric offices. *Archives of Pediatrics and Adolescent Medicine, 160*, 1018–1025. http://archpedi.jama network.com; links.com/index.php

Tolomeo, C., Shiffman, R., & Bazzy-Asaad, A. (2008). Electronic medical records in a sub-specialty practice: One asthma center's experience. *Journal of Asthma, 45*(9), 849–851. https://doi.org /10.1080/02770900802380803

Turkelson, C., Aebersold, M., Redman, R., & Tschannen, D. (2017). Improving Nursing Communication Skills in an Intensive Care Unit Using Simulation and Nursing Crew Resource Management Strategies: An Implementation Project. *Journal of nursing care quality, 32*(4), 331–339. https://doi.org/10.1097/NCQ.0000000000000241

Implementation Science, Team Science, and Translational Science: The Value for Improvement Projects

Clista Clanton
Linda Roussel

CHAPTER OBJECTIVES

1. Provide an overview of implementation and team science.
2. Discuss a variety of implementation science theoretical frameworks.
3. Describe the importance of compiling evidence-based implementation strategies to facilitate fidelity of translation.
4. Identify key characteristics for successful teamwork through implementation science.
5. Describe implications of project management through an implementation science lens.

KEY TERMS

Implementation science
Interprofessional Education
    Collaborative (IPEC)
Knowledge translation

National Center for Advancing
    Translational Science (NCATS)
Science of Team Science (SciTS)
Translational science

ROLES

Healthcare researcher

Healthcare team member

PROFESSIONAL VALUES

Evidence-based practice   Teamwork
Patient-centered care

CORE COMPETENCIES

Cultural competency and awareness   Resilience
Emotional intelligence   Shared problem-solving
Flexibility   Team building skills
Interprofessional collaboration

Introduction

The complexity of health care has led to the development of disciplines such as translational, team, and implementation sciences. Although interrelated and complementary, each discipline is distinct. This chapter will focus primarily on implementation and team sciences, yet it is helpful to place all three disciplines into context, because the development of each is directly related to specific needs and events within research and healthcare systems. An examination of how each area has developed gives a snapshot in time to some of the challenges healthcare professionals currently face in their day-to-day roles within practice settings, as well as ways to meet these challenges. Implications for project planning and management will be described.

It is estimated that it takes 17 years for research evidence to make an impact on clinical practice (Morris et al., 2011), which highlights the significant time lags in the conversion of basic science into practices that benefit patients. This process of conversion is referred to as *translation*, and each phase of the translational research process has activities that contribute to these time lags, including securing financing in the form of grants, receiving approvals from institutional review boards (IRBs), conducting clinical trials, presenting, publishing research results, and developing practice guidelines. Furthermore, there are different phases in the translational research process, and the activities contributing to these time lags may occur in more than one phase:

T1: involves processes that bring ideas from basic research through early testing in humans.

T2: involves the establishment of effectiveness in humans and clinical guidelines.

T3: primarily focuses on implementation and dissemination of research.

T4: focuses on outcomes and effectiveness in populations.

T0: involves research, such as genome-wide association studies, that wraps back around to basic research (Fort et al., 2017).

The term *translational research* first appeared in health science literature in the early 1990s. Given the relative newness of the field of translational science, it makes sense that formal definitions continue to evolve. The National Center for Advancing

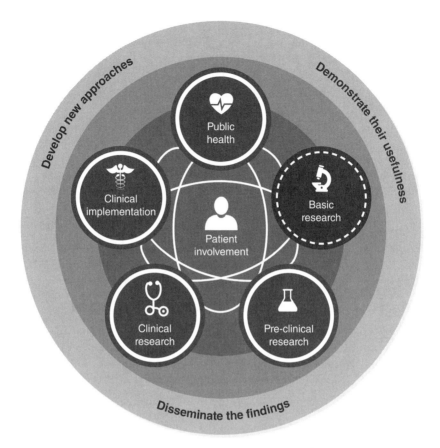

Figure 3-1 NCATS Translational Science Spectrum

Translational Science (NCATS) of the National Institutes of Health (NIH) currently describes a Translational Science Spectrum (**Figure 3-1**), which "represents each stage of research along the path from the biological basis of health and disease to interventions that improve the health of individuals and the public. The spectrum is not linear or unidirectional; each stage builds upon and informs the others." Patient involvement is considered a critical feature of all the stages of the translation process (NCATS, 2021c). The Clinical and Translational Science Awards (CTSA) Program operates under the leadership of NCAT to support a national network of medical research institutions known as *hubs*. In 2021, over 50 medical research institutions in the United States received CTSA program funding, with the hubs collaborating at both the local and regional level to develop and promote training, research tools, and processes designed to get more evidence into practice as quickly as possible and to make a positive impact on patient care (NCATS, 2021a, 2021b).

The T3 and T4 phases of the translational research process introduce us to implementation science, which is "the study of methods to promote the adoption and integration of evidence-based practices, interventions and policies into routine health care and public health settings" (Fogarty International Center, 2017).

The synthesis of research findings into digestible formats for inclusion in systematic reviews, practice guidelines, and other evidence-based resources is one of the strategies to help healthcare professionals implement relevant evidence into clinical practice (Straus et al., 2009). There are multiple conceptual frameworks that provide structure to the implementation of evidence into practice. Several online tools are available to researchers interested in identifying an appropriate theory, model, or framework for their implementation project, including the Theory, Model, and Framework Comparison and Selection Tool (T-CaST) (https://impsci.tracs.unc.edu/tcast/) and the Dissemination & Implementation Models Webtool (https://dissemination-implementation.org/index.aspx). Brief overviews of the Promoting Action on Research Implementation in Health Sciences (PARiHS); the Consolidation Framework for Implementation Research (CFIR); the Knowledge to Action (KTA) framework; the Reach, Effectiveness, Adoption, Implementation, and Maintenance (RE-AIM) framework, and the Aims, Ingredients, Mechanism, Delivery (AIMD) framework are included in the text that follows.

Promoting Action on Research Implementation in Health Sciences

PARiHS is a multidimensional framework designed to represent the complexity of the change processes involved in implementing research into practice and includes three elements: evidence, context, and facilitation. In the PARiHS framework, evidence includes research, clinical experience, patient experience, and local data or information. The PARiHS framework is outlined as: SI = f (E, C, F). Specifically, SI is successful implementation; E denotes evidence; C relates to context; F is facilitation; and f denotes the function of the change process. In the PARiHS, the factor of evidence, context, and facilitation consists of subelements that can be scored (rated) on a scale from low to high. According to researchers, high ratings on each factor are more likely to produce successful implementation results (Kitson et al., 1998; Kitson et al., 2008).

Implementation processes are likely to be more successful when research, as well as clinical and patient experiences, are located toward high. For research, high includes studies that are rigorous and have received consensus. High for clinical experiences are those that have been made explicit and verified via critical reflection, critique, and debate. Patient experience is considered at a high level when patient preferences have been used as part of the decision-making process. For local data and information to be considered high, they should have been systematically collected and evaluated.

Context in the PARiHS framework refers to the environment or setting where people receive health care as well as the environment or setting in which the proposed changes are to be implemented. Successful implementation of evidence into practice is influenced by three broad themes: culture, leadership, and evaluation. Organizations that create learning cultures are potentially able to facilitate change more easily, as attention is paid to individuals, group processes, and organizational systems. Transformational leaders are those who can transform cultures and create contexts that are more conducive to the integration of evidence into practice. They do this through inspiring staff to have a shared vision and by establishing clear roles, effective teamwork, and organizational structures. Evaluation is a key component in the environment, as measurement generates evidence on which to base practice and demonstrates if changes to practices have been successful.

Facilitation in the PARiHS framework refers to the process of enabling or making easier the implementation of evidence into practice. This is achieved by an individual with the appropriate role, skills, and knowledge who acts as a facilitator to help individuals, teams, and organizations apply evidence into practice. High facilitation in the PARiHS framework is holistic (sustained partnerships, developmental, adult learning approaches, high intensity or limited coverage) and with an appropriate level of facilitation, whereas low facilitation is more task oriented (episodic contact, practical or technical help, didactic approach to teaching, low intensity or extensive coverage) and would correspond to either absent or inappropriate facilitation (Rycroft-Malone, 2004).

For the PARiHS conceptual heuristic to become a truly useful and integrated framework for practitioners of implementation science, three areas have been identified that need further work: conceptual development, empirical testing and refinement, and the development of reliable measures to diagnose and evaluate readiness to change and the effectiveness of that change within an organization (Kitson et al., 2008). Subsequent studies have reinforced the need for development in these three areas and have suggested other issues to consider, such as the role that individuals play in the implementation process. To that end, the integrated or i-PARiHS has been proposed as a more integrated approach. In addition to the key constructs of evidence, context, and facilitation, a new construct has been suggested: the recipient, or the people who are affected by and influence implementation at both the individual and collective team level. This new construct recognizes the importance that groups, or teams of individuals, have in influencing the adoption of evidence into practice. The i-PARiHS also makes a distinction between the inner context of the immediate local setting versus the outer context of the wider health system that the organization is a part of, including the policy, social, regulatory, and political infrastructures surrounding the local context. The facilitation construct is also positioned as the active ingredient of implementation, with networks of novice, experienced, and expert facilitators who help structure the process while engaging and managing relationships with key stakeholders as well as identifying and negotiating the barriers to implementation within their settings (Harvey & Kitson, 2016).

Consolidation Framework for Implementation Research

The lack of consistent terminology and definitions in implementation theories as well as no one theory containing all the key constructs needed for successful implementation has been identified as a problem in the science of implementation, leading to the development of the Consolidated Framework for Implementation Research (CFIR; CFIR Research Team n.d.). This meta-theoretical framework contains the common constructs identified from published implementation theories and is designed to embrace, rather than replace, the already existing significant research related to implementation science. The CFIR's goal is to help advance the field by providing consistent taxonomy, terminology, and definitions and to allow researchers to select the constructs from the CFIR that are the most relevant for their setting and needs.

The CFIR is composed of five major domains which interact with each other to influence the effectiveness of implementation. **Table 3-1** briefly describes the

Table 3-1 Consolidated Framework for Implementation
Research Constructs

	Construct	Short Description
I. Intervention Characteristics		
A	Intervention Source	Perception of key stakeholders about whether the intervention is externally or internally developed
B	Evidence Strength and Quality	Stakeholders' perceptions of the quality and validity of evidence supporting the belief that the intervention will have desired outcomes
C	Relative Advantage	Stakeholders' perception of the advantage of implementing the intervention versus an alternative solution
D	Adaptability	The degree to which an intervention can be adapted, tailored, refined, or reinvented to meet local needs
E	Trialability	The ability to test the intervention on a small scale in the organization and to be able to reverse course (undo implementation) if warranted
F	Complexity	Perceived difficulty of implementation, reflected by duration, scope, radicalness, disruptiveness, centrality, and intricacy and number of steps required to implement
G	Design Quality and Packaging	Perceived excellence in how the intervention is bundled, presented, and assembled
H	Cost	Costs of the intervention and costs associated with implementing the intervention, including investment, supply, and opportunity costs
II. Outer Setting		
A	Patient Needs and Resources	The extent to which patient needs, as well as barriers and facilitators to meet those needs, are accurately known and prioritized by the organization
B	Cosmopolitanism	The degree to which an organization is networked with other external organizations
C	Peer Pressure	Mimetic or competitive pressure to implement an intervention, typically because most or other key peer or competing organizations have already implemented, or are in a bid for, a competitive edge
D	External Policy and Incentives	A broad construct that includes external strategies to spread interventions, including policy and regulations (governmental or other central entity), external mandates, recommendations and guidelines, pay-for-performance, collaboratives, and public or benchmark reporting

Construct		Short Description
III. Inner Setting		
A	Structural Characteristics	The social architecture, age, maturity, and size of an organization
B	Networks and Communications	The nature and quality of webs of social networks and the nature and quality of formal and informal communications within an organization
C	Culture	Norms, values, and basic assumptions of a given organization
D	Implementation Climate	The absorptive capacity for change; shared receptivity of involved individuals to an intervention; and extent to which use of that intervention will be rewarded, supported, and expected within their organization
1	Tension for Change	The degree to which stakeholders perceive the current situation as intolerable or needing change
2	Compatibility	The degree of tangible fit between meaning and values attached to the intervention by involved individuals; how those align with individuals' own norms, values, and perceived risks and needs; and how the intervention fits with existing workflows and systems
3	Relative Priority	Individuals' shared perception of the importance of the implementation within the organization
4	Organizational Incentives and Rewards	Extrinsic incentives such as goal-sharing awards, performance reviews, promotions, and raises in salary, as well as less tangible incentives such as increased stature or respect
5	Goals and Feedback	The degree to which goals are clearly communicated, acted upon, and fed back to staff, and alignment of that feedback with goals
6	Learning Climate	A climate in which (1) leaders express their own fallibility and need for team members' assistance and input; (2) team members feel that they are essential, valued, and knowledgeable partners in the change process; (3) individuals feel psychologically safe to try new methods; and (4) there is sufficient time and space for reflective thinking and evaluation
E	Readiness for Implementation	Tangible and immediate indicators of organizational commitment to the decision to implement an intervention
1	Leadership Engagement	Commitment, involvement, and accountability of leaders and managers with the implementation

(continues)

Table 3-1 Consolidated Framework for Implementation
Research Constructs   *(continued)*

Construct		Short Description
2	Available Resources	The level of resources dedicated for implementation and ongoing operations, including money, training, education, physical space, and time
3	Access to Knowledge and Information	Ease of access to digestible information and knowledge about the intervention and how to incorporate it into work tasks
IV. Characteristics of Individuals		
A	Knowledge and Beliefs About the Intervention	Individuals' attitudes toward, and value placed on, the intervention as well as familiarity with facts, truths, and principles related to the intervention
B	Self-Efficacy	Individuals' belief in their own capabilities to execute courses of action to achieve implementation goals
C	Individual Stage of Change	Characterization of the phase an individual is in as they progress toward skilled, enthusiastic, and sustained use of the intervention
D	Individual Identification with Organization	A broad construct related to how individuals perceive the organization and their relationship with and degree of commitment to that organization
E	Other Personal Attributes	A broad construct to include other personal traits such as tolerance of ambiguity, intellectual ability, motivation, values, competence, capacity, and learning style
V. Process		
A	Planning	The degree to which a scheme or method of behavior and tasks for implementing an intervention are developed in advance, and the quality of those schemes or methods
B	Engaging	Attracting and involving appropriate individuals in the implementation and use of the intervention through a combined strategy of social marketing, education, role modeling, training, and other similar activities
1	Opinion Leaders	Individuals in an organization who have formal or informal influence on the attitudes and beliefs of their colleagues with respect to implementing the intervention
2	Formally Appointed Internal Implementation Leaders	Individuals from within the organization who have been formally appointed with responsibility for implementing an intervention as coordinator, project manager, team leader, or other similar roles

Construct		Short Description
3	Champions	Individual dedicated "to supporting, marketing, and driving through an implementation, overcoming indifference or resistance that the intervention may provoke in an organization" (Powell et al., 2015, pg. 9)
4	External Change Agents	Individuals who are affiliated with an outside entity who formally influence or facilitate intervention decisions in a desirable direction
C	Executing	Carrying out or accomplishing the implementation according to plan
D	Reflecting and Evaluating	Quantitative and qualitative feedback about the progress and quality of implementation accompanied by regular personal and team debriefing about progress and experience

domains, but more comprehensive information on each is available at https://cfirguide.org/constructs/. These constructs are meant to provide a beginning foundation for understanding implementation as well as provide a guide for formative evaluations of intervention studies and programs. The CFIR can also be used to organize and promote the synthesis of implementation research findings and studies, because the constructs included in the framework can be used to explain the concepts more clearly in a consistent manner across studies (Damschroder et al., 2009). Damschroder et al. (2009) provide commentary on fostering health services research implementation (findings into practice) aligning the CFIR framework for advancing the science.

Knowledge-to-Action (KTA) Framework

The KTA framework is meant to help conceptually clarify key elements involved with moving knowledge into action. Recognizing that the multiple terms used in the KTA field were only contributing to confusion, the creators of the KTA framework reviewed multiple interdisciplinary planned action theories about the process of change and developed a framework focused on the concepts of knowledge creation and the action cycle that leads to the implementation or application of knowledge. Knowledge creation is represented as a funnel and consists of the knowledge or research types used in health care. As the knowledge moves through the funnel, it becomes more synthesized or refined (synopses, practice guidelines, clinical care pathways) and feasibly more usable by stakeholders. Action cycles contain the activities needed for knowledge implementation and are dynamic, influencing each other as well as being influenced by the knowledge creation phases. Commonalities within the various planned action theories reviewed are represented by the following phases:

- Identify a problem that needs addressing.
- Identify, review, and select the knowledge or research relevant to the problem.
- Adapt the identified knowledge or research to the local context.
- Assess barriers to using the knowledge.
- Select, tailor, and implement interventions to promote the use of knowledge.
- Monitor knowledge use.
- Evaluate the outcomes of using the knowledge.
- Sustain ongoing knowledge use (Graham et al., 2006).

The KTA framework is one of the most frequently cited conceptual frameworks for knowledge translation, but is being used in practice with varying degrees of completeness and theory exactness when integrated into an implementation process. Many of the studies that have utilized the KTA framework were conducted in Canada, no doubt a reflection of the association of the KTA framework with the Canadian Institutes of Health Research and the subsequent adoption by Canadian research funding organizations. These studies reported and gave examples of how the KTA framework was integral to the design, delivery, and evaluation of their implementation activities, with enactment of the KTA framework ranging from informing to full integration, indicating a flexibility of use for local needs and circumstances (Field et al., 2014).

Reach, Effectiveness, Adoption, Implementation, and Maintenance

RE-AIM has been used most frequently in public health and health behavior change research; however, it has been noted in more diverse content areas and within clinical, community, and corporate systems. The RE-AIM framework was created as a primary focus of translation of scientific advances into practice, and specifically into public health impact and policy which have been slow and inequitable (Glasgow et al., 1999). RE-AIM and other frameworks create a balance between the traditional focus on internal over external validity. The uniqueness of RE-AIM illuminates a focus on dimensions and steps in the design, implementation, and dissemination processes that facilitate or impede success in achieving broad and equitable population-based impact (Glasgow et al., 2019). Current emphasis on RE-AIM centers on the value of better understanding costs and adaptations to programs and expanding the use of qualitative methods to understand "how" and "why" results came about (Glasgow et al., 2019).

To better understand the steps or stages in the RE-AIM framework, it is useful to know the steps and phases. Each letter of RE-AIM has a purpose. For example, Reach is described as those who participate in a specific program, initiative, or program and the exact number, proportion, and representativeness of those engaged in the project and reasons for their involvement. Representativeness delineates if participants have features that reflect the target population's characteristics. For example, if the goal is to increase physical mobility in sedentary people between the ages of 50 and 75, you would not include individuals younger than 50 who are actively engaged in an exercise test in your program. *Effectiveness* or *Efficacy* refers to the impact of an intervention on significant outcomes such as potential negative effects, quality of life, and cost–benefit outcomes. It is also necessary to address variability across subgroups (heterogeneity) and why they exist. *Adoption* (referring to *Reach*) highlights absolute numbers, proportion, and representativeness of resources (settings, people) who want to start a program or approve a policy, and the pros and cons for decisions made. Settings and individuals involved may be multidimensional and on a continuum. *Implementation* refers to how closely individuals involved follow the program that the team creates and includes consistency of delivery as intended, adaptations made to the intervention or implementation strategies, and the time and cost of the program. *Maintenance* is described as the extent to which a program or policy becomes embedded in routine organizational practices and policies. Updated and newer guidance focuses on tailoring the timeline of maintenance to specific issues and programs, as well as evaluation of adaptations made for spread and sustainability. At the individual level, maintenance relates to the longer-term effects of a program on outcomes after the most recent intervention(s) (Glasgow et al., 2019).

Aims, Ingredients, Mechanism, Delivery

To address the issue of multiple terminologies and frameworks within the field of implementation science, an international collaboration of scholars met in 2012 to develop a simplified framework to describe interventions that promote and integrate evidence into health practices, systems, and policies. Their goal was to create a "meta-framework" that would accommodate the use of existing frameworks in the field and was thus designed to be "terminology agnostic." To that end, the working research group was composed of members from the fields of quality improvement, evidence synthesis, policy, information science, public health, patient safety, and behavior change. The framework developed as a result of these initial efforts was composed of four components: (1) intended targets, or the intended effects of the intervention or its beneficiaries; (2) active ingredients, or the critical components that define the intervention and are required to initiate change; (3) causal mechanisms, or the proposed pathways or policies by which an intervention will effect change; and (4) mode of delivery or application, or the ways in which active ingredients are applied.

The original framework went through a validation project and further refinement over the next 3 years, resulting in the validated and revised version of the simplified framework version 1, now called the AIMD framework (**Table 3-2**). The AIMD framework still contains the four original components, but the concepts and associated descriptions were made simpler and clearer. As a result, intended targets became aims, active ingredients became ingredients, causal mechanisms became mechanisms, and mode of delivery or application became delivery.

The creators of AIMD believe it can serve as a framework for effective communication between team members of implementation interventions as well as serve as a guide for the development of intervention designs and reporting toolkits (Bragge et al., 2017).

Selecting the appropriate implementation framework to guide local projects may be confusing, and some recommendations to help improve the process include using methods such as concept mapping, group model building, conjoint analysis,

Table 3-2 The AIMD Framework

Component	Description
Aims	What do you want your intervention to achieve and for whom?
Ingredients	What comprises the intervention?
Mechanism	How do you propose the intervention will work?
Delivery	How will you deliver the intervention?

Reproduced from Bragge, P., Grimshaw, J. M., Lokker, C., & Colquhoun, H. (2017). AIMD: A validated, simplified framework of interventions to promote and integrate evidence into health practices, systems, and policies. *BMC Medical Research Methodology*, *17*, 38. https://doi.org/10.1186/s12874-017-0314-8

and intervention mapping (Powell et al., 2017). Checklists for identifying the determinants of practice, including one tool with a focus on behavior change in health professionals, are available and may prove useful for those who are designing, conducting, evaluating, or reporting implementation projects (Flottorp et al., 2013). For those who are involved in implementation research, the Standards for Reporting Implementation Studies (StaRI) initiative developed a 27-item checklist that provides a guideline for the transparent and accurate reporting of implementation studies. The StaRI standards are registered with the EQUATOR Network (http://www.equator-network.org), where the checklist is available as a download (Pinnock et al., 2017).

Implementation Strategies

Theories, models, and frameworks are important to providing context to strategies and they can be implemented and evaluated. Powell et al. (2015) in their project on developing Expert Recommendations for Implementing Change (ERIC) focused on identifying, developing, and testing implementation strategies that are critical to the overall goals of implementation science. The authors note their efforts were complicated by inconsistent language and inadequate descriptions of implementation strategies in the research literature. Through the ERIC study, the authors further aimed to refine a published compilation of implementation strategy terms and definitions. This was accomplished through systematic gathering of input from a wide range of stakeholders with expertise in implementation science and clinical practice.

Powell and his associates' research advanced the implementation science field by improving the conceptual clarity, relevance, and comprehensiveness of implementation strategies (2015). These strategies can be employed in isolation or combination in implementation research and practice. The authors provide a table in their research study that includes a list of strategies and definition, respectively. For example, the strategy *conduct local needs assessment* is identified as the collection and analysis of data related to the need for the innovation. *Conducting ongoing training* as a strategy is described as planning and conducting training in the clinical innovation in an ongoing way. Another example, *create a learning collaborative*, is described as facilitating the formation of groups of providers or provider organizations and fostering a collaborative learning environment to improve implementation innovation (Powell et al., 2015). The ERIC project advances translational science by proffering a rigorously developed list of implementation strategies that can be employed in practice and tested. The authors describe future phases of ERIC that will center on creating conceptually distinct categories of strategies as well as ratings for each strategy's importance and feasibility. Secondly, the expert panel will advance multifaceted strategies for hypothetical yet real-world scenarios that vary by sites' engagement of evidence-based programs and practices and the strength of contextual supports that surround the effort.

Value of Implementation and Team Science for Sustainable Clinical Projects

Team science applies conceptual and methodological approaches from multiple disciplines and health professions to address complex clinical problems. Although there is a growing emphasis on interprofessional training for health professions students to prepare them for team-based clinical practice, training for researchers who are team- or interprofessional-based has traditionally been lacking. It is also increasingly being recognized that truly effective patient care requires a combination of both interprofessional medical practice and transdisciplinary scientific knowledge, which necessitate clinical practice guidelines that consider team-based care and that integrate knowledge from multiple disciplines (Begg et al., 2014; Croyle, 2008). The NIH recognizes the importance of cross-disciplinary science, in which team members with training and expertise in different fields work together to combine or integrate their perspectives in a single research endeavor, which is seen as a promising approach to accelerate both scientific innovation and the translation of scientific findings into effective policies and practices (National Cancer Institute, n.d.). The National Institute for Mental Health (NIMH) has made team science a priority and has designed a 2-year training institute in mental health implementation science called the Implementation Research Institute (IRI). Both mentoring and collaboration are emphasized in the training program, and an analysis of the IRI has demonstrated a significant impact of the mentoring relationships on future scientific collaborations, as evidenced by increases in grants, presentations, and publications produced by IRI attendees and their mentors in a posttraining 2-year time span (Luke et al., 2016).

A team science academic–industry hybrid model, the multidisciplinary translational team (MTT), is a combination of several team types adapted for an academic setting and includes an interprofessional group of scientists who are working together to solve a common translational problem. The CTSA has provided support for MTTs in the form of infrastructure and team development training, including orientation meetings to the CTSA for team members, assistance with producing team and individual objectives and tasks, the development of team leadership councils which functioned as a peer mentoring network, and hosting a team-building workshop. An evaluation of MTTs showed four different team type trajectories, which indicates the need for team-specific interventions in the areas of leadership and resources to help them reach their maximum potential: (1) teams with traditional leadership;

(2) teams focused on basic science; (3) stable, high-functioning teams with junior project managers; and (4) teams with inexperienced leaders. The teams that were identified as having effective team processes developed interdisciplinary concepts and publications that most likely would not have happened without the interaction between the team members (Wooten et al., 2015).

The Science of Team Science (SciTS) is a rapidly growing field that has the potential to positively impact both translational and implementation science and to improve health care. Interprofessional teams are not limited to just translational or research teams, as the complexity of providing optimal patient care within our modern healthcare system necessitates well-functioning teams composed of healthcare providers, administrative leaders, support staff, patients, industry members, and community agencies and their members. The composition of these teams will fluctuate depending on the task at hand, the need for different types of expertise, access to resources and personnel, or any other number of variables inherent in healthcare organizations. Many of the skills identified in the SciTS literature apply as much to clinical teams as they do to research teams, and strengthening teamwork has been identified as a top priority for improving health care, especially when it comes to patient safety (Clancy & Tornberg, 2007). The argument can be made that "soft skills" are integral for effective collaboration and team functioning and may not have received adequate emphasis in the health sciences curriculum during professional training. Many of these soft skills are addressed in the Interprofessional Education Collaborative (IPEC) Core Competencies for Interprofessional Collaborative Practice, which focus on four domains: (1) values/ethics: work with individuals of other professions to maintain a climate of mutual respect and shared values; (2) roles/responsibilities: use the knowledge of one's own role and those of other professions to appropriately assess and address the needs of healthcare patients and to promote and advance the health of populations; (3) interprofessional communication: communicate with patients, families, communities, and professionals in health and other fields in a responsive and responsible manner that supports a team approach to the promotion and maintenance of health and the prevention and treatment of disease; and (4) teams/teamwork: apply relationship-building values and the principles of team dynamics to perform effectively in different team roles to plan, deliver, and evaluate patient/population-centered care and population health programs and policies that are safe, timely, efficient, effective, and equitable (IPEC, 2017). Each domain includes subcompetencies that further identify the skills and actions needed to achieve the IPEC Core Competencies. These skills and actions can also be thought of in broader categories, such as cultural and diversity awareness, emotional intelligence, strategic thinking, conflict resolution, persuasion, resilience, flexibility, and the ability to inspire moral- and competence-based trust and have been identified for contributing to the ability to successfully collaborate with others in a variety of disciplines (Gibert et al., 2017).

Data from interviews with NIH researchers who were part of five teams that ranged from successful (defined as teams that developed a reasonable level of cohesiveness and were able to pursue their missions) to groups that ended because of conflict indicate that the following characteristics contribute to an effective team: effective leadership, self and other awareness, established trust among team members, open communication strategies, shared expectations, clear definition of roles and responsibilities, a shared vision, appropriate recognition and credit given to team members, allowing for disagreement while mitigating conflict, learning each other's languages, enjoying the science, and working together (Bennett et al., 2010). Trust has been identified as one of the most critical elements for successful teams and therefore should not be left to chance. Specific steps that can be taken to proactively build trust within teams include having explicit conversations where partnership expectations are discussed regarding what the roles within the team will be; on how information, data, or resources will be shared; on how decisions will be made; and on how disagreements or conflicts will be handled (Bennett & Gadlin, 2012).

Key contributing characteristics for successful teamwork such as the development of a common understanding of both the roles of team members and the structure of the work have been referred to as a shared mental model (SMM) (Canon-Bowers et al., 1993). The SMM construct, as it relates to clinical teamwork and health professions learners to date, has not been well defined, with interventions to foster or measure SMM in clinical teams being not well represented in the published literature (Floren et al., 2018). There are a variety of tools that can be used to measure teamwork, however, including those that measure the teamwork of individuals working within teams, the teamwork of teams, and those that assess both individuals and teams. One of the more well-known tools is the TeamSTEPPS Teamwork Attitudes Questionnaire, which is designed to assess the teamwork attitudes, knowledge, and skills of learners who have gone through the TeamSTEPPS curriculum (Agency for Healthcare Research and Quality, 2016). Another validated tool that has been associated with improved patient outcomes is the Team Climate Inventory, which was originally designed to measure a team climate for innovation using five scales related to: (1) participative safety, (2) support for innovation, (3) vision, (4) task orientation, and (5) social desirability (Anderson & West, 1996). Over 70 unique tools designed to quantitatively measure teamwork in an internal medicine setting have been identified in the literature, indicating no lack of resources for those looking to assess teamwork in their local setting (Havyer et al., 2014). Clearly, the behavior of healthcare professionals and healthcare organizational culture are key variables that impact the quality of patient care and the sustainability of clinical projects. Staying abreast of research findings in the fields of both implementation and team science can equip those who are part of clinical care teams or who are conducting quality improvement and research projects with strategies and tools that will better enable successful outcomes.

Implications for Project Planning and Management

Understanding implementation science models and the various tools and strategies for moving evidence into true practice and sustained improvement provides the "next steps" in the uptake of evidence-based practice. Common language and terminology provide a beginning to the effective spread and scale-up of successful projects. Incorporating the SciTS and working together as interprofessional teams can also be facilitative in the process. Being able to "diagnose" teamwork attitudes, knowledge, and skills of learners using assessment tools will be an important starting point in developing an SMM. Trust is a cornerstone of team success and positive outcomes. Evaluation of the structure, processes, and outcomes of the actual implementation and the team's effectiveness advances real-time improvement and sustainability for population health management.

Summary

- Strategies to address the real-world needs of patients and the providers who care for them are the impetus behind translational, implementation, and team science in health care.
- Advances in the fields of implementation science and team science are identifying effective strategies for healthcare providers to take the evidence produced from these research studies and apply them to improve the health of patients in their local settings.
- Although the challenges of working in multidisciplinary or interprofessional teams can be great, the benefits of increased opportunities for new scientific knowledge, mentorship, and innovation can provide great rewards that will benefit patients, practice settings, organizations, and healthcare systems.

Reflection Questions

1. What role do you see for yourself in the more efficient and timelier implementation of evidence into practice to help improve the health of patients?
2. What are some of the characteristics essential to fostering a productive team environment?
3. How can you contribute to an organizational culture that promotes and rewards collaboration?
4. Consider your last project. How did you use (or could use) an implementation model and team science principles?

Learning Activities

1. Identify a program or clinical project that would benefit from the structure provided by an implementation science theory or framework. Which theory or framework would you use and why?
2. What characteristics or strategies do you believe would best work for promoting team cohesiveness in your practice environment? How would you go about improving teamwork in your environment?

References

Agency for Healthcare Research and Quality. (2016, May 20). *TeamSTEPPS*. https://www.ahrq.gov/teamstepps/index.html

Anderson, N., & West, M. (1996). The Team Climate Inventory: Development of the TCI and its applications in teambuilding for innovativeness. *European Journal of Work and Organizational Psychology, 5*(1), 53–66. https://doi:10.1080/13594329608414840

Begg, M. D., Crumley, G., Fair, A. M., Martina, C. A., McCormack, W. T., Merchant, C., & Umans, J. G. (2014). Approaches to preparing young scholars for careers in interdisciplinary team science. *Journal of Investigative Medicine: The Official Publication of the American Federation for Clinical Research, 62*(1), 14–25. https://doi:10.231/JIM.0000000000000021

Bennett, L. M., & Gadlin, H. (2012). Collaboration and team science: From theory to practice. *Journal of Investigative Medicine: The Official Publication of the American Federation for Clinical Research, 60*(5), 768–775. https://doi.org/10.2310/JIM.0b013e318250871d

Bennett, L. M., Gadlin, H., & Levine-Findley, S. (2010). *Team science and collaboration: A field guide*. Department of Health and Human Services. https://ccrod.cancer.gov/confluence/download/attachments/47284665/TeamScience_FieldGuide.pdf

Bragge, P., Grimshaw, J. M., Lokker, C., & Colquhoun, H. (2017). AIMD—A validated, simplified framework of interventions to promote and integrate evidence into health practices, systems, and policies. *BMC Medical Research Methodology*, *17*, 38. https://doi.org/10.1186/s12874-017-0314-8

Canon-Bowers, J., Salas, E., & Converse, S. (1993). Shared mental models in expert team decision-making. In N. J. Castellan (Ed.), *Individual and group decision making: Current issues* (pp. 221–246). Lawrence Erlbaum Associates.

Clancy, C. M., & Tornberg, D. N. (2007). TeamSTEPPS: Assuring optimal teamwork in clinical settings. *American Journal of Medical Quality: The Official Journal of the American College of Medical Quality*, *22*(3), 214–217. https://doi.org/10.1177/1062860607300616

Consolidated Framework for Implementation Research Team. (n.d.). *Consolidated Framework for Implementation Research (CFIR)*. https://cfirguide.org/

Croyle, R. T. (2008). The National Cancer Institute's transdisciplinary centers initiatives and the need for building a Science of Team Science. *American Journal of Preventive Medicine*, *35*(suppl-2), S90–S93. https://doi.org/10.1016/j.amepre.2008.05.012

Damschroder, L. J., Aron, D. C., Keith, R. E., Kirsh, S. R., Alexander, J. A., & Lowery, J. C. (2009). Fostering implementation of health services research findings into practice: A consolidated framework for advancing implementation science. *Implementation Science*, *4*, 50. https://doi.org/10.1186/1748-5908-4-50

Field, B., Booth, A., Ilott, I., & Gerrish, K. (2014). Using the Knowledge to Action framework in practice: A citation analysis and systematic review. *Implementation Science*, *9*, 172. https://doi.org/10.1186/s13012-014-0172-2

Floren, L. C., Donesky, D., Whitaker, E., Irby, D. M., Ten Cate, O., & O'Brien, B. C. (2018). Are We on the Same Page? Shared Mental Models to Support Clinical Teamwork Among Health Professions Learners: A Scoping Review. *Academic Medicine*, *93*(3), 498–509. https://doi.org/10.1097/ACM.0000000000002019

Flottorp, S. A., Oxman, A. D., Krause, J., Musila, N. R., Wensing, M., Godycki-Cwirko, M., Baker, R., & Eccles, M. P. (2013). A checklist for identifying determinants of practice: A systematic review and synthesis of frameworks and taxonomies of factors that prevent or enable improvements in healthcare professional practice. *Implementation Science: IS*, *8*, 35. https://doi.org/10.1186/1748-5908-8-35

Fogarty International Center. (2017, July 27). *Implementation science information and resources*. https://www.fic.nih.gov/researchtopics/pages/implementationscience.aspx

Fort, D. G., Herr, T. M., Shaw, P. L., Gutzman, K. E., & Starren, J. B. (2017). Mapping the evolving definitions of translational research. *Journal of Clinical and Translational Science*, *1*(1), 60–66. https://doi.org/10.1017/cts.2016.10

Gibert, A., Tozer, W. C., & Westoby, M. (2017). Teamwork, soft skills, and research training. *Trends in Ecology & Evolution*, *32*(2), 81–84. https://doi.org/10.1016/j.tree.2016.11.004

Glasgow, R. E., Harden, S. M., Gaglio, B., Rabin, B., Smith, M. L., Porter, G. C., Ory, M. G., & Estabrooks, P. A. (2019). RE-AIM planning and evaluation framework: Adapting to new science and practice with a 20-year review. *Frontiers in Public Health*, *7*, 64. https://doi.org/10.3389/fpubh.2019.00064

Glasgow, R. E., Vogt, T. M., & Boles, S. M. (1999). Evaluating the public health impact of health promotion interventions: The RE-AIM framework. *American Journal of Public Health*, *89*(9), 1322–1327. https://doi.org/10.2105/ajph.89.9.1322

Graham, I. D., Logan, J., Harrison, M. B., Straus, S. E., Tetroe, J., Caswell, W., & Robinson, N. (2006). Lost in knowledge translation: Time for a map? *The Journal of Continuing Education in the Health Professions*, *26*(1), 13–24. https://doi.org/10.1002/chp.47

Harvey, G., & Kitson, A. (2016). PARiHS revisited: From heuristic to integrated framework for the successful implementation of knowledge into practice. *Implementation Science: IS*, *11*. https://doi.org/10.1186/s13012-016-0398-2

Havyer, R. D. A., Wingo, M. T., Comfere, N. I., Nelson, D. R., Halvorsen, A. J., McDonald, F. S., & Reed, D. A. (2014). Teamwork assessment in internal medicine: A systematic review of validity evidence and outcomes. *Journal of General Internal Medicine*, *29*(6), 894–910. https://doi.org/10.1007/s11606-013-2686-8

Interprofessional Education Collaborative. (2017). *Resources*. http://ipecollaborative.org/resources
.html

Kitson, A., Harvey, G., & McCormack, B. (1998). Enabling the implementation of evidence-based
practice: A conceptual framework. *Quality in Health Care*, 7, 149–158. https://doi.org/10.1136
/qshc.7.3.149

Kitson, A. L., Rycroft-Malone, J., Harvey, G., McCormack, B., Seers, K., & Titchen, A. (2008).
Evaluating the successful implementation of evidence into practice using the PARiHS framework: Theoretical and practical challenges. *Implementation Science: IS*, 3(1). https://doi
.org/10.1186/1748-5908-3-1

Luke, D. A., Baumann, A. A., Carothers, B. J., Landsverk, J., & Proctor, E. K. (2016). Forging a
link between mentoring and collaboration: A new training model for implementation science.
Implementation Science, 11, 137. https://doi.org/10.1186/s13012-016-0499-y

Morris, Z. S., Wooding, S., & Grant, J. (2011). The answer is 17 years, what is the question:
Understanding time lags in translational research. *Journal of the Royal Society of Medicine*,
104(12), 510–520. https://doi.org/10.1258/jrsm.2011.110180

National Cancer Institute. (n.d.). *What is team science?* https://www.teamsciencetoolkit.cancer.gov
/public/WhatisTS.aspx

National Center for Advancing Translational Sciences. (2021a, May 25). *About the CTSA program*.
https://ncats.nih.gov/ctsa/about

National Center for Advancing Translational Sciences. (2021b, February 24). *CTSA program hubs*.
https://ncats.nih.gov/ctsa/about/hubs

National Center for Advancing Translational Sciences. (2021c, April 16). *Translational science spectrum*. https://ncats.nih.gov/translation/spectrum

Powell, B. J., Beidas, R. S., Lewis, C. C., Aarons, G. A., McMillen, J. C., Proctor, E. K., & Mandell, D. S.
(2017). Methods to improve the selection and tailoring of implementation strategies. *The
Journal of Behavioral Health Services & Research*, 44(2), 177–194. https://doi.org/10.1007
/s11414-015-9475-6

Powell, B. J., Waltz, T. J., Chinman, M. J., Damschroder, L. J., Smith, J. L., Matthieu, M. M., Proctor,
E. K., & Kirscher, J. (2015). A refined compilation of implementation strategies: Results from
the Expert Recommendations for Implementing Change (ERIC) project. *Implementation Science*.
10(21). https://doi.org/10.1186/s13012-015-0209-1

Rycroft-Malone, J. (2004). The PARiHS framework: A framework for guiding the implementation of evidence-based practice. *Journal of Nursing Care Quality*, 19(4), 297–304. https://doi
.org/10.1097/00001786-200410000-00002

Straus, S. E., Tetroe, J., & Graham, I. (2009). Defining knowledge translation. *CMAJ: Canadian
Medical Association Journal*, 181(3–4), 165–168. https://doi.org/10.1503/cmaj.081229

Wooten, K. C., Calhoun, W. J., Bhavnani, S., Rose, R. M., Ameredes, B., & Brasier, A. R. (2015).
Evolution of multidisciplinary translational teams (MTTs): Insights for accelerating translational innovations. *CTS: Clinical & Translational Science*, 8(5), 542–552. https://doi.org/10.1111
/cts.12266

Case Exemplar

Collaboration and Implementation Science

Linda Roussel

Building on the concept of collaboration from an implementation science perspective has been the focused work of the CTSA hubs on a multisite research platform perspective. The partner CTSA hubs became aware of the limited study on the implementation process, specifically noting the chasm between evidence generated and actions taken to implement evidence into routine clinical and public health practice (Kerner et al., 2005). Effective interventions "tested" under controlled research settings do little to illuminate the challenges and barriers to translating findings into real-world settings. The translational perspective is essential to reaching the longer-term goal of improving research's impact to the broader population, resulting in value-added returns on scientific investments. The National Implementation Research Network (NIRN, 2015) defines implementation science as the study of factors that impact the full and effective use of innovations in practice. The aim is not to answer factual questions about what is but rather to determine what is required to make the change or improvement. The NIH has made implementation science (T3–T4 research) a priority, launching CTSAs in 2006. We have noted growth in implementation science, specifically moving from a set of studies chronicling the many barriers and facilitators to successful adoption, uptake, and sustainability. The past decade has experienced the movement toward comparing implementation strategies to implementation as a matter of course and more recently to the comparison of multiple active strategies (Proctor et al., 2013). In tandem, researchers have been advancing the methods and measures of implementation science by focusing on greater rigor and robustness of complex processes (Neta et al., 2015). With this backdrop, CTSA hubs have conceptually developed a platform using implementation science and collaboration to advance frontline engagement and nursing-sensitive outcomes. Through a robust virtual collaboratory, the CTSA hubs and their clinical teams would focus on sharing implementation strategies to improve key critical patient care and systems outcomes, such as reducing readmission rates, reducing length of stay, improving transitions of care, and reducing hospital-acquired conditions (HACs).

Reflection Questions

1. What is the process for building a virtual collaboratory from an implementation science perspective?
2. How may one address challenges associated with partner hubs within a virtual environment?

References

Kerner, J. F., Guirguis-Blake, J., Hennessy, K. D., Brounstein, P. J., Vinson, C., Schwartz, R. H., Myers, B. A., & Briss, P. (2005). Translating research into improved outcomes in comprehensive cancer control. *Cancer Causes Control, 16*, 27–40. https://doi.org/10.1007/s10552-005-0488-y

National Implementation Research Network. (2015). *Implementation science defined.* http://nirn.fpg .unc.edu/learn-implementation/implementation sciencedefined

Neta, G., Glasgow, R. E., Carpenter, C. R., Grimshaw, J. M., Rabin, B. A., Fernandez, M. E., & Brownson, R. C. (2015). A framework for enhancing the value of research for dissemination and implementation. *American Journal of Public Health, 105*, 49–57. https://doi.org/10.2105 /AJPH.2014.302206

Proctor, E. K., Powell, B. J., & McMillen, J. C. (2013). Implementation strategies: Recommendations for specifying and reporting. *Implementation Science, 8*, 139. https://doi.org/10.1097 /00001786-200410000-00002

CHAPTER 4

Forming and Managing a Synergistic Interprofessional Improvement Team

James L. Harris
Kathryn M. Ward-Presson
Patricia L. Thomas
Janet E. Winter

CHAPTER OBJECTIVES

1. Identify strategies and methods used to create and manage synergistic interprofessional teams for project planning, management, and person-centered programs.
2. Discuss the importance of team development stages, synergy, creativity, appreciative inquiry (AI), transformational leadership, and innovation for interprofessional project/program team outcomes.
3. Explore the importance of a common language and potential barriers shared by clinical and administrative project improvement planners and leaders for successful outcomes.
4. Translate the characteristics of coaching interprofessional teams in planning, initiating, and evaluating phases of projects.
5. Describe the significance of team leadership and needs of interprofessional teams in order to maintain continuous performance imposed from accrediting agencies, regulations, and stakeholders.
6. Identify key areas associated with measuring team effectiveness and value.

KEY TERMS

Advocate
Appreciative inquiry (AI)
Brainstorming

Collaboration
Communication
Decision-making

Diversity and inclusivity
Innovation
Interprofessional
Interprofessional team
Language
Management
Multidisciplinary team
Organizational culture
Performance
Project management

Situation, background, assessment,
    and recommendation (SBAR)
    communication
Synergy
Task force
Team
Team leader effectiveness
TeamSTEPPS
Team synergy
Transdisciplinary team
Transformational leader

ROLES

Advocate
Coach
Communicator

Integrator
Leader
Manager

PROFESSIONAL VALUES

Accountability
Advocacy
Patient-centered care

Quality
Value-driven

CORE COMPETENCIES

Assessment
Communication
Coordination
Design
Diversity
Emotional intelligence

Evaluating
Innovation
Interpersonal relationships
Leadership
Management

Introduction

Health care remains at a crossroads as patients' medical conditions become increasingly more complex, reimbursement and regulatory mandates intensify, and knowledge emerges from a series of catalyzing changes that challenge care delivery globally. As innovative quality projects are planned and initiated, engagement of interprofessional team members and their continuous management are vital to success. Speaking a common language and understanding the meaning of each term and concept translates into significant outcomes, value, and team synergy.

Knowledge gleaned from projects requires mobilization of the evidence through continuous communication and consciousness-raising if innovation is to be sustained (Crisp, 2014). Healthcare organizations have unprecedented opportunities to assume the challenges to innovate and leverage knowledge and change. When various disciplines engage in interprofessional projects, education, and collaborative practice, high-quality, safe, and efficient care is realized as evidence-based knowledge is spread (Interprofessional Education Collaborative [IPEC] Expert Panel, 2016; World Health Organization [WHO], 2013).

This chapter discusses the essentials in forming and managing synergistic interprofessional teams that are engaged in clinical and quality projects. The importance of team stages, transformational leadership, creativity, innovation, and a common language in all phases of projects, their management, and collaborative efforts is emphasized. The value of coaching interprofessional project improvement teams is also addressed as a means to capitalize on team performance given the changing healthcare landscape being driven by new and existing accrediting, regulatory, and stakeholder demands. Measuring team effectiveness and value using different metrics is discussed.

Interprofessional Teams: Overview and Management

Much has been written to stress the importance of interprofessional learning, forming and developing interprofessional teams, and the implementation of innovative interprofessional collaborative practices across care systems. Although several distinct models have been developed to emphasize changes needed in the practice and academic settings, implementation of these models and sustained outcomes have been slow, sporadic, and inconsistent. Landmark reports from the Institute of Medicine (IOM) and the Robert Wood Johnson Foundation provide keen perspectives by discussing how healthcare providers claim to value teamwork, communication, collaboration, and shared outcomes. However, they are often inundated by professional assumptions, definitions, habitual use of language, and power structures.

In addition to dissonance around role and identity across various professions, the IOM's *To Err Is Human* report attributed preventable errors to organizational structures, incomplete information, failures in communication, and faulty systems and processes (IOM, 1999). Similarly, the IOM's *Crossing the Quality Chasm* report (2001) emphasized that healthcare systems are not able to translate knowledge into practice related to quality and safety in large part because resources are not used effectively in fragmented systems where gaps and redundancies create waste and fail to achieve desired outcomes.

The Robert Wood Johnson Foundation and IOM published the *Future of Nursing: Leading Change, Advancing Health* (2010) report and made recommendations about how to transform the nursing workforce through education, leadership development and competencies, and use of data and information to address the gaps apparent in our current delivery systems. The recently released *2020–2030 Future of Nursing* report (National Academies of Sciences, Engineering, and Medicine, 2021) advanced many areas from the 2010 report discussing new paths of improvement dedicated to a culture of health, reduced disparities, and improved health and well-being of society. In light of these reports and recommendations, alignment and understanding of team dynamics, synergies that can be generated, and the need for creative and innovative models implemented by interprofessional teams remains a consistent theme in health care.

The six aims to improve patient care (safe, effective, patient-centered, timely, efficient, and equitable) are cornerstones to project management amid expectations for the delivery of cost-effective, high-quality care espoused in organizational mission, vision, and value statements. However, despite best efforts, these aims have not been accomplished consistently across the healthcare industry. Transformative change, leadership, investment in organizational capacity, expanding information infrastructure, and reconfiguration and retraining of care teams is needed (IOM, 2001).

Principles and constructs for teams and teamwork, team building, and team facilitation are extensive, spanning decades of work in nursing, business, and the social sciences. Alignment of safety, quality, and high-reliability organizations has catapulted the need for the implementation of effective team structure and processes through investment in project management team skills that ultimately drive optimum person-centered and culturally diverse care delivery.

Under the premise that project work can be accomplished through productive, high-functioning teams, key considerations in working with interprofessional as well as interdisciplinary team configurations during the project management processes of initiating, planning, executing, monitoring and controlling, and closing (Project Management Institute, 2013, p. 6) is pivotal to success. Integral to this approach is an appreciation for current accomplishments, recognition of any voids or gaps, and an understanding of how new strategies and competencies should be leveraged to optimize team performance around project work.

Achieving optimal outcomes is a hallmark of any team effort. However, sustaining those outcomes requires professionalism, ongoing engagement, commitment, collaborative interprofessional practice, and management. Each professional must work independently and in parallel with one another. Drinka and Clark (2000) reiterated the need to function interdependently as solutions are generated collaboratively. The concepts of interprofessional teams and collaborative practice are not foreign ideas to healthcare professionals. Zaccagnini and White (2014), for example, support the notion that effective interprofessional teamwork and collaboration include vested professionals, other stakeholders, and team members from various disciplines. A well-orchestrated and assembled project improvement team may require the inclusion of patients and consumers as well as professionals from technology, health policy management, and library science. Rigorously aligning and integrating the needs and interests of individuals collectively creates a transformative connection. Ideas can be generated, shared, and communicated toward a defined aim. This approach can guide projects, add value, and create avenues for managing processes and conflicts that may arise during any project improvement team effort. Value, whether directly or indirectly, indicates growth or improvement occurring within the team, system, or project (Dunevitz, 1997).

To provide a context for the remainder of this chapter and throughout the text, it is important to distinguish between interprofessional teams and interdisciplinary teams given that both terms are used—sometimes interchangeably—in the literature. These terms actually have quite different meanings. Zaccagnini and White (2014) distinguish "interprofessional" as signaling the inclusion of representatives from a particular discipline or knowledge branch with differing experiences, education, values, roles, and expectations. By comparison, "interdisciplinary" is more specific to a particular discipline. Generally, "interprofessional" is associated with a broader definition and context as related to projects, collaborative efforts, and their management.

Forming, Understanding, and Managing a Synergistic Improvement Team

The rapidity of change in the healthcare industry has necessitated support of understanding and integrating management and leadership, as interprofessional project improvement teams generate novel approaches for meeting the increasing demands made by consumers and the healthcare industry itself. Managing a successful team that is dedicated to improvement and practice change requires the development of reciprocal trust and continuous interpersonal relationships among team members (Kouzes & Pozner, 2007).

Having an awareness of the different team member compositions can be helpful to consider when forming a team. Although terms are often used interchangeably, each composition offers nuances around member composition (see **Table 4-1**). For example, depending on the discipline or specialty, in the healthcare literature there is a distinction between a multidisciplinary team and an interdisciplinary team. Interdisciplinary teams recognize the interdependence of members who come together to understand complex situations or solve complex problems that require the knowledge, skills, and abilities of diverse individuals who cannot be successful without one another. As teams form, recognition of overlapping roles is common and unraveling the distinctions between them leads to an understanding of how each member's contributions could be woven together in a unique way to bring a new or different result. In contrast, multidisciplinary teams engage the knowledge, skills, and abilities of the members who work in parallel with distinct

Table 4-1 Team Compositions

Interdisciplinary	A group of healthcare professionals from diverse fields who work in a coordinated fashion toward a common goal for the patient.
Multidisciplinary	A team of professionals including representatives of different disciplines who coordinate the contributions of each profession, which are not considered to overlap, in order to improve patient care.
Intraprofessional	A team of professionals who are all from the same profession, such as three physical therapists collaborating on the same case.
Interprofessional	The inclusion of representatives from a particular discipline or knowledge branch with differing experiences, education, values, roles, and expectations (Zaccagnini & White, 2014).
Transdisciplinary/ Transprofessional	A team composed of members of a number of different professions cooperating across disciplines to improve patient care through practice or research.

responsibilities to accomplish a shared goal. The former creates synergy and new possibilities, whereas the latter reinforces consistency in defined disciplinary outcomes (Nancarrow et al., 2013; Walters, 2012). However, although unique characteristics exist across team configurations, perhaps most importantly, each team composition represents a purpose that aligns with any or all of the IOM's six aims.

Team composition can promote unique interactions with regard to whether an individual's role interests or knowledge support a team (interdisciplinary); when a professional's insights build from the conversations in a varied team (interprofessional); or when disciplines, professionals, and team members from seemingly unrelated fields come together to innovate to achieve a desired outcome (transdisciplinary or transprofessional) (Armstead et al., 2016; Hewitt et al., 2014; Mueller, 2016).

Having a working knowledge of the differences between teams and groups is foundational to project or program success aimed at promoting inclusive and diverse person-centered care. Groups and teams hold attributes in common, but differentiation between attributes can explain why projects or programs derail. Groups and teams hold in common groups of individuals who gather to accomplish work. What distinguishes groups from teams is the degree of interdependence, how they are led, and who has ownership of the end product of the members' interactions. Groups have individual accountability to complete work, come together to share information, and complete individual work or tasks based on their role. A leader directs the group members' purpose and goals while they remain focused on their own challenges and interests. In contrast, teams have individual and mutual accountability; gather for discussion, problem solving, and planning; and collectively focus on achieving goals and outcomes. The leader shapes the team members' purpose, work, and goals with the members (Armstead et al., 2016; Braithewaite, 2015).

Analogies are often offered using sports examples to showcase the differences between groups and teams. For example, marathon runners would serve as an example of a group. They have met for the same purpose, want to win, and share common interests. In terms of teams, thinking about baseball, soccer, or football teams, individual players come together but have to rely on each other to win. They have common goals but have to rely on the direction of the coach and the decisions and actions of their team members to ultimately achieve the "win." An individual could have a "great game" but still lose. For the purposes of project and program management, building teams rather than groups is the desired state.

Using a person-centered approach, the IPEC Practice Expert Panel (2016) distinguished teamwork from team-based care (**Table 4-2**).

Determination about when the efforts of an individual versus the efforts of a team are needed is pivotal to success. There are times when individual choices, decisions, or actions enable success. Historically, the belief was held that individual actions, decisions, and accountability alone brought results. From this, silos of information and action were created, resulting in inconsistent and fragmented results, ineffective communication, and poor outcomes.

Throughout history much has been learned about how success coming from collective efforts in complex systems rests in the ability to draw distinctions between when an individual's effort (commitment, participation, and actions) versus facilitated team efforts bring greater efficiency, effectiveness, and consistency aimed toward desired results. This tension between the individual team members'

Table 4-2 Interprofessional Teamwork versus Interprofessional Team-Based Care

Interprofessional Teamwork	The levels of cooperation, coordination, and collaboration Characterizing the relationships between professions in delivering patient-centered care.
Interprofessional Team-Based Care	Care delivered by intentionally created, usually relatively small work groups in health care, who are recognized by others as well as by themselves as having a collective identity and shared responsibility for a patient or group of patients (e.g., rapid response team, palliative care team, primary care team, operating room team).

Reproduced from Interprofessional Education Collaborative. (2016). *Core competencies for interprofessional collaborative practice: 2016 update.* Author.

productivity and the team's overall productivity requires sensitivity among members on how their level of engagement affects the dynamics of the team in achieving desired goals. For example, timeliness in providing information integral to the workflow keeps the project moving forward, as does conveying only pertinent information needed for team decision-making. Conversely, an overabundance of extraneous information may overwhelm or distract team members, and inability to produce assigned work can contribute to delays in workflow.

As further expanded upon in the chapter, the role of the project manager or team leader involves systematically guiding the tension between individual and team productivity toward synergy over shared goals and shared language. In this, the unspoken assumption is that goals and desired outcomes held by people in the same organization are the same because individuals care for the same patients and rely on a common mission and vision statement to guide work. To encourage team productivity, time is spent on setting team expectations and confirming the perceived meaning behind written, verbal, and nonverbal team member communications. This proactive approach clarifies and informs the use of communications that one may assume hold common meaning; however, in reality, because of education and experiences, they have shaped underlying assumptions in ways that are not consistent with others. Confluence over shared goals using shared language better positions a team to achieve successful outcomes integral to quality person-centered care.

Whereas the definitions for team configurations provide insight on member composition and focus, words used to describe the structure of teams provide perspective on the duration of work the team has been charged to accomplish. Committees, task forces, ad hoc teams, and councils represent common structures (and language) in healthcare organizations. Their permanency, charter, and purpose often determine how and why a team is established and guide the relevance attributed to organizational work. Committees and councils may result from expectations held by regulators (such as The Joint Commission or state regulations) or governing boards and have defined responsibility and authority directed toward ongoing work. Task forces and ad hoc teams are often created to address an issue or need that has arisen. As such, their work is typically geared toward making recommendations aimed at an issue with the intent of informing leaders and disbanding (or transitioning into a newly created committee or council) (Danna, 2013; Walters, 2012).

Building a team is critical to the success of any project and often is the first challenge of executives, sponsors, and team leaders. Critical success of the compiled team members resides in the selection process, as each individual team member can provide knowledge, insight, and energy to the accomplishment of work or become an obstacle in attaining project goals.

Central to team selection are diversity, the attitude and skill of contributors, the ability of the team leader to build trust, and the balance between differing viewpoints and conflict management (Bennett & Gadlin, 2012). A shared purpose, mutual goals, and professional knowledge and maturity embodied in emotionally intelligent participants are desired. However, contrarians and novices are also needed. Likewise, those who know the process should work alongside those who indirectly contribute to the process and those impacted by the outcomes of the process. Selection criteria begin with the role or position someone holds in an organization or the skill set the participant would contribute. Coupling this with a team inventory of desired attributes related to communication, flexibility, openness to differing ideas, and motivation can enhance the selection process to support achievement of desired outcomes (Bennett & Gadlin, 2012; Ryan, 2017).

Danna (2013) identified six rules to synergy and team building pivotal to interprofessional team effectiveness and management. The six rules are as follows:

1. Define a clear purpose. All team members must clearly be knowledgeable about the reason they are coming together. They must also be able to articulate the goals, objectives, and purpose of the team.
2. Actively listen. Each team member must be focused on each individual and listen to what is being said. Active listening is not judgmental and means being completely absorbed and attentive to the speaker.
3. Maintain honesty. Each team member must be objective in providing feedback to the speaker. No one should make the speaker feel belittled or that their view is not correct or important.
4. Demonstrate compassion. Each team member should listen in a caring manner to the other's viewpoint.
5. Commit to resolution of conflicts. Each team member must agree to disagree even though their view or opinions are not the same. Team members must work toward a common understanding and acceptance of the issue at hand.
6. Be flexible. Each team member must be open and flexible to another individual's perspective. Everyone works together to accomplish the goal or objective.

Stages of Team Development

Irrespective of team purpose, composition, or expected duration, there are stages of development that can be anticipated and observed in teams. The interactions between team members reflect the dynamic interplay between intrapersonal and interpersonal behaviors that contribute to the identity of the team. A commonly cited model in anticipating the evolutions within a team comes from the work of Bruce Tuckman (1965) and the revisions by Tuckman and Jensen in 1977. The model is helpful in understanding team dynamics that begin as teams form and progress toward cohesiveness and synergy, produce outcomes, and culminate. The stages are as follows:

Forming: Members define interpersonal boundaries and task behaviors.

Storming: Members resist group influence or task requirements; this stage is characterized by interpersonal conflict.

Norming: Resistance declines and cohesion emerges as expectations and roles are accepted. Members feel free to share thoughts and ideas.

Performing: Members are productive and work for the common goal of the group. Interpersonal relations drive activities and results (Tuckman, 1965).

Adjourning: The team dissolves because the tasks have been completed and the goals are achieved (Tuckman & Jensen, 1977).

During forming, the team members discover themselves and want to preserve their uniqueness or individuality. The goals and tasks for the team are provided, and individuals establish why they may have been selected for the team and their contributions. The focus is on individual interests, and testing comes in the form of establishing acceptable behaviors. The exchange of information is high as the team members establish ground rules. As the team forms, selection of content experts and recognition of those who have implemented solutions in the past is common practice. Attention to different problem-solving styles and ensuring equal numbers of sensing/thinking versus intuitive/feeling members is key. This will benefit the group in the performing stage (but may be a source of conflict expressed in the storming stage). The team leader or project manager develops the explicit norm of constructive conflict by addressing disagreement, multiple definitions, minority opinions, the role of the "devil's advocate," and a "group wins" psychology (Antai-Otong, 2013; Bennett & Gadlin, 2012; Danna, 2013; Walters, 2012).

In the storming stage, members of the group jockey for position, control, and influence. Competition becomes apparent, and leadership struggles ensue. The honeymoon phase of orientation has ended, and work requirements become evident. Resistance to team influence emerges, and intrateam conflict may arise. During this stage, team members have low levels of trust and often display anger and resentment. Although turf battles may ensue, the foundations for trust and respect may be further developed during this stage as a result of how conflicts are resolved. The leader supports the team by assisting with assignments, team roles, and conflict resolution and abiding by the ground rules that were developed in the forming stage (Antai-Otong, 2013; Bennett & Gadlin, 2012; Danna, 2013; Walters, 2012).

During norming, team cohesion develops as roles and norms are established to promote decision-making through consensus. Members have a common understanding of the opportunity to reach team goals, and there is openness to alternative definitions and multiple views. Morale and trust are high, and negativity is suppressed. Open communication during this stage facilitates constructive discussions and the sharing of personal and professional insights (Antai-Otong, 2013; Danna, 2013; Walters, 2012).

In the performing stage phase, team members work with deep involvement, greater disclosure, and unity. Linked by common goals, productivity is high, and team synergy is evident as members rely on the talents of the team members to accomplish work. Loyalty to the team is evident, and efforts revolve around the quality of the team product. This is the phase where work is completed, and the leader may be less involved (Antai-Otong, 2013; Danna, 2013; Walters, 2012).

In the adjourning stage, team tasks and goals have been completed. The outcomes of the work often lead to self-evaluation by the team, both on an individual and collective basis. Some team members may experience sadness and mourning related to the absence of team interaction, routine, and sense of purpose (Antai-Otong, 2013; Danna, 2013; Walters, 2012).

The stages of team development are described as if sequential in nature. However, because of various factors, team development is not always linear. Phases may be repeated, interrupted, or skipped. With the entering of a new team member, the departure of a team member, new leadership, or revised goals and deliverables, the team may shift to an earlier or later stage to find new equilibrium along a continuum of performance (Antai-Otong, 2013; Danna, 2013; Walters, 2012).

As a project or program leader, having an understanding and awareness of these stages helps explain team member behaviors across the life span of the team. This knowledge prompts proactive approaches in guiding interprofessional teams composed of individuals with diverse backgrounds (educationally) and experiences (in terms of tenure and previous work on teams) to work through each developmental milestone. For example, recognizing that conflict during certain phases may actually bring harmony and productivity, the project manager who understands storming as a developmental stage can channel team conflict into positive energy and high performance. If the conflicts arise and persist in the performing stage, the project manager might intervene using a different approach that relies on the established interpersonal relationships of the team members to find a resolution (Antai-Otong, 2013; Tuckman, 1965; Walters, 2012). Overall, when seeking to create synergistic interprofessional teams that are dedicated to effective project planning, management, and diverse person-centered programs, the project leader remains focused on ensuring that the team reaches the performing stage where team members are most productive.

Synergy and Creativity

Although the essence of project or program management is a systematic and disciplined approach to leading people through change and the completion of tasks, it also provides the opportunity to bring new ideas, relationships, and enthusiasm to an organization. The confidence of the team leader in navigating pitfalls and deliberately moving members through the achievement of milestones is expected. What may be overlooked is the opportunity for creativity and transformation, often displayed by teams led by experienced project managers. In times of great change or uncertainty, it is easy to reflect and use knowledge from past experiences and conform to rules or practices that resulted in success. Appreciative inquiry (AI), coupled with project management skills and quality improvement structures, advances teams from transactional interactions to transformational results and warrants attention given the expectations during the era of health reform and rapid change.

Although difficult to define, synergy is a product of effective teams, and the experience is commonly cited by team members as one of the benefits and personal satisfiers of working in a highly effective team. As individuals become members of a team and successfully work through the developmental stages, an energy, respect, and anticipation of positive outcomes sustains the members as they experience the benefits of productively working well together. While sharing experiences and implementing change, team members' synergistic influence is expanded by inciting enthusiasm and the spirit of possibility with individuals outside the work team (Gottlieb & Gottlieb, 2017; Lewis et al., 2017).

In consideration of professional development and team identity, synergy is experienced by those working in teams and is often described as growth derived from relationships, feedback, and insights gained from the experience. Attributes that contribute to synergy come through the interactions of team members supported by active listening, contributing, motivation, and cognition (Porter-O'Grady & Malloch, 2015). A team-level phenomenon of synergy has been described as an unconscious process of the team that manifests in individual team member actions that create collective positive or negative outcomes very different from the outcomes that would have been achieved by simply adding up the contributions of the individuals. Part of the synergy comes from the active listening and openness of team members as they explore options that may have been dismissed by an individual, lending to the creativity. Another part of the synergy originates from the self-correcting function of teams to counteract undesired outcomes and position the team to use individual and team creative assets.

Appreciative Inquiry

Although often thought of as a strategic lever for leadership and change, appreciative inquiry (AI) has applications relevant to project planning and management central to preserving clinical outcomes and quality metrics. At its core, AI is the art and practice of asking questions that strengthen a systems capacity to apprehend, anticipate, and heighten positive potential. Focused on what is working rather than what is not, it shifts thinking away from our typical "what is not working" focus and guides us to greater acknowledgment and preservation of those things that do work well. Rather than finding deficits and gaps, AI brings attention to strengths within teams or organizations and those things that can be replicated.

Cooperrider's (1990) seminal work in AI describes four stages: discovery, dream, design, and destiny. Discovery is the mobilization of the team or system into a positive change core. The dream stage occurs when a transparent, results-oriented vision is created through discovering potential and questions that provide a higher purpose. Design occurs when possibilities are realized with regard to the ideal state and people feel capable of expanding the positive core, making new dreams and concepts. Destiny evolves from the strengthening of the positive capabilities and capacities of the system, building hope and momentum focused on deeper purpose. Because members of the organization feel safe and energized, a space for learning, adjustment, and improvisation is created (Stratton-Berkessel, 2016; Thomas & Roussel, 2013).

AI is an intervention that heightens imagination and innovation by mobilizing a spirit of inquiry. The language of AI is different from a current state, given that critical analysis and identification of what is not working assumes more time and attention than the celebrations of what is working.

Hubbard (1998) views AI as a conscious evolution for realities in the new century. AI recognizes social construction focusing on metaphor, ways of knowing, and language producing a generative theory and advancement in action research. AI has been used in organizational development practice, as part of strategic planning, and as a framework to move from problem-based management to transformative leadership and human development (Thomas & Roussel, 2013).

Transformational Leadership

Given the need for engagement, honesty, innovation, trust, creativity, and recognition of things valued by members of teams, AI as a framework to generate solutions merits consideration. Underlying the success of AI are strong leaders with clarity, vision, and the ability to influence the thinking of others. Transformational leadership has been recognized as a style of leadership that extends beyond transactions. Transformational leadership includes a change or transformation of both the leader and the follower when leaders broaden, extend, and transcend the interests of employees, generate awareness and acceptance of the purposes and mission of the team, and encourage employees to expand ideas and thoughts beyond individual self-interests for the benefit of the group (Bennis & Nanus, 1985; Northouse, 2015; Roussel & Ratcliffe, 2013). As a result, leaders are agents of change who influence and inspire others and are also transformed.

Transformational leaders motivate followers to perform beyond normal expectations by transforming their thoughts and attitudes and by enlisting the vital support of the vision while striving for its fulfillment. This is accomplished through attributed charisma or modeling behaviors that gain admiration and trust; inspirational motivation or the ability to envision and articulate a future; intellectual stimulation involving questioning assumptions and reframing problems from a new perspective; and individualized consideration by delegation and empowerment while attending to individual needs, abilities, and aspirations (Avolio & Bass, 2002; Bass, 1990; Weberg, 2017). The theory of transformational leadership implies people need a sense of mission that extends beyond transactions and interpersonal relationships. This is especially true in health care, where the speed of and demand for change often exceed our perceived capacity.

For project and program leaders, transformational leadership provides a framework that promotes the synergistic interprofessional teamwork required for effective project planning, management, and diverse person-centered care. Empowerment of others, clarity in vision, and expectations of transformative change through the leadership of teams generate synergy around creative possibilities not previously considered. Transformative leadership brings extraordinary results through its capacity to influence others, build trust, and support teams as work is accomplished to meet identified goals.

Innovation

Much has been published on the need to hardwire evidence-based practices. Recently, attention has shifted from evidence to innovation with opportunities to form discipline and team identity with endeavors that are outcome-based (Lalley & Clouthier, 2017). Porter-O'Grady and Malloch (2015) pointedly stated, "Innovation is not merely a process. It is a dynamic. Innovation offers new meaning and direction and challenges the historic, the expected, and the routine. It calls for innovators to adopt an attitude that reflects that all work processes and activities are subject to the discipline of constant inquiry and reassessment" (p. 155).

The challenge for the interprofessional team is not how to generate new ideas and opportunities, but to make innovation a deeply entrenched aptitude and competency in any project endeavor (Gibson, 2014). The innovative project improvement team should ensure that the integrity and sustainability of the projects' outcomes are adaptable to the changing supply and demands of both the internal and external environment, and that the collective interests of the organization are advanced through those outcomes. Producing value in a singular innovative improvement project can create opportunities for additional value-based opportunistic projects. Sustained project outcomes and effective teams are the goal of and standard for high-functioning innovative systems where a culture of innovation is valued and respected. Missed opportunities occur daily in clinical settings and life in general. Connecting the energy and talents of an interprofessional team will turn missed opportunities into an innovative pipeline that produces high-quality, safe, and effective outcomes that benefit diverse populations and communities.

Common Language: A Driver for Interprofessional Project Improvement Team Successful Outcomes

Interprofessional project improvement teams are composed of individuals from diverse backgrounds, both clinically and culturally. Developing and adopting a mutually agreed-upon common language and shared purpose can only benefit the improvement project and function as a driver for team success and measurable outcomes (Chichirez & Purcarea, 2018; Kouzes & Pozner, 2007; Suter et al., 2009). Central to the improvement team leader's role is an understanding of the importance of communication among generations and use of commonly used tools, strategies, and models to elicit ideas from project improvement team members (Martin & Tulgan, 2006).

Table 4-3 identifies various communication preferences by generation that may benefit the outcome of any improvement team project.

Beyond generational and diverse communication differences, the use of standardized communication tools, strategies, and models that support teamwork and outcomes have been explored in the literature. The findings include supporting evidence specific to improved decision-making and increased safety (AHRQ, 2015; Danna, 2013; Stewart & Hand, 2017). Improvements can be credited to brainstorming; nominal grouping; situation, background, assessment, and recommendation (SBAR) communication, and TeamSTEPPS.

Brainstorming sessions are used to generate a large number of ideas through interaction among team members. In this strategy, the objective of the brainstorming is established and is often directly related to the team goals. One individual is selected to record ideas (generally on a board or flip chart) to avoid duplications. Individuals in the group then state ideas until they are saturated and, conversely, no new ideas emerge. The essential rules of brainstorming are that everyone participates and that no discussion, critique, or evaluation of the ideas takes place

Table 4-3 Communication Preferences by Generation

Generation	Spoken Preference	Written Preference
Traditionalists (Veterans, Silent, Moral Authority, Radio Babies, The Forgotten Generation) (Birth years: 1900–1945)	Formal linear thinkers, direct and to the point, no foul or offensive language, no small talk, proper grammar.	Well organized, proper grammar and punctuation, to the point, likes written communication for future reference.
Baby Boomers ("Me" Generation, Moral Authority) (Birth years: 1946–1964)	Like small talk to reach consensus and foster teamwork.	Written word for later reference and creation of paper trail preferred.
Generation X (Gen X, Xers, The Doer, Post Boomers, 13th Generation) (Birth years: 1965–1980)	Informal and direct with little to no small talk. Focus is on what things mean for them.	Little preference for reading; desire concise bullet points with outcomes clearly delineated. Little focus on grammar and punctuation.
Millennials (Generation Y, Gen Y, Generation Next, Echo Boomers, Chief Friendship Officers, 24/7's) (Birth years: 1981–2000)	Prefer spoken communication if the message is very important; desire others to show respect through language spoken; prefer action verbs with important messages; desire use of language to portray visual pictures; not skilled at personal communication because of the technical ways of communicating used during their life span.	Use positive, respectful, motivational electronic communication style; portray pictures through language; use action verbs. May need direction or written communication formats.

during the session. Following the creative thinking session, each idea is clarified to facilitate subsequent discussion on feasibility (Goldenberg & Wiley, 2011; Levine et al., 2015).

In a similar manner, the nominal group process begins with the establishment of an objective, but proceeds with each member generating an individual list of possible solutions. When sufficient time has been allowed, members take turns calling out ideas to the group. As with the brainstorming session, ideas are not discussed until all have been presented, and clarification occurs only after the team's entire list of ideas has been compiled (McMillan et al., 2014).

Once ideas are generated using brainstorming or nominal group processes, the team can then proceed to reduce the number of ideas on the list by voting to eliminate ideas that are not feasible, identifying items that may be readily implemented, and ranking/ordering related alternatives. Once individual team members rank each idea, then idea percentage distributions or average score calculations can be performed to determine the degree of agreement among team members. Clarification and discussion of the internal strengths and weaknesses within the organization as well as external opportunities and threats outside the organization that are useful for a SWOT analysis (discussed in Chapter 5) that currently or potentially support or mitigate actualization of the idea can be undertaken by the team. Additionally, an affinity diagram or Q-sort, in which ideas are written on cards and placed randomly on a table or chart, can be generated. Similar or related ideas are then organized by the silently working team members. When cards are no longer being moved, the team then discusses the ideas and generates a title for each grouping. Each method is useful in exploring alternative plans of action toward goal attainment.

SBAR communication was developed at Kaiser Permanente and is among the techniques useful in teamwork for communicating essential information using a standardized format (Stewart & Hand, 2017). In this strategy, communication is provided using the SBAR format (situation, background, assessment, and recommendation). The communication begins with a brief summary outline describing the situation. This is followed by background information about the situation or the context of the issue. The assessment component presents a statement of what the individual has identified as the problem and is followed by a recommendation of what corrective action is needed. Originally developed to facilitate communication between nurses and physicians, the use of a standardized format within team communication dynamics provides a succinct method of communicating information rapidly.

Created by the Agency for Healthcare Research and Quality and the Department of Defense, TeamSTEPPS is an evidence-based teamwork model developed to describe necessary skills and behaviors for team outcomes. The model includes skills for leadership, mutual support, situation monitoring, and communication. Attention to team composition, leadership, communication strategies and skills, standardization, and shared purpose underpin effectiveness. Feedback cycles are used with specific tools for communication to plan, deliver care, and evaluate care. Tools such as briefings, team huddles, and SBAR communication are the foundation from which fewer errors and improved outcomes flow (AHRQ, n.d.-a, n.d.-b, 2015; Danna, 2013).

The work of an improvement team to improve processes can be both challenging and rewarding. All members of the team facilitate effective leadership through the use of structures, tools, and models to ensure participation. However, barriers to the team's effectiveness do exist and must be considered.

Barriers to Team Effectiveness

Although the most effective communication knowledge and tools are used with any improvement team, there are times when barriers arise that decrease the effectiveness. Common pitfalls include an inability to trust or rely on team members, fear, unresolved conflict, lack of commitment, low standards, and the avoidance of accountability, as well as attention to personal gain rather than the results of the team. Each of these pitfalls can be avoided with effective leadership (Ulrich & Crider, 2017). The project improvement leader's role is to assist the team in developing trusting relationships by demonstrating reliance on the improvement team members to overcome limitations of knowledge, skills, or abilities that may be demonstrated by an individual team member. The improvement team leader can demonstrate vulnerability and identify team members to satisfy gaps. Fear and fear of conflict require improvement team leaders to support constructive debates and demonstrate the ability to manage it by establishing group norms for dealing with issues in a manner that is respectful to all team members (Bennett & Gadlin, 2012; Ulrich & Crider, 2017).

When team members avoid assuming a clear position on issues, the improvement team leader must work to provide critical information and a mechanism that considers all points of view before decisions are made. Similarly, assisting the team to focus on goals, continually tracking team progress, and communicating frequently through meetings and status reports may counter a lack of accountability.

Inattention to the results of the improvement team can be minimized through the selection of measures that clearly define success for the team effort (not individual interests) and the development of a tracking mechanism to monitor team progress. Success and failures must be equally shared within the team and used to reinforce progress toward goal achievement (AHRQ, 2015; Ulrich & Crider, 2017).

Unintentional and various jargon used by improvement team members can also hinder the progress of the team. It is not uncommon to observe different disciplines or individuals with personal agendas from a specific discipline that have priorities that compete with the project aim. For example, on a pain management project team, different disciplines or individuals may differ in terms of their preferred pain assessment techniques, observations, and descriptors; in turn, these differences may create a barrier to accomplishing the aim of developing a mutually agreeable language and process for documenting and describing a patient's pain experience.

Communication barriers are created when others do not comprehend the language, which then limits opportunities for mutual idea and knowledge sharing. As discussed, tools provide a method for ensuring team information exchange among others.

Project teams may also benefit from other shared, common language as projects are envisioned and implemented. For example, the National Patient Safety Goals and the IOM's Six Safety Aims highlight contributions by interprofessional teams in achieving desired, measurable collaborative goals (IOM, 2001; The Joint Commission, 2018). Many projects today focus on quality, safety, efficiency, and opportunities in an effort to demonstrate sustainable outcomes with replicable measurement and generation of empirical data. Language included in Lean, Six Sigma, and other methodologies offers a sustainable means of engaging in projects that emphasize the continuum of care, care coordination, pay for performance, and at-risk contracting for payment (Naylor, 2012).

An organization's culture plays an important role in how information is communicated and language is used, and both of these factors influence every project plan and activity. Organizational culture also plays an important role in all healthcare processes and the interchanges between patients and providers. Organizations that engender ingenuity of project improvement teams and remove an entrenched "culture of blame" in favor of a "just culture" will prevail in these turbulent times. Notably, safer practices will follow when the just culture approach is adopted

(Scott-Cawiezell et al., 2006). Just cultures foster supportive environments in which staff can question practices, express concerns, and admit mistakes without punishment (Kennedy, 2016; Tucker et al., 2007). A supportive environment is the cornerstone for a successful organization where employees are engaged and eager to be innovators (Hoying, 2017).

If an organization is able to promote interprofessional project teams that invest their efforts in advancing practice and creating empirical evidence, it is likely to have fewer incidents and system failures than an organization that holds on to the traditional "culture of blame" (Khatri et al., 2009). Incorporating the language of just culture and being true to its meaning will continuously foster positive team function and sustainability. Hence, high-reliability organizations are realized in which care is safe and errors are minimized while achieving exceptional performance in quality, safety, and efficacy (LaPorte, 2006; Ledema et al., 2019).

Coaching Interprofessional Project Teams

Teams are the driving force to success in any organization. Whether they form a functional team, a team of managers, or a specific project team, people collaboratively working together produce effective outcomes. As part of interprofessional team socialization, coaches assist members throughout all phases of a project. Coaches act as connectors who know lots of people. Their importance extends beyond the *number* of people they know to the *kinds* of people they know (Gladwell, 2002). A coach uses this information when working with teams to assist them in recognizing the value of all members and the importance of demonstrating interprofessional respect toward one another. Otherwise, the performance and productivity of a project suffer.

Hanson and Spross (2009) posit that a paradox of the current healthcare system is the existence of both incentives and disincentives for interprofessional team members and organizations to collaborate. Both the incentives and the disincentives play powerful roles, such that motivation to collaborate is eliminated by a counterforce. Recognizing this paradox will assist interprofessional project teams in seizing opportunities for strategic and sustainable collaboration in supportive environments.

Team coaching can be a powerful tool as teams work together to accomplish a specific aim. Coaching is a method used for support, encouragement, and career development (Finkelman & Kenner, 2010). Equally important is showing teams how to reduce conflict and improve working relationships for achievement of an identified aim.

Coaching a team requires this leader to focus on skills and interactions versus individual development. Interactions with team members and their communication are central to effective performance. One of the initial characteristics of a successful coach is understanding the team dynamics and translating this information throughout the phases of the project so as to attain the desired outcomes. Identifying how team members relate to one another is important for decision-making and productivity. Indeed, member behavioral assessments often prove beneficial for improving a team's productivity. As a coach, encouraging group discussion of behavioral assessments assists members to see one another differently, understand other people's perspectives, and adapt individual behavior for improved results. To realize this outcome, the team coach must ensure that a clear set of behavior expectations is mutually established and maintained to eliminate individual preferences that might otherwise obscure the project aim. Defining processes for team members to follow will support this endeavor.

Recognizing the need to evaluate reward and recognition systems and support individual development are the final roles of a team coach. When team members have personal goals that do not match with the goals of the team, problems may potentially arise. In such a case, the coach needs to identify sources of competing values and ensure that reward systems align correctly with individual performance. Being supportive of individual development is important for the coach as well, because members ideally will gain insights and attain new skills that ultimately benefit them individually in future team activities as well as the current project (Edmonson, 1999; Hall & Weaver, 2001).

In summary, Hackman and Wageman (2005, p. 283) suggest that team coaching will foster effectiveness only when four conditions are present:

1. The group performance processes that are key to performance effectiveness (i.e., effort, strategy, and knowledge and skill) are relatively unconstrained by task or organizational requirements.
2. The team is well designed, and the organizational context within which it operates supports rather than impedes teamwork.
3. Coaching behaviors focus on salient task performance processes rather than members' interpersonal relationships or on processes that are not under the team's control.
4. Coaching interventions are made at times when the team is ready for them and able to deal with them—that is, at the beginning for effort-related (motivational) interventions, near the midpoint for strategy-related (consultative) interventions, and at the end of a task cycle for (educational) interventions that address knowledge and skills.

Leading Interprofessional Project Teams Based on Needs and Mandates

Despite widespread agreement in disciplines about the centrality of clinical experiences to knowledge acquisition, extensive findings about the teaching practices or learning opportunities that foster interprofessional healthcare teams' outcomes remain limited. Such knowledge will benefit acquisition of the knowledge and skills needed to design and implement interprofessional projects resulting in safe, quality care. The extent to which individuals are best positioned to lead effective clinical or administrative project teams reflect needs, competencies, and competing mandates.

The 21st-century technologies, accreditation standards, and stakeholder demands for teamwork, communication, and coordination rely heavily on evidence to inform processes and care delivery. Identifying the needs of interprofessional project teams highlights the importance of leading them to engage in continuous improvement. Likewise, leaders and teams who possess interprofessional competencies and understand the interrelationships between patients and the team will facilitate project completion and satisfaction of the mandates that often drive management actions and decisions (IPEC Expert Panel, 2016).

Leaders at all levels must be action oriented and are challenged to shape new clinical environments and create a culturally sensitive environment that incorporates diversity and change (Brooks et al., 2019; Hall, 2009). Unlike management that seeks to control and manage, leaders seek to create and inspire change (Kotter, 1990). This change will be influenced, managed, and ultimately evaluated as it spreads to other environments. The call to create environments and core competencies sensitive to interprofessional team needs, strengths, and cultural diversity recognizes this reality. Globalization has promoted team inclusivity and ethnic diversity, resulting in multiple improvements (American Association of Colleges of Nursing, 2015, 2021). But one may ask, "Why now, and which core competencies should be adopted and utilized that maximize leader performance and preference?"

The IPEC Practice Competencies Panel is one group that has accepted the call to action and attempted to answer this question. This panel suggested the following steps as a response:

1. Create efforts across professions to ensure content is included in curricula.
2. Guide curricular development toward outcomes.
3. Provide foundations for a learning continuum across professions that embrace and engender lifelong learning.
4. Acknowledge that evaluation and empirical inquiry strengthen scholarship related to interprofessional competencies.
5. Prompt dialogue to identify goodness of fit between core competencies, practice, needs, and mandates (IPEC Expert Panel, 2011, p. 7).

In addition, the IPEC panel identified four domains of interprofessional collaborative practice (**Table 4-4**) and desired principles of the interprofessional competencies (**Box 4-1**).

Although the competency domains and specific competencies are general in nature and function, there is mutual agreement that they can position leaders of interprofessional teams to be successful. As teams accomplish project aims, mandates posed internally and externally will be met. However, project leaders must ensure

Table 4-4 Interprofessional Collaborative Practice Domains

Competency Domain 1:	Values and Ethics for Interprofessional Practice
Competency Domain 2:	Roles and Responsibilities
Competency Domain 3:	Interprofessional Collaboration
Competency Domain 4:	Teams and Teamwork

Reproduced from Interprofessional Education Collaborative. (2016). *Core competencies for interprofessional collaborative practice: 2016 update.* Author.

Box 4-1 Desired Principles of Interprofessional Competencies

- Patient centered
- Community and population oriented
- Relationship focused
- Process oriented
- Developmental learning activities, strategies, and behavioral assessments specific to the learner
- Integration across the continuum of learning
- Sensitive to systems and the applicability across all care settings
- Applicable across professions
- Stated in common and meaningful language across professions
- Outcome driven

---

that the team is aware of the realities inherent in any change and recognize that adaptation is even more important than anticipation (Porter-O'Grady & Malloch, 2015).

Managing any team, whether a clinical project team or a systems change team, requires leaders to keep in mind that the membership of the interprofessional team is a partnership among professionals, individuals, families, and communities. Team leadership and management are based on expertise and competencies that match the needs of the team. Decision-making and problem-solving are a shared responsibility, where information provided by patients and various disciplines is key for the success of any project endeavor (Simpson et al., 2001). Although there is no assurance that a leader can manage a project team with 100% effectiveness, these ideas can turn the interprofessional project team into an energetic and productive enterprise.

Measuring Interprofessional Project Leader Effectiveness and Value

Researchers have argued that the effective leader is a key analyst of organizational function success or failure (Madanchian et al., 2017). This can easily be transferred when applied to measuring interprofessional project team leader effectiveness. Organizational learning requires that effectiveness be continuously assessed. This assists leaders to avoid pitfalls and strengthens their ability to manage interprofessional teams to be more effective.

Yukl (2008) argued that identifying leadership characteristics is paramount to improving leader and organizational effectiveness. Dhar and Mishra (2001) further advanced this idea by identifying outcomes used to assess leader effectiveness, which include subordinate effectiveness, job satisfaction, commitment and performance, decision-making skills, and group performance. Identifying if expectations were met and changes improved outcomes is one strategy to assess interprofessional project team leader effectiveness. This evidentiary approach strengthens the quality and reliability of how decisions were made, goals were communicated, and the value of actionable improvements and sustainable outcomes (Porter-O'Grady & Malloch, 2021).

Summary

- Interprofessional team engagement is pivotal to quality, safe, value-based, and effective improvement project outcomes.
- Effective improvement project and program management is dependent on the ability for leaders to facilitate teams and guide them toward successful goal attainment.
- Time spent in understanding team dynamics is well spent, followed by leadership development and coaching to support and sustain trust, satisfaction, and accomplishment of goals by creating a space where curiosity, diversity, inclusivity, and innovation become the norm.
- The five stages of team synergy and its development are forming, storming, norming, performing, and adjourning, the platform on which effective teams can be built to perform.
- The challenge to synergistic, interprofessional teams is to adopt an aptitude of creativity, innovation, AI, and leadership that is disciplined, diverse, inclusive, constantly inquiring, and reassessing.
- Strategies directed toward building trust, effective communication, curiosity, and innovation will provide organizations moving through the demands placed on the industry in care delivery redesign.
- Using a common language that interprofessional team members understand and endorse will advance care delivery and continuous improvement.
- Project improvement teams require leadership competencies as well as an understanding of interprofessional core competencies, the basic assumptions of team functioning, stakeholder requirements, and guiding principles to meet the project aim and create a productive enterprise.
- Measuring interprofessional project team effectiveness and value is pivotal to organizational learning for sustained growth and success as improvement is recognized and becomes a marker of success in any organizational culture.

Reflection Questions

1. For a member of an interprofessional project team, which characteristics are essential for efficient and effective management of the team toward accomplishing the identified aim? How could you use the leader characteristics to lead a project team to successful outcomes?
2. How can the use of a common language by project team members enhance or inhibit success?
3. What are two primary needs of successful interprofessional teams? Discuss how you might use this information to meet various mandates in the current healthcare environment.
4. The chief executive officer (CEO) has identified that the first priority is to prevent unnecessary readmissions from skilled nursing facilities and home care agencies that the health system owns. Whom would you request to be on this team, and why? What would be your first steps?
5. You have been asked to step in and chair a subcommittee of the Quality and Safety Committee of the Board. The subcommittee you will chair has been charged to create a patient safety program, and the leader of this group has been on leave for 3 months. The trends, by unit, evidence increased injury fall rates

and increases in medication errors despite new documentation requirements and bar-code scanning. After reviewing the team charter and the outcomes dashboard for the work of this committee, you realize that the team has stalled and that the metrics/measures of success have not changed for more than a year despite meeting monthly. You know you will need to make some changes to achieve the team charge. You have been asked to write your plan for a meeting with the CEO and chief nursing officer (CNO) tomorrow. What would you include in your plan? What recommendations might you make regarding selection of new team members or disbanding this team and starting with new members? To manage expectations, what would you emphasize to the senior executives in terms of the team composition, timing, and future meetings?

6. You have been asked to join a newly created organizational team tasked to create the strategy and processes to increase department-specific innovations to fulfill the Triple and Quadruple Aim. As you listened to the discussion, you walked away feeling as if the team did not have a clear definition of innovation. You decide to call the team chair to meet for lunch so that you can learn about how "innovation" will be defined. Knowing what you do about the discipline and rigor involved in project and team leadership, who else in the organization would you want to talk to before the next meeting? What approach might you take with the team to generate ideas? What resources would you tap to assess the organization's past successes with change and innovation?

References

Agency for Healthcare Research and Quality. (n.d.-a). *TeamSTEPPS national implementation*. http://teamstepps.ahrq.gov/about-2cl_3.htm

Agency for Healthcare Research and Quality. (n.d.-b). *TeamSTEPPS: Strategies and tools to enhance performance and patient safety*. https://psnet.ahrq.gov/issue/teamstepps-strategies-and-tools-enhance-performance-and-patient-safety

Agency for Healthcare Research and Quality. (2015). *TeamSTEPPS 2.0*. https://www.ahrq.gov/teamstepps/instructor/fundamentals/index.html

American Association of Colleges of Nursing. (2015). *Enhancing diversity in the workforce*. http://www.aacn.ache.edu/media-relations/fact-sheets/enhancing-diversity

American Association of Colleges of Nursing. (2021). *The essentials: Core competencies for professional nursing education*. AACN.

Antai-Otong, D. (2013). Effective communication and team collaboration. In J. L. Harris, L. Roussel, & P. Thomas (Eds.), *Initiating and sustaining the clinical nurse leader role: A practical guide* (2nd ed.).pp. 105–140. Jones & Bartlett Learning.

Armstead, C., Bierman, D., Bradshaw, P., Martin, T., & Wright, K. (2016). Groups vs. teams: Which one are you leading? *Nurse Leader, 14*(3), 179–182. https://doi.org/10.1016/j.mnl.2016.03.006

Association of American Medical Colleges. (2011). *Core competencies for interprofessional collaborative practice*. https://nexusipe-resource-exchange.s3-us-west-2.amazonaws.com /IPEC_Core Competencies_2011.pdf

Avolio, B., & Bass, B. (2002). *Developing potential across a full range of leadership: Cases on transactional and transformational leadership*. Lawrence Erlbaum Associates, Publishers.

Bass, B. (1990). *Bass & Stogdill's handbook of leadership: Theory, research, and managerial applications* (3rd ed.). The Free Press.

Bennett, L., & Gadlin, H. (2012). Collaboration and team science. *Journal of Investigative Medicine, 60*(5), 768. https://doi.org/10.2310/JIM.0b013e318250871d

Bennis, W., & Nanus, B. (1985). *Leadership: The strategies for taking charge*. Harper & Row.

Braithewaite, J. (2015). Bridging gaps to promote networked care between teams and groups in health delivery systems: A systematic review of non-health literature. *BMJ Open; London, 5*(9), 1–12. http://dx.doi.org/10.1136/bmjopen-2014-006567

Brooks, L. A., Manias, E., & Bloomer, M. J. (2019). Culturally sensitive communication in health-care: A concept analysis. *Collegian*, *26*(3), 383–392.

Chichirez, C. M., & Purcarea, V. L. (2018). Interpersonal communication in healthcare. *Journal of Medicine and Life*, *11*(2), 119–122. PMCID: PMC6101690

Cooperrider, D. (1990). Positive image, positive action: The affirmative basis of organization. In S. Srivastva & D. L. Cooperrider (Eds.), *Appreciative management and leadership* (pp. 91–125). Jossey-Bass.

Crisp, N. (2014). Mutual learning and reverse innovation: Where next? *Crisp Globalization and Health*, *10*(14), 1–4. https://doi.org/10.1186/1744-8603-10-14

Danna, D. (2013). Organizational structure and analysis. In L. Roussel (Ed.), *Management and leadership for nurse administrators* (6th ed., pp. 213–307). Jones & Bartlett Learning.

Dhar, U., & Mishra, P. (2001). Leadership effectiveness: A study of constituent factors. *Journal of Management Research*, *1*(4), 254.

Drinka, T., & Clark, P. (2000). *Healthcare teamwork: Interdisciplinary practice and teaching*. Auburn House. ISBN-13: 978-0865692985

Dunevitz, B. (1997). Perspectives in ambulatory care: Collaboration—in a variety of ways—creates health care value. *Nursing Economics*, *15*(4), 218–219.

Edmondson, A. C. (1999). Psychological safety and learning behavior in work teams. *Administrative Science Quarterly*, *44*, 350–383. https://doi.org/10.2307/2666999

Finkelman, A., & Kenner, C. (2010). *Professional nursing concepts: Competencies for quality leadership*. Jones & Bartlett Publishers.

Gibson, R. (2014). *The no. 1 challenge to innovation*. http://www.innovationexcellence.com/blog,2014/09/14/the-no-1-challenge-to-innovation

Gladwell, M. (2002). *The tipping point: How little things can make a big difference*. Back Bay Books /Little, Brown.

Goldenberg, O., & Wiley, J. (2011). Quality, conformity, and conflict: Questioning the assumptions of Osborn's brainstorming technique. *Journal of Problem Solving*, *3*(2), 96–118.

Gottlieb, L., & Gottlieb, B. (2017). Strengths-based nursing: A process for implementing a philosophy into practice. *Journal of Family Nursing*, *23*(3), 319–340. https://doi.org/10.1177/1074840717717731

Hackman, J. T., & Wageman, R. (2005). A theory of team coaching. *Academy of Management Review*, *30*(2), 269–287. https://doi.org/10.5465/amr.2005.16387885

Hall, P. (2009). Interprofessional teamwork: Professional cultures as barriers. *Journal of Interprofessional Care*, *23*(7), 188–196. https://doi.org/10.1080/13561820500081745

Hall, P., & Weaver, L. (2001). Interdisciplinary education and teamwork: A long and winding road. *Medical Education*, *35*, 867–875. https://doi.org/10.1046/j.1365-2923.2001.00919.x

Hanson, C. M., & Spross, J. A. (2009). Collaboration. In A. B. Hamric, J. A. Spross, & C. M. Hanson (Eds.), *Advanced practice nursing: An integrative approach* (4th ed., pp. 283–314). Saunders Elsevier.

Hewitt, G., Sims, S., & Harris, R. (2014). Using realist synthesis to understand the mechanisms of interprofessional teamwork in health and social care. *Journal of Interprofessional Care*, *28*(6), 501–506. https://doi.org/10.3109/13561820.2014.939744

Hoying, C. (2017). Creating a business case for innovation. In S. Davidson, D. Weberg, T. Porter-O'Grady, & K. Malloch (Eds.), *Leadership for evidence-based innovation in nursing and health professions*. (pp. 173–216). Jones & Bartlett Learning.

Hubbard, B. (1998). *Conscious evolution: Awakening the power of our social potential*. New World Library.

Institute of Medicine. (1999). *To err is human: Building a safer health system*. National Academies Press.

Institute of Medicine. (2001). *Crossing the quality chasm: A new health system for the 21st century*. National Academies Press.

Interprofessional Education Collaborative (IPEC) Expert Panel. (2011). *Core competencies for interprofessional collaborative practice: Report of an expert panel*. Interprofessional Education Collaborative.

Interprofessional Education Collaborative (IPEC) Expert Panel. (2016). *Core competencies for interprofessional collaborative practice: 2016 update*. Interprofessional Education Collaborative.

Kennedy, B. (2016). Toward a just culture. *Nursing Management, 46*(6), 13–15. doi: 10.1097/01
.NUMA.0000483125.70978.b5

Khatri, N., Brown, G. D., & Hicks, L. L. (2009). From a blame culture to a just culture in health
care. *Health Care Management Review, 34*(4), 312–322. doi: 10.1097/HMR.0b013e3181a3b709

Kotter, J. (1990). What leaders really do? *Harvard Business Review, 68,* 104. https://doi.org/10.1108
/bl.2000.17013aae.001

Kouzes, J., & Pozner, B. (2007). *The leadership challenge.* Wiley.

Lalley, K., & Clouthier, K. (2017). Emergence and disruption: Working on the edge of evidence. In
S. Davidson, D. Weberg, T. Porter-O'Grady, & K. Malloch (Eds.), *Leadership for evidence-based
innovation in nursing and health professions* (pp. 217–239). Jones & Bartlett Learning.

LaPorte, T. A. (2006). High reliability organizations: Unlikely, demanding and at risk. *Journal of
Contingencies and Crisis Management, 4*(2), 60–71. https://doi.org/10.1111/j.1468-5973.1996
.tb00078.x

Ledema, R., Greenhalgh, T., Russell, J., Alexander, J., Amer-Sharif, K., Gardner, P., Juniper, M.,
Lawton, R., Mahajan, R. P., McGuire. P., Roberts, C., Robson, W., Timmons, S., & Wilkinson,
Lorna. (2019). Spoken communication and patient safety: A new direction for healthcare communication policy, research, education and practice? *BMJ Open Quality, 8,* e000742. https://doi
.org/10.1136/bmjoq-2019-000742

Levine, J., Alexander, K., Wright, A., & Higgins, E. (2015). Group brainstorming: When regulatory
nonfit enhances performance. *Group Processes & Intergroup Relations, 19*(2), 257–271. https://
doi.org/10.1177/1368430215577226

Lewis, M., Fitzgerald, T., & Zulkiewicz, B. (2017). Identifying synergies in multilevel interventions: The convergence strategy. *Health Education & Behavior, 44*(2), 236–244. https://doi
.org/10.1177/1090198116673994

Madanchian, M., Hussein, N., Noordin, F., & Taherdoost, H. (2017). Leadership effectiveness
measurement and its effect on organizational outcomes. *Procedia Engineering, 181,* 1043–1048.
https://doi.org/10.1016/j.proeng.2017.02.505

Martin, C. A., & Tulgan, B. (2006). *Managing generational mix: From urgency to opportunity.* HRD
Press.

McMillan, S., Kelly, F., Sav, A., Kendell, E., King, M., Whitty, J., & Wheeler, A. (2014). Using the
nominal group technique: How to analyze across multiple groups. *Health Services & Outcomes
Research Methodology, 14*(3), 92–108. https://doi.org/10.1007/s10742-014-0121-1

Miller-Keane, B., & O'Toole, M. T. (2003). *Encyclopedia and dictionary of medicine, nursing, and allied
health* (7th ed.). Elsevier, Inc.

Mueller, S. (2016). Transdisciplinary coordination and delivery of care. *Seminars in Oncology Nursing, 32*(2), 154–163. https://doi.org/10.1016/j.soncn.2016.02.009

Nancarrow, S., Booth, A., Ariss, S., Smith, T., Enderby, P., & Roots, A. (2013). Ten principles
of good interdisciplinary team work. *Human Resources for Health, 11*(19), 1–11. https://doi
.org/10.1186/1478-4491-11-19

National Academies of Sciences, Engineering, and Medicine. (2021). *The future of nursing
2020–2030.* The National Academies Press. https://doi.org/10.17226/25982

Naylor, M. (2012). Achieving high value transition care: The central role of nursing and its leadership. *Nursing Administration Quarterly, 36*(2), 115–126. doi: 10.1097/NAQ.0b013e31824a040b

Northhouse, P. G. (2015). *Leadership theory and practice.* Sage.

Porter-O'Grady, T., & Malloch, K. (2015). *Quantum leadership: Building better partnerships for sustainable health.* Jones & Bartlett Learning.

Porter-O'Grady, T., & Malloch, K. (2021). *Quantum leadership: Building better partnerships for sustainable health* (4th ed.). Jones & Bartlett Learning.

Project Management Institute. (2013). *A guide to project management body of knowledge (PMBOK
guide)* (5th ed.). Author.

Robert Wood Johnson Foundation & Institute of Medicine. (2010). *The future of nursing: Leading
change, advancing health.* https://www.nap.edu/resource/12956/Future-of-Nursing-2010-Report
-Brief.pdf

Roussel, L., & Ratcliffe, C. (2013). Transformational leadership and evidence-based management
in a changing world. In L. Roussel (Ed.), *Management and leadership for nurse administrators*
(6th ed., pp. 729–756). Jones & Bartlett Learning.

Ryan, S. (2017). Promoting effective teamwork in the healthcare setting. *Nursing Standard*, *31*(30), 52. https://doi.org/10.7748/ns.2017.e10726

Scott-Cawiezell, J., Jones, K., Moore, L., & Vojir, C. (2006). Moving from a culture of blame to a just culture in the nursing home setting. *Nursing Forum*, *41*, 133–140. https://doi.org /10.1111/j.1744-6198.2006.00049.x

Simpson, G., Rabin, D., Schmitt, M., Taylor, P., Urban, S., & Ball, J. (2001). Interprofessional healthcare practice: Recommendations of the National Academies of Practice Expert Panel on healthcare in the 21st century. *Issues in Interdisciplinary Care*, *3*(1), 5–19.

Stewart, K., & Hand, K. (2017). SBAR, communication, and patient safety: An integrated literature review. *Medsurg Nursing*, *26*(5), 297–305.

Stratton-Berkessel, R. (2016). *Appreciative inquiry for collaborative solutions: 21 strength-based workshops.* Pfeiffer.

Suter, E., Arndt, J., Arthur, N., Parboosingh, J., Taylor, E., & Deutschlander, S. (2009). Role understanding and effective communication as core competencies for collaborative practice. *Journal of Interprofessional Care*, *23*(1), 41–51. doi: 10.1080/13561820802338579.

The Joint Commission. (2018). *National patient safety goals.* http://www.jointcommission.org/standards _information/npsgs.aspx

Thomas, P., & Roussel, L. (2013). Clinical nurse leadership: Creating the vision. In J. L. Harris, L. Roussel, & P. Thomas (Eds.), *Initiating and sustaining the clinical nurse leader role: A practical guide* (2nd ed., pp. 481–510). Jones & Bartlett Learning.

Tucker, A. L., Nembhard, I. M., & Edmondson, A. C. (2007). Implementing new practices: An empirical study of organizational learning in hospital intensive care units. *Management Science*, *53*, 894–907. https://doi.org/10.1287/mnsc.1060.0692

Tuckman, B. (1965). Developmental sequence in small groups. *Psychological Bulletin*, *63*, 384–399. https://doi.org/10.1037/h0022100

Tuckman, B., & Jensen, M. (1977). Stages of small group development revisited. *Groups and Organizational Studies*, *2*, 419–427. https://doi.org/10.1177/105960117700200404

Ulrich, B., & Crider, N. M. (2017). Using teams to improve outcomes and performance. *Nephrology Nursing Journal*, *44*(2), 141–151.

Walters, S. (2012). Team power and synergy: Project planning and program management essentials. In J. L. Harris, L. Roussel, S. Walters, & C. Dearman (Eds.), *Project planning and management: A guide for CNLs, DNPs and nurse executives* (pp. 39–50). Jones & Bartlett Learning.

Weberg, D. (2017). Innovative leadership behaviors: Starting the complexity journey. In S. Davidson, D. Weberg, T. Porter-O'Grady, & K. Malloch (Eds.), *Leadership for evidence-based innovation in nursing and health professions* (pp. 43–76). Jones & Bartlett Learning.

World Health Organization. (2013). *Interprofessional collaborative practice in primary health care: Nursing and midwifery perspectives: Six case studies.* Author.

Yukl, G. (2008). How leaders influence organizational effectiveness. *The Leadership Quarterly*, *19*(6), 708–722. https://doi.org/10.1016/j.leaqua.2008.09.008

Zaccagnini, M., & White, K. (2014). *The doctor of nursing practice essentials; a new model for advanced practice nursing* (2nd ed.). Jones & Bartlett Learning.

Case Exemplars

Emotional Intelligence: A Catalyst for Interprofessional Team Success

Margaret Mitchell

All behavior has purpose and consequences, whether recognized at a given moment or at a later time during self-reflection. Failure to recognize how one reacts to situations and subsequent interactions with others can be a detriment to individual and team success. Interactions among team members drive outcomes and successful change. If a member of a team is resistant or reactive during a situation and is unaware of this behavior, the entire team may suffer. A project's potential outcomes may therefore be unattainable or significantly reduced. The interactions, relationships, and emotional intelligence of team members become vital to individual (evolutionary) or team (revolutionary) change in today's chaotic healthcare environment. If these are overlooked, opportunities for both team synergy and the notion of mindfulness are reduced, if not lost. Being mindful of recurring situations, past reactions, and emotions can only improve the odds for interprofessional team synergy and success.

Numerous authors have recognized the importance of one's emotional intelligence as a determinant for achieving personal and team excellence (Bradberry & Graves, 2009; George, 2000; Goleman, 1998). According to Goleman, emotional intelligence determines the potential for learning the practical skills of emotional competence. Appreciation and governance of one's emotions and those of the team can help alleviate team conflict as team activities and interprofessional projects evolve (George, 2000). Bradberry and Graves (2009) and Goleman (1998) advocate for the reinvestment in beliefs and values as an opportunity to redirect disruptive impulses that are prone to suspend judgment and to think before acting. Failing to handle or even consider one's actions or consider the feelings of others limits team synergy and any sustainable outcomes. This may further diminish the commitment and motivation of any team in the immediate and long-range future (Porter-O'Grady & Malloch, 2015).

Throughout one's career, nurses and other professionals are required to interact with one another. Observing how individuals respond to members of their individual discipline, especially nurses, can be especially enlightening, as the phrase "we eat our own" is commonplace when listening to nurses in conversation. Being mindful of how another nurse responds to a new graduate nurse can be directly attributed to one's emotional intelligence and can directly impact this relationship. A negative response or action can create conflict, and when individuals are unaware of their own negativity or reactivity in such a situation, this behavior may be observed in interactions with others.

Although there are no guarantees to changing how one reacts to any situation or crisis, thought leaders have offered several insights into enhancing one's emotional intelligence and potentials for effective and sustainable interprofessional team synergy (Goleman, 1998; Porter-O'Grady & Malloch, 2015). These include the following:

- Openness to novel ideas
- Valuing the knowledge and expertise of others
- Compassion
- Resilience
- Passion toward accomplishing a team goal
- Impulse control

The value of emotional intelligence advances a team's function and outcomes. Team members who are attuned to self and use their emotional intelligence can be beneficial to outcomes and sustained success. Being open to serendipitous and developing influences that occur unexpectedly is a hallmark of an emotionally intelligent team member and an effective team. Such influences can improve care delivery and advance health care in the 21st century and beyond.

Reflection Questions

1. Which of your personal strengths and attributes advance team functioning?
2. How are these attributes used in your daily practice environment?
3. What skills or abilities do you want to develop to become a more effective interdisciplinary or interprofessional team member? Why did you select these skills or abilities?

References

Bradberry, T., & Graves, J. (2009). *Emotional intelligence 2.0*. TalentSmart.

George, J. (2000). Emotions and leadership: The role of emotional intelligence. *Human Relations*, *53*(8), 1027–1055. https://doi.org/10.1177/0018726700538001

Goleman, D. (1998). *Working with emotional intelligence*. Bantam.

Porter-O'Grady, T., & Malloch, K. (2015). *Quantum leadership: Building better partnerships for sustainable health* (4th ed.). Jones & Bartlett Learning.

Transforming Care with Engaged Teams

Kathryn M. Ward-Presson

Background

Visionary leadership and interprofessional collaboration among all members of the healthcare leadership team are essential to improve patient care outcomes and meet Triple Aim objectives (Bisognano & Kenney, 2012). As a member of the "C suite," the CNO routinely works with other executives such as the CEO, chief of staff (COS), chief operating officer (COO), and chief financial officer (CFO) to identify organizational goals and determine clinical outcome measures and commensurate targets requiring priority focus. Goals and outcome measures identified should be consistent with those established by the facility's board of directors. Achieving goal attainment and the sustainability of improved patient outcomes depends on the selection of healthcare leadership team members who demonstrate effective project management and collegial problem-solving competencies (American Nurses Association, 2009; American Organization of Nurse Executives, 2007; Harris et al., 2011).

Nursing's Role

The CNO and other nursing leaders hold pivotal roles that may positively influence the achievement of organizational quality improvement objectives. One example of that influence is seen with the successful execution of designated projects such as the implementation of clinical bundles to address patient outcome deficits. This is especially true when the organization's priority projects involve nurse-sensitive indicators such as rates of hospital-acquired pressure ulcers (HAPUs) and catheter-associated urinary tract infections (CAUTIs).

Facility Exemplar

The existence of higher-than-target (0%) HAPU and CAUTI rates in a large tertiary teaching and research healthcare facility provides an example highlighting strategies to improve these rates through the collaborative efforts of the facility's nursing staff and other members of the team. Creating effective senior and mid-level nursing leadership teams was essential to the nursing team's ability to work collegially with other disciplines and address unit-based (microsystem) and overall nursing (macrosystem) performance improvement (PI) initiatives. Any improvements achieved because of nursing interventions and partnerships with non-nurse colleagues also served to improve the organization's HAPU and CAUTI rates at the macrosystem level.

The CNO employed a variety of leadership assessment strategies (e.g., one-on-one sessions with each senior nursing leadership member, Strengths Finder 2.0 assessments [Rath, 2007], and small-group meetings) to determine senior nursing leadership team members' interests, strengths, challenges, and career goals. Each member's ability to work with all nursing staff and other disciplines was also examined. Individual professional development plans were implemented to assist with each member's growth and competency development. Similar strategies were adopted by senior nursing leaders when assessing and establishing development plans for their direct-report nurse managers.

Establishing a senior nurse leader role of "Performance Improvement and Practice" and identifying an individual to fill this position (someone who possessed the necessary advanced competencies in the application of evidence-based practice principles, data gathering, and analysis and staff engagement) was critical to providing oversight for nursing PI projects, a central repository for performance-related information, and the availability of a subject-matter expert to assist line staff with unit-based and global PI projects. The facility's existing nursing shared governance structure was also evaluated and strengthened to ensure staff participation reflective of all job categories throughout the continuum of care.

Nursing wound care specialists led the facility's wound care committee and engaged committee members from other disciplines (medicine, infection control, dietary, materials management, and pharmacy) to ensure the creation of an interprofessional forum to address needed improvements in policies, procedures, and processes related to the organization's pressure ulcer prevention program. The committee reviewed evidence-based HAPU bundles and led the rollout of the designated HAPU bundle on an organization-wide basis. This group also monitored HAPU bundle implementation progress and reported relevant outcomes data to the medical and nursing executive committees and the governing body. Similar interprofessional team creation and operational strategies were employed to address the facility's CAUTI bundle implementation and outcome monitoring/reporting project.

The facility's unit-based and overarching nursing PI committees and the Nurse Executive Council (NEC) were updated at least quarterly regarding progress toward meeting the 0% HAPU and CAUTI rate targets. Unit-based PI committees and NEC members evaluated the data, provided input regarding further opportunities to improve the efforts, and determined strategies that appeared to be more effective than others in decreasing either rate. Results and reports were presented visually in the form of graphs and run charts, and raw numbers with benchmarks were shared during small- and large-group meetings. Results were also posted on unit bulletin boards for all stakeholders to review. The information provided also included narrative discussions about the effectiveness of the interventions used. Summary information was incorporated in the organization's annual nursing report as well.

With the support of the organization's executive team, senior nursing leadership and the NEC developed another strategy to improve HAPU and CAUTI outcomes—the implementation of the clinical nurse leader (CNL) role. The CNL is a master's-prepared nurse who possesses the competencies necessary to address the lateral integration of care delivery in collaboration with other healthcare disciplines and leads PI initiatives designed to improve patient care outcomes such as HAPU and CAUTI rates at the microsystem (unit) level (American Association of Colleges of Nursing, 2007). A medical–surgical unit was selected as the target site for CNL role introduction, and a new graduate CNL (who had been a staff nurse on the designated unit) was selected. Although no statistically significant improvements were found within the first year of the CNL role implementation, clinical significance during the first year and zero unit HAPU and CAUTI rates were achieved 1 year after role implementation. Nursing leaders should consider the implementation of the CNL role as a strategy to foster interdisciplinary collaboration and clinical outcome improvements at the microsystem level. As noted previously, a healthcare facility's microsystem improvements may favorably impact macrosystem patient care outcomes and overall improvements to care delivery.

Reflection Questions

1. Consider a unit/organization and the IOM's Triple Aim objectives. What are the priority clinical outcome improvement projects in the area? How and why were they selected?
2. Reflect upon an improvement conducted on a unit/organization. What was the outcome of the improvement project? How would you describe the effectiveness of those leading the project in ensuring collaboration among the key stakeholders? What did the leaders (formal and informal) do well to encourage team member engagement, and which suggestions do you have to improve full team-member participation?
3. Think about a unit or organization. How would the introduction of a different position, such as the clinical nurse leader, clinical educator, or clinical nurse specialist role, potentially impact team engagement and interprofessional collaboration to achieve project improvement success and positive outcomes? Which strategies would you use to introduce a new nursing role and ensure interprofessional collaboration and engagement?

References

American Association of Colleges of Nursing. (2007). *White paper on the role of the clinical nurse leader*. http://www.aacn.nche.edu/publications/white-papers/ClinicalNurseLeader.pdf

American Nurses Association. (2009). *Nursing administration scope and standards of practice*. Nursesbooks.org.

American Organization of Nurse Executives. (2007). *AONE guiding principles for the role of the nurse executive in patient safety*. http://www.aone.org/resources/role-nurse-executive-patient-safety.pdf

Bisognano, M., & Kenney, C. (2012). *Pursuing the Triple Aim*. Jossey-Bass.

Harris, J. L., Roussel, L., Walters, S. E., & Dearman, C. (2011). *Project planning and management: A guide for CNLs, DNPs and nurse executives*. Jones & Bartlett Learning.

Rath, T. (2007). *Strengths finders*. Gallup Press.

Making the Case for a Project: Organizational and Needs Assessment

Carolyn Thomas Jones
Linda Roussel

CHAPTER OBJECTIVES

1. Identify the primary components of a clinical needs assessment.
2. List the steps to take when completing a needs assessment.
3. Compare a clinical needs assessment and a community needs assessment.
4. Apply principles for project planning needs assessments.

KEY TERMS

Business case	Quantitative
Clinical needs assessment	Reliable
Community needs assessment.	Replicable
Institutional review board (IRB)	Stakeholders
Population	Transparent
Qualitative	Validity

ROLES

Clinician	Researcher
Project leader	

PROFESSIONAL VALUES

Advocacy	Quality
Confidentiality	

CORE COMPETENCIES

Advocacy	Design
Assessment	Development
Coordination	Stewardship
Data management	SWOT analysis

Introduction

The identification of a need is the cornerstone of project planning when an organization is starting a new clinical program, or a community is considering enhancing existing services. Unmet needs motivate the formation of laws, policies, innovative practices, learning, treatment, and health service funding (Harrison et al., 2013). Developing and conducting a needs assessment for a healthcare "project" is a project in itself. As described in Chapter 1, a project cycle evolves from initiation, to planning, to executing the project, to analysis and closure. A needs assessment requires determining the factors that may systematically identify specific need, the development of tools to measure those factors, carrying out the assessments using defined qualitative and quantitative methods, analysis of results, and closure. This then leads to the next steps in project or program management. This chapter identifies what a clinical needs assessment evaluates, answers the question of why one completes a needs assessment, and outlines steps followed when completing the assessment.

The Institute of Medicine (IOM), in its pivotal report *Crossing the Quality Chasm* (2001), identified six specific aims and observable metrics required for the delivery of quality care (**Figure 5-1**). Each of these six aims can provide direction in developing a needs assessment. A healthcare practitioner could apply several of the primary aims in one overarching project design, or just focus on a single element. In 2018, a subsequent publication focused on the "quality chasm" from a global perspective (National Academies of Sciences, Engineering, and Medicine, 2018) including the six aims described by the IOM, but also incorporating principles of systems thinking, optimizing technology, transparency, co-design of care delivery (inclusive of patient groups), and items that were evidence-based, anticipatory, and predictive at all system levels (environment, organization, and frontline care).

Figure 5-1 Six Aims and Metrics for Delivering Quality Care

Data from Institute of Medicine. (2001). *Crossing the quality chasm: A new health system for the 21st century.* Author.

Consider the importance of rapid diagnosis and treatment for ST-segment-elevation myocardial infarction (STEMI) through the emergency department (ED). Diagnostic confirmation to initiation of treatment (e.g., ED administration of antiplatelet agents, antithrombotic agents, and glycoprotein IIb/IIIa inhibitors) and transport to percutaneous coronary intervention (PCI) timeliness impact morbidity and mortality in those patients (Niccoli et al., 2019; Zughaft & Harnek, 2019). In addition to adhering to evidence-based practice standards, other factors can impact quality and equitable care. The COVID-19 pandemic revealed issues of health equity, prompting a potential need to evaluate recent trends and metrics for the purpose of defining sustainable improvements (Rashid et al., 2021).

For EDs, it is important to understand how well the STEMI program is operating and managing care by measuring several outcome factors based on the IOM's six aims, especially considering COVID-19 and new initiatives to address health equity concerns:

- *Safe:* In the year before the COVID-19 pandemic and the initial year of the COVID-19 pandemic, what were the percentage of patients who presented to the ED with STEMI, treatments used, and times to PCI according to demographic groups (gender, age, race/ethnicity)? What were the mortality rates for this care?
- *Effective:* What are the mortality and morbidity rates for STEMI care in the ED (pre- and during COVID-19)? Have there been any STEMI protocol changes for the two time periods? Are the protocols being carried out correctly?
- *Efficient:* How many staff are trained to deliver STEMI care? Has the COVID-19 pandemic affected staffing levels? Are there budget issues for STEMI treatments?
- *Timely:* Are STEMI diagnoses, treatments, and time from admission (door) to PCI similar or different during the two time periods? Are there time differences based on gender, age, race, or ethnicity? Do language issues interfere with timeliness?
- *Patient-centered:* What are the STEMI patient and family satisfaction scores, and how do they compare to scores for pre-COVID and during COVID time periods?
- *Equitable:* Are there disparities in how and to whom STEMI care is being delivered? Are patients with insurance treated differently than those who are uninsured? What other health equity issues negatively impact care?

These are skeletal examples of how to use the IOM's six aims and metrics for delivering quality care. Applying this rubric to project planning will aid in focusing the development of a robust needs assessment.

The World Health Organization (WHO, 2020) has defined a needs assessment as the collection and analysis of information that relates to the needs of affected populations and that will help determine gaps between an agreed standard and the current situation (p. 314). A needs assessment can be a systematic review of the way things are and the way they should be (Rouda & Kusy, 1995). Wright et al., (1998) stressed that health needs assessments are systematic measures that identify unmet needs of health and the system that can lead to actionable change.

Similar to any other research methodology, a needs assessment should be transparent, reliable, and replicable. Needs assessments are also dynamic processes. Although the assessment may measure "need" or identify "unmet needs" at one point in time to establish a baseline reading, it also provides a means to identify positive or negative shifts, changes, and improvements. Needs assessments can use a combination of qualitative and quantitative data collection techniques. The steps and considerations for conducting a needs assessment are summarized in **Box 5-1**.

Box 5-1 **Steps to Planning a Needs Assessment**

Step 1: Purpose
- What is known about the issue?
- What do you want to know?
- What will you do with the information?
- What are your biases?

Step 2: Population
- Who is being assessed: A community? A patient population? An institution? A department? A service? A treatment provider?
- What do stakeholders say about this population and approaches to measuring need? (Conduct focus groups or expert panels.)
- Will private health information be collected? How is confidentiality maintained?
- Will an informed consent form be needed?

Step 3: Method
- Will a survey be used?
- Will it be anonymous?
- Will it be observational?
- Will data collected be quantitative or qualitative?
- Which kind of sampling method will be used?

Step 4: Instrument
- Are reliable and valid tools being used?
- Will new tools be developed?
- Are questions or queries clearly stated and without bias?
- How will responses be recorded or measured?
- How easy is it to use the instrument?
- Does it include culturally competent language?
- Can results be easily summarized and analyzed?
- Will institutional review board (IRB) review and approval be required? Which type?

Step 5: Data Collection
- Is there a data management system for collecting and organizing data?
- Data dictionaries?
- Key data categories?
- Calculation methods?
- Missing or incomplete data?

Step 6: Analyses
- What are the results?
- What are the assessment's limitations?

Step 7: Use the Results
- Short-term and long-term goals
- Resource allocation
- Summarized findings
- Dissemination plans

The University of Kansas created the Community Toolbox (n.d.) as a publicly available resource for completing a needs assessment survey. Specifically, questions that are important to consider are as follows:

1. What is the purpose (or goal) for doing this needs assessment survey?
   Focusing on the goals can help the team clarify reasons for doing the needs assessment and planning for the project. Other considerations include how the results may be used and how aligned the goals are with the overall purpose. Asking this question gives the team the opportunity to be clearer as a collective and have dialogue from all perspectives.
2. Is the timing right for the needs assessment?
   The team questions the preparation needed to do the work with high-quality effort. It is important that timing and resources are in tandem and that resources are available. The team needs to be assured that the timing necessary to do the needs assessment survey from start to finish has been thought through at every step.
3. Has the team considered the number of individuals who need to be involved in taking the needs assessment survey? Has the team considered the kinds of people (consumers, stakeholders) who will offer the most relevant information to inform decisions about the overall purpose of the project?
   Following the purpose (goals) and timing, individuals and groups germane to the needs assessment can be asked to offer insights, feedback, and perspectives that will provide a more robust conceptualization of the need and project.
4. Who (on the team) is best suited to ask the questions (needs assessment survey/interview)?
   Considering the community and insider perspective, individuals "closest" to the individuals who will be impacted by the project would be best suited to connect the purpose with the plan.

In 2000, the WHO identified three evaluation components that should be considered and/or adopted in the needs assessment process for healthcare services for a given population:

- *Capacity of services* in relation to prevalence and incidence of a syndrome or disease in a specific area
- *Combination of services* required or desired for a syndrome or disease
- *Coordination of services* in a healthcare delivery system whereby entry, transition, and follow-up occur and are standard practice (WHO, 2000)

Purpose of Needs Assessment

When assessing needs and capacity within an organization, a SWOT analysis is often used. This assessment identifies the strengths, weaknesses, opportunities, and threats impacting an organization at a point in time. SWOT analyses have been used for assessing needs and performing strategic planning in healthcare organizations (van Wijngaarden et al., 2012). They unpack the dichotomies between external developments (opportunities or threats) and internal capabilities (strengths and weaknesses). A proposed model for SWOT analysis includes a three-pronged approach for its implementation:

- Stakeholder expectations: demands and standards
- Contextual factors: trends and network developments
- Resources: capabilities, people, finance, and means

The goals for a project needs assessment should be clearly identified and should provide a guide for data collection. The basic components of a needs assessment address the differences between what is known about the idea and what is still unknown. A tenet for all scholarly work, including needs assessment, is, "If you do not need to know the answer, then do not ask the question." Therefore, all known and unknown elements and their impact must be assessed to determine their fit with the project. The goal of any project is to produce usable results that will positively impact functions and deliverables within the organization. If not, then one must ask, "Why did you do it?"

An important element in identification of purpose and need is the identification of biases within the project team, the stakeholders, and the organization. The needs assessment data can also serve as a guide to project financial impact, justify the allocation of funding by the funding source, and provide support for the business case. Business cases are guided by data that validate inefficiencies, the unpredictable nature of organizations, occupational differences, and interdependencies within and across systems and how improvements will impact service quality and costs.

Another method of assessing quality-associated care and the planning of new projects is to apply the semi-qualitative method developed by Donabedian (1998). This approach is based on three key components: structure, process, and outcomes. Each of these components has direct influence on the others, in a sequential fashion. *Structure* refers to the healthcare setting: personnel (staff expertise), material resources (e.g., electronic health records), organizational structure (hospital, clinic), and leadership. *Process* refers to what is done at the microsystem level, for instance, interventions and care coordination. *Outcomes* refer to health-related outcomes and improvements. Assembling data into these three "buckets" (**Figure 5-2**) can assist in better understanding the next steps in identifying key needs and proposed project plans for evolving improvements.

Population

The population of interest must be described whether the project is focused on an organization, a patient population, or a community. The purpose of the project will guide identification of the population.

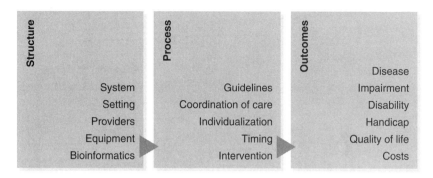

Figure 5-2 Donabedian Model: Structure, Process, and Outcomes

Once the population is identified, the project leader and/or team must determine the stakeholders' perception of the problem that the project is designed to address. Project team members must collect information from all stakeholders to facilitate an effective problem resolution. Stakeholders may include the following groups: (1) patients or those experiencing the need, (2) health and human services providers, (3) government officials, (4) influential people, (5) people whose jobs are impacted by the proposed actions that would result from the assessment, (6) community activists, and (7) affected local businesses.

Population assessment methods can include expert panels, focus groups, surveys, and interviews, among others. The method selected should fit both the population and the project. During this assessment phase, project team members should also determine the level of data that will be collected. For example, if private health information is needed to carry out the project and produce a viable product, then the project team must determine how that information will be collected, protected, stored, and used.

Questions related to maintenance of confidentiality, anonymity, and informed consent must be considered. Will data be reported, individually or in aggregate format? How will the research or project team assure security of all information? Inherent in these considerations is "goodness of fit": Do the data fit the purposes of the project, and will they yield the desired results? These and other questions provide much context for the project and are also considerations when measuring community needs. Methods of assessing stakeholder needs are illustrated in **Figure 5-3**. The increasing availability of digital and secondary data should also be considered.

Recruiting stakeholder participants requires preplanning. It is common to use more than one method to contact existing and potential stakeholders.

Organization and Systems

In any project, there is always the possibility of uncovering potential problems in an organization at the micro-, meso-, or macro-level when one is completing a needs assessment. Understanding the organizational culture (e.g., what are the norms? What guides behaviors, readiness for innovations?) and organizational climate (e.g., what do the employees think? What are their perceptions

Figure 5-3 Sources and Methods for Measuring Community Needs

of role? Do they have work satisfaction, exhaustion, frustration?) can provide insights to best approach needs assessments of factors related to systems and organizational structures (Aarons et al., 2009, Aarons et al., 2011; Autin et al., 2019). Loo (2003) proposed two methods that organizations may consider using when problems or issues are identified: an issues analysis chart and an issues impact assessment. An issues analysis chart assists in describing the problem, its impact, and required actions. It complements an issues impact assessment by identifying how the problem(s) may become a barrier to initiating the project and which negative impacts may arise if the problems occur as the project is being completed.

Oliva and Rockart (1997) suggested three other considerations to be considered when an organization is conducting a clinical needs assessment: (1) interprogram complementarities, (2) interprogram competition, and (3) interactions among and between programs and services. First, whether a project or program was successfully implemented and sustained, organizations must assess how previous projects and programs might have benefited the current endeavor. It is important to determine if tools can be used again or modified for future use. Moreover, if shifts in knowledge, organizational culture, performance, or attitudes occur, those shifts should be measured. Second, organizations should assess the benefits or challenges associated with interprogram competition. Conflicts across programs or competitive programs can become barriers rather than facilitators of the organization's mission, vision, and purpose. Barriers can result in fragmented roles and performance outcomes and ultimately erode employee motivation, resulting in a domino effect of mounting cynicism and deterioration

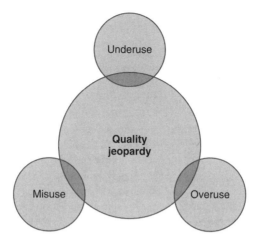

Figure 5-4 Three Categories for Healthcare Quality

of management's leadership. Finally, organizations must consider the interactions within and between programs and services and examine each program's contributions to the overall success of each unit, the broader organization, and quality of care that will follow.

The IOM (1999) suggests that problems associated with quality of care can be organized into the three categories illustrated in **Figure 5-4**. Underuse, overuse, and misuse may stem from clinical guidelines, policies, equipment, staffing, informatics, authority, funding sources, and many other elements that are at play in structuring and managing a healthcare facility in acute care, long-term care, ambulatory care, or community care. These factors can jeopardize quality care.

An example of underuse may occur with electronic medical record (EMR) data. Nurses and staff who input data into EMRs spend a tremendous amount of time on this task. Some of those data are redundant, however; other data are not accessed or used on a routine basis to deliver care. Consequently, the time spent documenting in the electronic record may not correspond directly to those data's ultimate utility.

Another example is *workarounds*. Nurses often use workarounds to facilitate the daily activities involved in performing their jobs. For example, some may employ personal mobile devices that aid in getting the job done but which may be a violation of institutional policy and could jeopardize patient privacy. Such workarounds may represent overuse or misuse issues that impact quality performance and care.

Innovative and creative problem solving can lead to improvements in care delivery; however, it is important to collect data on the utility and risks/benefits of such initiatives. In doing so, it can be useful to consider the underuse, overuse, and misuse issues that are observable and measurable in the organization. Closing gaps in those areas can have a strong positive impact on both quality care and cost savings. The needs assessment is a first step toward planning a project that can address those gaps.

Methods and Instruments

Project personnel should select the method of data collection and either locate or develop instruments that will best fit the project and the methods. Surveys, for example, are a popular method of gathering information from larger groups. When developing survey questions, it is important to be concise, clear, and measurable. The phrasing of stem questions and selections can impact the intended assessment. Questions that fall into categorical (or nominal) level categories should be separated from those that fall in ordinal levels (**BOX 5-2**). Consider the potential respondent.

Other considerations related to methods of data collection include determining whether the data are best captured through a qualitative or quantitative approach. Likewise, the sampling method to be used is an important consideration. Samples are groups of individuals that represent the target population and must be sufficient in number to support the findings.

Instruments

The validity (Does the instrument measure what it is designed to measure?) and reliability (Does the instrument measure the concepts/constructs consistently in different settings, populations, or projects?) of an instrument are integral in determining the usefulness of the project outcomes. If existing tools are available that fit the project, the project team must determine the validity and reliability of those instruments. Traditionally, the validity and reliability of an instrument are described in the original and subsequent research studies that were used to establish them.

If instruments exist but must be altered, the project team must contact the author(s) of the tool and seek permission to use and modify it. Once modified, the

---

Box 5-2 Example Questions

An example of a nominal-level question is:
Categorize your highest educational level:

a. Some high school
b. High school graduate/GED
c. Some college
d. Associate's degree
e. Baccalaureate degree
f. Postbaccalaureate degree

An example of an ordinal-level question would be:
    Protected learning time for ED staff members should be increased to 1 hour per month:

a. Strongly agree
b. Agree
c. Disagree
d. Strongly disagree

    These types of questions can be incorporated into surveys, questionnaires, and interviews.

instrument must be subjected to procedures to establish the validity and reliability of the modified sections.

If an instrument does not exist that will effectively measure the concepts and constructs of the project, then the researcher or project team may develop a new instrument for use with the project. All researcher- or project team-developed instruments must have their validity and reliability established. Most research texts provide a clear description of the processes and procedures involved in establishing validity and reliability. The reader is encouraged to review such a text for further discussion of this topic.

Instruments must be applicable to the project, expedient, and easy to use. These characteristics are essential not only in collecting data but also in collating, analyzing, and summarizing the data and disseminating the findings.

Before launching a survey or data collection system, it is important to first conduct a pilot run using members of the team or other volunteers to quality check the tool (spelling, grammatical errors, confusing questions, or ambiguous instructions). A pilot will also provide insights on the time the assessment will take to complete. This will ensure that the assessment is not launched before it is ready.

Data Collection

Whether the assessment is lengthy or small, a data management plan that defines the system for collecting and organizing data and how data will be analyzed will be helpful. Data management systems can be as simple as a web-based Qualtrics^{XM} survey instrument that can be easily accessed by respondents online using a personal computer or a digital device. Introductions and informed consent can be embedded in initial sections. Data will be summarized through their report mechanism and can also be downloaded to a statistical software program or Excel. An Excel spreadsheet is a simple method of reviewing or inputting data. The grid shown in **Figure 5-5** is a simple method of managing key data categories.

A data dictionary or glossary is another essential tool, especially if different members of the team are involved with collecting, categorizing, and entering data. Internal consistency of team usage will facilitate "clean" data collection and entry. For instance, the method of documenting the date can vary (mm/dd/yyyy–01/15/2021 or dd/mon/yyyy–15 Jan 2021) or weight (lbs. or kgs), if well defined, can reduce data management hurdles. Adverse side effects may be collected using a drop-down menu from the MEDRA system, to ensure further consistency in data collection and greatly ease data retrieval and analysis.

The final steps in data collection are determining consistent calculation methods and retrieving missing or incomplete data. Preliminary planning as to how

Participant ID number	Informed consent	Instrument 1	Instrument 2	Data input complete
	Date out/received	Date out/received	Date out/received	

Figure 5-5 Data Collection Grid

partial and incomplete responses will be incorporated in the findings will assist with these processes.

Analysis and Use of Findings

Once the data have been collected, they must be analyzed and applied within the organization/system. Any findings must be clearly described and linked back to the original short- and long-term goals and objectives of the project.

Once findings are published, at least internally, resource allocation processes for full implementation can begin. Dissemination of findings to a broader audience will be directly linked to organizational goals and objectives. Dissemination may also take the form of poster and podium presentations at international, national, and local conferences, as well as professional organizational meetings. Many doctor of nursing practice (DNP) programs require that scholarly projects be digitally submitted—for example, through an eRepository. At this point, the current study and project are considered to have ended, and another problem identification and needs assessment cycle begins.

Summary

- Needs assessments are the cornerstones for project planning.
- Clinical, organizational, and community needs assessments provide the rationale and support for the project's business case.
- A series of steps are followed when completing a clinical needs assessment and a community needs assessment.
- A variety of tools can assist the project team when completing a needs assessment.

Reflection Questions

1. Which elements are part of successful clinical needs assessment?
2. How are community needs assessments similar or different?
3. Conduct a CINAHL (Cumulative Index of Nursing and Allied Health Literature) search for the term *health needs assessment*. Note the variety of needs assessments published. Focus your search on needs assessments in a population of interest to you. Begin to formulate best approaches for conducting a needs assessment for that population.

Learning Activities

1. Using Box 5-1 (Steps to Planning a Needs Assessment), describe ways this tool provides foundational information in planning a project.
2. The Donabedian model (structure, process, outcome) (Figure 5-2) can provide a framework for any project. Using the model, describe each concept in your current project.

References

Aarons, G. A., Fettes, D. L., Flores, L. E., & Sommerfeld, D. H. (2009). Evidence-based practice implementation and staff emotional exhaustion in children's services. *Behaviour Research and Therapy, 47*(11), 954–960. https://doi.org/10.1016/j.brat.2009.07.006

Aarons, G. A., Hurlburt, M., & Horowitz, S. M. (2011). Advancing a conceptual model of evidence-based practice implementation in public service sectors. *Administration Policy and Mental Health, 28,* 4–23.

Autin, K. L., Duffy, R. D., Blustein, D. L., Gensmer, N. P., Douglass, R. P., England, J. W., & Allan, B. A. (2019, March). The development and initial validation of need satisfaction scales within the psychology of working theory. *Journal of Counseling Psychology, 66*(2), 195–209. https://doi.org/10.1037/cou0000323. Epub 2019 Feb 4. PMID: 30714744

Donabedian, A. (1988). The quality of care. How can it be assessed? *Journal of the American Medical Association, 269*(12), 1743–1748. https://doi.org/10.1001/jama.260.12.1743

Harrison, J. D., Young, J. M., Butow, P. N., & Solomon, M. J. (2013). Needs in healthcare: What beast is that? *International Journal of Health Services, 43*(3), 567–585. https://doi.org/10.2190/HS.43.3.1

Institute of Medicine. (1999). *To err is human.* National Academies Press. http://nationalacademies.org/hmd/reports/1999/to-err-is-human-building-a-safer-health-system.aspx?_ga=2.48614627.439078995.1520992418-1302790904.1520992418

Institute of Medicine Committee on Quality in Healthcare in America. (2001). *Crossing the quality chasm: A new health system for the 21st century.* National Academies Press. PMID: 25057539.

Loo, R. (2003). Project management: A core competency for professional nurses and nurse managers. *Journal of Nurses in Staff Development, 19*(4), 187–193.

National Academies of Sciences, Engineering, and Medicine. (2018). *Crossing the global quality chasm: Improving health care worldwide.* The National Academies Press. https://doi.org/10.17226/25152

Niccoli, G., Montone, R. A., Ibanez, B., Thiele, H., Crea, F., Heusch, G., Bulluck, H., Hausenloy, D. J., Berry, C., Stiermaier, T., Camici, P. G., & Eitel, I. (2019). Optimized treatment of ST-elevation myocardial infarction. *Circulation Research, 125*(2), 245–258. https://doi.org/10.1161/CIRCRESAHA.119.315344. Epub 2019 Jul 3. PMID: 31268854.

Oliva, R., & Rockart, S. (1997). *Dynamics of multiple improvement efforts: The program life cycle model.* https://citeseerx.ist.psu.edu/viewdoc/download?doi=10.1.1.17.8458&rep=rep1&type=pdf

Rashid, M., Timmis, A., Kinnaird, T., Curzen, N., Zaman, A., Shoaib, A., Mohamed, M.O., de Belder, M. A., Deanfield, J., Martin, G. P., Wu, J., Gale, C. P., & Mamas, M. (2021). Racial differences in management and outcomes of acute myocardial infarction during COVID-19 pandemic. *Heart, 107*(9), 734–740. https://doi.org/10.1136/heartjnl-2020-318356. Epub 2021 Mar 8. PMID: 33685933.

Rouda, R. H., & Kusy, M. E. (1995). *Needs assessment: The first step.* https://www.achievemission.org/wp-content/uploads/2021/03/Needs-Assessment%E2%80%93First-Step.pdf

University of Kansas. (n.d.). Chapter 3, Section 7. Conducting needs assessment surveys. In: University of Kansas, *Community toolbox.* https://ctb.ku.edu/en/table-of-contents

Van Wijngaarden, J. D. H., Scholten, G. R. M., & van Wijk, K. P. (2012). Strategic analyses for healthcare organizations: The suitability of the SWOT-analysis. *International Journal of Health Planning and Management, 27,* 34–49. https://doi.org/10.1002/hpm.1032

World Health Organization. (2000). *Needs assessment: Workbook 3.* http://whqlibdoc.who.int/hq/2000/WHO_MSD_MSB_00.2d.pdf

World Health Organization. (2020). Chapter 10 needs assessment. In World Health Organization, *Health cluster guide: A practical handbook* (pp. 314–353). World Health Organization. License: CC BY-NC-SA 3.0 IGO

Wright, J., Williams, R., & Wilkinson, J. R. (1998). Development and importance of health needs assessment. *British Medical Journal, 316*(7140), 1310–1313. https://doi.org/10.1136/bmj.316.7140.1310

Zughaft, D., & Harnek, J. (2014). A review of the role of nurses and technicians in ST-elevation myocardial infarction (STEMI). *EuroIntervention, 10*(suppl T), T83–T86. https://doi.org/10.4244/EIJV10STA13. PMID: 25256539.

Case Exemplars

Project Planning and Management in Antimicrobial Stewardship

Carolyn Thomas Jones

Core elements and guidelines for a hospital-based antimicrobial stewardship (AMS) program have been described by the Centers for Disease Control and Prevention (CDC, 2014). The impact of antibiotic resistance continues to rank as one of the rising unmet medical needs. "The CDC (2019) estimates that more than 2.8 million antibiotic-resistant infections occur in the United States, resulting in the deaths of more than 35,000 Americans" (p. vii). Moreover, antibiotic prescribing is inappropriate in 20% to 50% of such prescriptions and is contributing to the rising levels of resistance.

Although the primary goal of AMS programs is to improve patient care and public health, a by-product of implementing and tracking these measures is huge financial savings to institutions and the healthcare enterprise, not to mention mitigating local and global healthcare threats. The aim is to use the correct diagnosis, correct agent, correct dose, and appropriate duration of dosing for desired outcomes in cure or prevention, minimization of toxicity, and prevention of development of resistant organisms. Institutional costs of implementing an antimicrobial resistance program (whether in an inpatient or ambulatory setting) are minimal compared with the resulting health and financial savings. Building and maintaining sustainability in managing an AMS program is, therefore, an essential challenge for healthcare organizations. The CDC and the ANA (2017) co-published a white paper on the role of nurses in hospital antibiotic stewardship practices (**Figure 5-6**).

Components of Hospital-Based Antibiotic Stewardship Programs

Supporting a business case for ongoing measures requires continuous assessment of need, impact, and resource requirements. Manning (2014) discusses the urgent need for nurse practitioners (NPs) to lead AMS programs in ambulatory care settings and estimates that NPs in those settings write an average of 19 prescriptions per day, many of which are for antibiotics. Bedside nurses and infection control nurses have an increasing role in every aspect of AMS. Olans et al., (2017) describe specific AMS nursing functions at hospital admission, during the hospital stay, and at discharge, stressing that AMS is a hallmark of good nursing care.

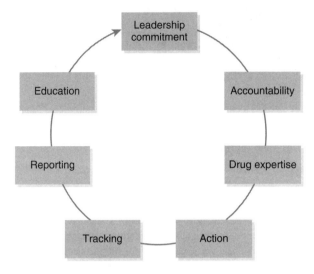

Figure 5-6 Seven Case Exemplars

Project planning and management of a variety of facets of AMS are ripe for advanced practice nurse involvement, whether as a clinician, a nurse executive, or a program manager. After developing a focused approach for problem identification in AMS, the NP should consider how to assess needs from clinical, pharmaceutical, financial, and resource perspectives. A key challenge in such a broad topic will be to focus attention on one population, specific organisms, or specific settings. Such a focused approach can bring about stepwise improvements.

References

American Nurses Association & Centers for Disease Control and Prevention. (2017). Redefining the antibiotic stewardship team: Recommendations from the American Nurses Association/Centers for Disease Control and Prevention Workgroup on the Role of Registered Nurses in Hospital Antibiotic Stewardship Practices. https://www.cdc.gov/antibiotic-use/healthcare/pdfs/ANA-CDC-whitepaper.pdf

Centers for Disease Control and Prevention. (2014). *Core elements of hospital antibiotic stewardship programs.* U.S. Department of Health and Human Services. http://www.cdc.gov/getsmart/healthcare/implementation/core-elements.html

Centers for Disease Control and Prevention. (2019). *Antibiotic resistance threats in the United States, 2019.* U.S. Department of Health and Human Services, CDC.

Manning, M. L. (2014). The urgent need for nurse practitioners to lead antimicrobial stewardship in ambulatory health care [Editorial]. *Journal of the American Association of Nurse Practitioners, 26* (8), 411–413. https://doi.org/10.1002/2327-6924.12150

Olans, R. D., Olans, R. N., & Witt, D. J. (2017). Good nursing is good antibiotic stewardship. *American Journal of Nursing, 117*(8), 58–63. https://doi.org/10.1097/01.NAJ.0000521974.76835.e0

Establishing Medical Emergency Response Teams (MERT) in a School System

Kimberly Goins

Health care within a school system is vastly different from that offered in acute care facilities; however, the skills and goals needed to provide quality, efficient, and equitable care are constant. Although historically considered a minimally trained position by many, contemporary school nurses must be prepared to provide acute care to a diverse group of students. The school nurse is an advocate for improved care to patients, families, and communities through education, awareness, and system-wide changes necessary for care (Willgerodt & Yonkaitis, 2021). The changes in a school system must be compliant with the federal law (Title IX), the state's Department of Public Health and Department of Education, and the local education association.

In 2003, the American Heart Association advised all schools to begin instructing educators in first aid and CPR (Hazinski et al., 2003). In 2015, the American Academy of Pediatrics recommended that, at a minimum, school health services should be authorized to provide and administer to students with special needs and related health issues any medications needed that might affect their education (American Academy of Pediatrics, 2016). These recommendations provided the impetus o consider establishing Medical Emergency Response Teams (MERT) that then qualified the entire school to be designated as a Heart Safe Certified environment.

Within many school systems, the only staff members required to possess CPR certification were the physical education instructor, coaches, and school nurses. Consider that, in a student body that includes 3,500 students (200 of which may require emergency intervention), 45 staff members would require the certification.

A needs assessment, underpinned by a process map consisting of five domains (define, measure, analyze, improve, and control), helped the staff form a committee of administrators and school nurses to examine documented occurrences in the system, review current responsiveness to emergencies, and develop an improvement plan. The committee was provided responses from a survey of 117 respondents that included administrators, educators, and other school nurses who had experienced the need for first aid and CPR knowledge. Upon approval from administrators and support of the lead school nurse, MERT classes were conducted. After the training, all employees interested in MERT classes were approved and received an advanced first aid kit. MERT will be fully implemented during the 2021–2022 school year, followed by Heart Safe Certification. Automated external defibrillator (AED) drills, as well as a follow-up survey, are planned for future dissemination of information to other school systems throughout the states.

Reflection Questions

1. What requisite tools are useful when forming an improvement team within a school system?
2. Who are the stakeholders necessary to include in a school system improvement?

References

American Academy of Pediatrics. (2016). Role of the school nurse in providing school health services. (2016). *Pediatrics, 137*(6), e20160852–e201608852. https://doi.org/10.1542/peds.2016-0852

Hazinski, M. F., Markenson, D., Neish, S., Gerardi, M., Hootman, J., Nichol, G., Taras, H., Hickey, R., O'Connor, R., Potts, J., van der Jagt, E., Berger, S., Schexnayder, S., Garson, A., Doherty, A., & Smith, S. (2003). Response to cardiac arrest and selected-life-threatening medical emergencies: The medical emergency response plan for schools. A statement for healthcare providers, policymakers, school administrators, and community leaders. *Pediatrics, 113*(1), 155–168. https://doi.org/10.1542/peds.113.1.155

Willgerodt, M. A., & Yonkaitis, C. (2021). School nurses: Keeping children, families, and communities. *American Nurse Journal, 16*(2), 44–47. https://doi.org/10.1177/1059840517752456

Evaluation of a Policy Change for Discontinuation of Contact Precautions for Endemic Methicillin-Resistant *Staphylococcus aureus* and Vancomycin-Resistant *Enterococcus*

Carolyn Thomas Jones

Review the study by Schrank et al. (2020) that evaluated the impact of an evidence-based policy in 2016 to discontinue contact precautions for endemic methicillin-resistant *Staphylococcus aureus* (MRSA) and vancomycin-resistant *Enterococcus* (VRE).

Using a retrospective, quasi-experimental design, the study team sought to determine the true impact of the policy change in terms of hospital savings, patient satisfaction, wait times, and patient adverse events. The policy change was evidence based, but the impact of the new policy had not been measured for effectiveness and quality improvement and there were mixed results from other published studies prompting local study.

Nursing Implications: Approximately 15% of hospitalized patients with MRSA or VRE are in contact precautions. Active MRSA and VRE infections are serious bacterial infections that are resistant to multiple antibiotics, are contagious nosocomial infections, and require lengthy treatments and contact precautions. However, prior hospital policies required contact precautions for all patients with a history of MRSA or VRA, even when they are simply colonized. Being colonized with MRSA or VRE means that patients have no signs or symptoms of infection, but the bacteria can be detected. Those patients do not have active infection. Hospital policies differ on the use of contact precautions inclusive of colonized patients.

Issues to Explore: After reading the published case (Schank et al., 2020), consider the following:

1. What was the defined study period?
2. Which nursing units were evaluated and excluded?
3. Is this an accurate assessment?
   Impact was measured by blocked beds, occupancy, lost hospital revenue, ED admission wait times, gown and glove expenditures, patient satisfaction, time series analyses, nosocomial MRSA and VRE rates, patient falls, and nosocomial pressure ulcers.
4. Why were patient safety issues (falls, pressure ulcers) included?
5. Were there differences in MRSA and VRE nosocomial rates before or after policy activation?
6. What was the overall hospital cost savings using the policy?
7. Should the hospital sustain the new policy guidelines or modify them?

Using Tools to Meet Patient Needs

Carolyn Thomas Jones

Review a study published by Cianetti et al. (2020) entitled "Oral Health Knowledge Level of Nursing Staff Working in Semi-Intensive Heart Failure Units."

Nursing Implications: Intensive care nursing is fraught with daily challenges in addressing the clinical needs of patients with high acuity and managing diagnostic, pharmaceutical, and technological elements of care. Often lacking is attention to the basic oral care needs of patients. Consider the impact of poor oral hygiene in critically ill populations and preventable morbidity outcomes.

Issues to Explore:

1. What poor oral health disease risks were identified in the published article?
2. What was the evidence base for exploring ICU nurses' patient oral health practices?
3. Discover the tools used to measure attitudes and educational needs.
4. What might be the next steps in project planning and management based on the findings of this small needs assessment?

Using a Mixed-Methods Approach to Assess Chronic Disease Needs in Low-Resource Countries

Carolyn Thomas Jones

The WHO (2001, p. 1) defines community health needs assessment as a process that "describes the state of health of local people; enables the identification of major risk factors and causes of ill health; and enables the identification of actions needed to address these." Studies of chronic disease epidemiology and practices in low-resource countries are limited. To provide care in these settings requires an understanding of disease rates and the facilitators of and barriers to appropriate management and patient healthcare educational needs. Effecting change in these settings requires a stakeholder approach to best identify future healthcare and research needs.

Exemplar Issues

Review a published study by Dekker et al. (2017) that used a mixed-methods approach to determine chronic disease care gaps for diabetes mellitus and hypertension among rural populations in the district of Toledo, Belize.

1. How did this study use a stakeholder approach to identifying gaps?
2. Characterize the healthcare system and patient population under study.
3. The study used a mixed-methods approach. What were the multitiered levels of assessment in this study? Which were quantitative and which were qualitative?
4. What gaps were identified that could lead to future research and care?
5. Generate a research question that might evolve from these study results.
6. Compare and contrast this study and other needs assessments performed in low-resource countries for chronic disease management and resources.

References

Cianetti, S., Anderini, P., Pagano, S., Eusebi, P., Orso, M., Salvato, R., & Lombardo, G. (2020, February 12). Oral health knowledge level of nursing staff working in semi-intensive heart failure units. *Journal of Multidisciplinary Healthcare*, 13, 165–173. https://doi.org/10.2147/JMDH.S224453. PMID: 32103976; PMCID: PMC7024767.

Dekker, A. M., Amick, A. E., Scholcoff, C., & Doobay-Persaud, A. (2017). A mixed method needs assessment of adult diabetes mellitus (type II) and hypertension care in Toledo, Belize. *BMC Health Services Research*, 17(1), 171. https://doi.org.proxy.lib.ohio-state.edu/10.1186/s12913-017-2075-9

Schrank, G. M., Snyder, G. M., Davis, R. B., Branch-Elliman, W., & Wright, S. B. (2020). The discontinuation of contact precautions for methicillin-resistant *Staphylococcus aureus* and vancomycin-resistant *Enterococcus*: Impact upon patient adverse events and hospital operations. *BMJ Quality & Safety*, 29(10), 1–2. https://doi.org/10.1136/bmjqs-2018-008926. Epub 2019 Jul 18. PMID: 31320496.

World Health Organization. (2001). *Community health needs assessment: An introductory guide for the family health nurse in Europe*. http://www.euro.who.int/__data/assets/pdf_file/0018/102249/E73494.pdf

Using Findings from Organizational Analysis and Clinical Needs Assessment to Frame Improvement Projects and Implementation

Linda Roussel
Shea Polancich

CHAPTER OBJECTIVES

1. Describe the steps in using a clinical needs assessment for building the case for value-based projects and their management.
2. Delineate how findings from a rigorous organizational analysis support project planning and management.
3. Describe the life cycle of a project plan.
4. Identify the anticipated project risks and methods for addressing these risks.
5. Analyze the value and pitfalls of various tools, surveys, methods, measures, and strategies used in developing sustainable projects and within clinical microsystems, mesosystems, and macrosystems.
6. Identify leverage and capacity and explain their relationship in maintaining project and program efficacy.
7. Describe the stakeholders' role in clinical projects and strategies for their engagement throughout the project life cycle.

KEY TERMS

Agility   Metrics
Evidence

ROLES

Decision-maker   Leader
Implementation project manager   Risk anticipator

PROFESSIONAL VALUES

Accountability   Evidence-based
Commitment

CORE COMPETENCIES

Assessment   Management
Leadership

Introduction

Developing, implementing, and managing a project can be a challenging experience, from moving the original idea to planning, carrying out the project, studying the results, and acting on outcomes. Simply stated, these steps put the planned work into an actionable framework. The importance of project management is underscored by the research conducted by the Project Management Institute (PMI), which has conducted a global survey of project management practitioners since 2006. The PMI's survey, *Pulse of the Profession*, charts the major trends for project management now and in the future. The *Pulse* provides original market research that reports feedback and insights from project, program, and portfolio managers, along with an analysis of third-party data. The survey represents feedback and insights from 3,234 professionals globally at different levels within organizations from diverse industries (PMI, 2020).

The 2020 *Pulse of the Profession* research noted a positive change in the methods organizations are employing to manage projects and programs. Specifically, the *Pulse* reported that for the first time in 5 years, more projects were completed within budget and were on target for original goals and business intent. Also, important to project planning and management, the *Pulse* described a significant decline in dollars lost. That is, organizations were wasting an average of $97 million for every $1 billion invested, because of poor project performance—a 20% decline from 2019 (PMI, 2020). The survey results also revealed an average 11.4% of investment was wasted because of poor project performance. Additionally, organizations that considered project management as a low priority and not a strategic competency for driving change reported an average of 67% more of their projects failing (PMI, 2020).

The 2020 *Pulse* described a new way of doing business, reporting that organizational leaders face complex issues that require rethinking the nature of work as well as the strategies needed to accomplish the tasks at hand. Executive leaders delineated factors they considered to be of importance in achieving successful outcomes in the future. The top three factors were organizational agility (35%), choosing the right technologies to invest in (32%), and securing relevant skills (31%) (PMI, 2020). Other noteworthy findings revealed that actively engaged executive sponsors remained a top driver for projects in meeting their original goals. That fact did not go unrecognized by survey respondents, who revealed an increase in the percentage of their organizations' projects with actively engaged sponsors compared with 2019—an average of 62% compared with 59%, respectively. The PMI noted that the percentage of organizations providing training and development have been stable for the period of 2015 to 2020. Three in five organizations support training on project management tools and techniques; under half have a formal process to develop project manager competency and a tailored career path for project managers. Organizations that are considered champions prioritize development of technical skills (76% vs. 19% of underperformers), leadership skills (76% vs. 16% of underperformers), and strategic and business management skills (65% vs. 14% of underperformers) (PMI, 2020).

Through their 2020 research, PMI noted that organizations are on a quest for ways to be more agile, customer focused, and competitive. Specifically, a large majority of organizations described greater agility over the period from 2015 to 2020. More than half of the organizations ascribe this improvement to significant change factors, including innovation, leadership, and shifting customer demands. Nearly half of the organizations also credited their greater agility to enhanced skills and experience of project managers (PMI, 2020). Delineating and fine-tuning skills needed to plan and manage projects are value-added strategies that are worth the time, effort, and resources necessary to achieve organizational goals to meet the mission.

Understanding how to use a value equation and value proposition statement is essential to any possible success. Without a deep dive into understanding the organization's overall mission and goal, a project may squander resources, deliver poor financial returns, create substandard operating processes, compromise products and services to patients, and reduce stakeholders' returns. Despite improved project management methodologies, software development methodologies, and training in those methodologies, there has not been an appreciable increase in the success rate for project implementation over the past 20 years (Phelan & Stockwell, 2014).

The importance of using findings from a needs assessment to inform the developing, planning, and implementing phases of a project cannot be understated. The role of the implementation project manager is essential to this accomplishment, particularly from an interprofessional, collaborative perspective. When managing projects, it is important to have a leader who possesses strong communication skills, is results oriented, understands organizational dynamics, and is committed to the system's values. A close and mutually reinforcing (supportive) relationship exists between developing, planning, implementing, and monitoring. This chapter discusses the value of understanding the organization, collaboration in a project's life cycle, and the role of the implementation project manager. A description of a systems change model is provided as an example that can assist readers in answering key questions that support project implementation and sustainability in practice settings.

Organizational Analysis: Deep Dive to Determine Needs

A thorough understanding of the organizational system and its performance are foundational to completing a needs assessment and developing strategic initiatives to address gaps in executing the mission and vision of the system. An organizational analysis is the cornerstone to project planning, development, and analysis. Tools that guide assessment of the healthcare system are useful in collecting data (qualitative, quantitative) and provide ways to think through analysis and evaluation. One such resource is the Baldrige Excellence Builder, which provides key questions to assess organizational performance (Baldrige Excellence Builder, 2019–2020). The Baldrige Excellence Builder, along with the Baldrige Excellence Framework, are built on core values and concepts including a systems perspective, visionary leadership, customer-focused excellence, valuing people, organizational learning, and agility, focusing on success, managing for innovation, management by facts, societal contributions, ethics, and transparency, as well as delivering value and results. For each of the key concepts, questions are posed that the team can explore for a deeper understanding of structure, leadership, strategy development, culture, and communication (Baldrige Excellence Builder, 2019–2020).

The Baldrige Excellence Builder includes questions on essential qualities of organizational excellence, starting with a full organizational profile. For example, organizational learning incorporates both continuous improvement of existing approaches and any change or innovation leading to new or revised goals, approaches, products, and markets. Organizational learning must be agile, which is the capacity for rapid change and flexibility in operations. Another example, ethics and transparency, focuses on ethical behavior by the workforce in all stakeholder transactions and interactions. This core concept would also require organizational leaders to serve as role models of ethical behavior, to include transparency, illustrated by frank and open communication of leadership and management and exchanging accurate information. Key questions for discussion around ethics and transparency may include the following: How do leaders set their organization's vision and values? How do leaders' personal actions demonstrate their commitment to legal and ethical behavior? How do leaders initiate action-oriented behavior that seeks to address the organization's mission and value (Baldrige Excellence Builder, 2019–2020)?

Another example, management by fact, considers the significance of measuring and analyzing the organization's performance within the organization and its competition. Also, it is essential to think carefully about performance measures and indicators that reinforce organizational evaluation, alignment, and decision-making. This is key to how the organization measures, analyzes, and improves the system's performance. Probing questions to address measurement, analysis, and improvement of organization performance may include the following: describe how data and information are tracked on daily operations and overall organizational performance; identify how the organization selects comparative data and information (benchmarks) that support fact-based decision-making; realize how findings are used from performance reviews to determine priorities for improvement and opportunities for innovation; and note how the organization projects future performance and what this might mean for project planning (Baldrige Excellence Builder, 2019–2020). By asking questions, tracking, and analyzing data, team members can collaborate on best practices for project planning and development.

Organizational analysis also includes attention to the community and population-based care. The Centers for Disease Control and Prevention (CDC) delineates the benefits of a community needs assessment, which may include the following: better organizational and community coordination and collaboration, greater awareness of public health and the interconnectedness of activities, improved partnerships within and between state and local community health systems, recognition of strengths and weaknesses to target continuous quality improvement initiatives, and identifying benchmarks for public health practice improvements (CDC, n.d.).

The CDC describes overall steps and phases in community assessment and planning frameworks. These actions include the need to organize and plan for the assessment, engaging the community through focus groups, and community outreach to develop a vision, building on relationships to conduct a community health assessment to prioritize health issues. As needs are prioritized, the next steps include developing community health improvement plans, implementing and monitoring the plans, and lastly evaluating the processes and outcomes. Assessment and planning are both cornerstones to identifying relevant needs and issues and proceeding accordingly. Although there are similarities and overlapping actions, there are differences. For example, analysis tools may differ in the types of data; recommended sources; and specific indicators for each (quantitative, qualitative, primary, secondary) need or issue, the level of community engagement, the particular model (context) and length of time necessary to undertake the process, and whether the framework is broadly comprehensive or more focused directly on particular types of data and issues; for example, chronic disease, environmental health, poverty, crime, and similar issues (CDC, n.d.).

A deep understanding of organizational and community analysis involves the ability to compare information and data in such a way as to explain, analyze, and interpret what requires priority attention. Translation and application allow reflection and creation of best practices for overall project planning and management of relevant needs and issues.

Project Life Cycle: Role of the Clinical Needs Assessment

The project life cycle consists of four phases: initiation, planning, execution, and evaluation (Gido & Clements, 2015). In the *initiation* phase of the project life cycle, the scope, purpose, objectives, resources, deliverables, timescales, and structure of the project are defined. These definitions are guided by the results of a clinical needs assessment, which considers information (data) from a variety of sources. These data are quantified—for example, length of stay, cost of a day in the intensive care unit, and infection rates. Qualitative data obtained through interviews, focus groups, and observations can add further depth to the needs assessment. A microsystem analysis using the five P's (purpose, population, processes, patterns, and providers) is a helpful assessment tool for obtaining internal data related to the organization and the larger system. With a thorough microsystem analysis, gaps can be identified—for example, between benchmarks and actual infection and falls rates—and further drilled down through a root cause analysis (RCA) and a failure mode effects analysis (FMEA):

- RCA gets at the core of a complication or problem and considers all aspects of why a particular work process or patient care intervention has not worked as intended, perhaps leading to a fatal event. This type of analysis is generally done after the adverse event.

- FMEA is a proactive risk mitigation tool that identifies areas of potential failure and considers the severity and probability that a failure will occur. Hazard scores are then assigned based on the severity and frequency of the misstep (failed action) in the process.

RCA and FMEA are tools and processes that give the project team direction when considering the level of information needed to improve the overall process. Their results, which are considered internal data, are essential in determining the need to move forward to improve quality of work and care delivery. Internal data provide the necessary evidence and often baseline information for developing a business case, which often includes solutions and a cost–benefit analysis for each possible action for improvement. The feasibility of any one intervention (or a bundle of actions) should be thoroughly considered to ensure that the solution is realistic and has an acceptable level of risk. A project team is chartered to assure that all aspects of the initial plan (the business case) have been thoughtfully considered and to collectively step through the process to assure consensus and investment in the project plan's success (Gido & Clements, 2015).

The American Society for Quality (ASQ) provides robust tools to further advance the clinical needs assessment (ASQ, n.d.). For example, the cause analysis tool, also called the cause-and-effect diagram or Ishikawa diagram, can be useful when delineating possible causes for an effect or problem. It is a constructive tool when structuring a brainstorming session, which can serve to quickly sort ideas into meaningful categories. This tool can also be employed when a team's thinking is at a standstill and new perspectives are needed to stimulate innovative ideas and strategies. Another tool, the checklist, also called a defect concentration diagram, is a structured, prepared form for collecting and analyzing data. The checklist tool can be applicable when data can be observed and gathered repeatedly by the same person or at the same location. The team may consider the checklist when collecting data on the patterns of events, problems, defects, defect location, and defect causes. The checklist can also serve as a data collection tool from a production process perspective. ASQ provides a wide variety of resources, including templates that are beneficial for the project team to apply as they explore the needs and issues within the system for a greater clarity. The ASQ website also includes an excellent list of articles, books, and case studies (ASQ, n.d.).

Internal data collection can also include the use of a variety of assessment tools. For example, the Institute for Healthcare Improvement (IHI, 2017) provides an Improvement Capability Self-Assessment Tool created to help organizations in assessing their capability in six key areas that support improvement:

- Leadership for Improvement
- Results
- Resources
- Workforce and Human Resources
- Data Infrastructure and Management
- Improvement Knowledge and Competence

The tool describes levels of capability and is intended as a baseline indication of the improvement capability of a healthcare system in several domains associated with overall improvement success. The levels are Just Beginning, Developing, Making Progress, Significance Impact, and Exemplary. For example, Leadership for Improvement, at a Just Beginning level, might be described as leadership not co-ordinated across departments or services with very little, if any, learning from improvement activities shared across the healthcare system. This level could serve as a baseline when you begin this assessment. Moving from Just Beginning to Exemplary would indicate progress and an ongoing measure of improvement. The information on the tool can be confidential, and the more honest the assessment, the greater the opportunities that the initiatives selected will be aligned with current ability and probability of success. This tool can be used by hospital leaders and staff in a few ways, including stimulating discussion about areas of strength and weakness, to better understand current improvement capability, and to reflect on and evaluate specific improvement efforts (IHI, 2017).

Collecting internal data is important in the *planning* phase, which includes a detailed project plan created and monitored by the project manager and referred to throughout the life of the project. The monitoring aspect includes examining results such as costs and quality of expected outcomes. Aspects of the project plan include specific information on resources (staffing, equipment, supplies), finances (cost–benefit analysis, return on investment), quality (benchmarks, dashboard, key indicators for effective outcomes), risks (what could go wrong and how to mitigate or minimize such events), and deliverables (executive summary, manuscript, presentations). It is important to know what to expect to deliver before the team goes too far into implementing the plan (acting). Accountability for deliverables must be established early in the planning phase to assure that dissemination of results and sustainability are as important as implementing and evaluating the overall results (Gido & Clements, 2015).

Execution involves staying on task when implementing the action plan. The project manager and the team consider monitoring time (tracking and recording time spent on the various aspects of the plan), cost (under/over budget), quality (indicators, outcomes), change (was there enough preparation in readying the environment for the change?), risks (were strategies taken to minimize risk and eliminate barriers?), buy-in (is there acceptance of the intervention strategies taken?), and communication (does information flow freely; is there transparency in how the project is going?). A communication plan is important to ensuring that all stakeholders are kept apprised of the actions taken, any complications or risks mitigated, and success (or failure) in realizing the expected outcomes. Sharing this information is essential to the success of the project and to future dissemination of its learnings, extension of its scope, and sustainability (Gido & Clements, 2015).

Evaluation involves reviewing overall project outcomes, performance of the project team, and stakeholder involvement. Did the project deliver the benefits, meet the objectives, produce the deliverables on time and within budget, and use resources wisely? Did the action plan follow the expected pathway (management processes)? Was the project team able to determine key project achievements, failures, and lessons learned to inform future direction? Referring to the initiation and planning phases, the project team considers how the project performed relative to the description in the business case, objectives (outcomes), quality targets, timelines, budget, and resources. Did the internal and external (research) evidence used to support the interventions (action) work as anticipated? How does this contribute to the larger system? What are the implications for spread and dissemination?

Within the overall summary (executive summary), key elements to include are the major achievements (positive effects/benefits), failures (what did not go as planned), and lessons learned and recommendations (next steps). A successful project management plan and model can inform future projects, serving as a guide (template) for ongoing deliberate work of the project team (Gido & Clements, 2015). Cost–benefit strategies are important to long-term gains and sustainability.

Planning for Implementation

A successful implementation begins with the creation of an executable work plan. The implementation project manager is responsible for crafting the details of this plan—an activity that includes defining goals, objectives, and strategies; developing a timeline; establishing project milestones; and matching project tasks with resources. During the planning process, it is also important to consider overall aims, goals, outcomes, costs, and budgets simultaneously.

Developing a Project Charter

Developing a written charter is one method of providing clarity regarding the goals, objectives, and timelines for a project plan. In addition, a charter is a key aspect of improvement in that it establishes the written plan for an improvement intervention and defines the small test-of-change methods that will be used. In health care and specific to improvement teams, the elements of the charter provide the framework or scaffold for the project plan and the improvement team that will be responsible for initiating the plan (Richter & Scudder, 2014).

To create a functional written charter, the first step is to form an interprofessional team whose members will work together cohesively to meet the improvement plan or project goals. A team is formed based on the needs of the project to be completed. The skills of the members selected are those necessary to provide insight into the most efficient and effective methods to meet the project goals.

The team's initial composition may be expanded over time as the project goals and objectives are fleshed out and if additional representation is deemed necessary. However, it is essential that those persons involved in the work be the individuals most directly affected by the work to be accomplished as well as those who have the authority and responsibility to effect change.

Once a team is formed, the members of the group operationally define all aspects of the project plan and establish the written charter. A written charter may be developed using an established template that provides a "checklist" of all essential elements for developing, implementing, and evaluating an intervention or improvement project (Richter & Scudder, 2014). Key elements of a written charter may include items such as a project title that clearly articulates the context of the project, dates of project initiation and completion, a listing of team members who will participate in the project, and executive sponsors and team leaders to address the "demographics" of the project. Other sections of the charter may include, but are not limited to, a methodological framework for completing the project; a section providing data and operational definitions for metrics used; a section on literature appraisal and synthesis for concepts relevant to the topic and the interventions envisioned; a section for process mapping and any other analyses performed to provide context or direction for the project (e.g., analyses such as policy assessments and strengths, weaknesses, opportunities, and threats [SWOT] assessments); and a defined project plan with numbered "steps," resources needed, timelines (for initiation and completion of steps), assigned accountabilities, interventions, and evaluations for the steps and the overall plan. Additional items that are relevant to the charter may include items such as evaluation and recommendation sections as well as a plan for dissemination and sustainability of improvements or interventions.

In summary, the charter should clearly articulate the goals and objectives of the defined improvement effort or project. With a written, clear, well-defined charter, there is less room for ambiguity of goals and interpretation errors of the project plan. Moreover, a clearly defined charter assists in decreasing project scope creep. Therefore, it is recommended that a written charter be clearly defined using some degree of standardization and consistency of elements (Richter & Scudder, 2014).

Model for Improvement

One methodological framework that may be used in project planning and as the underpinnings of the written charter is the Model for Improvement (MFI; Langley et al., 2009). The MFI provides a strong foundation and plan for any improvement effort or intervention. Using the three guiding questions of the MFI may assist the project team in clearly articulating the goals, aims, and/or objectives of the project:

1. What am I trying to accomplish?
2. How will I know a change is an improvement?
3. Which changes can I implement that will result in an improvement?

These three questions provide clarity of purpose and form the central components for a project plan (Langley et al., 2009).

The initial guiding question is central to providing the goal of the project. What is the overall goal or objective that the group should work toward? Sometimes answering this question is more difficult than one would imagine. Indeed, projects that are broad in scope may have many smaller subprojects that need to be completed before a goal representing a broader perspective may be accomplished. The reverse may also occur. A smaller project may mushroom into one with a broader, more global view of, or perspective on, a process. For example, a team may form to understand the transfer of a patient with a pain pump through a hospital, but upon better understanding the elements of the project, the goal may change to become standardizing "pain management processes" throughout a facility. Clearly defining the goal is central to developing a project plan that will meet that goal.

The second question of the MFI provides the evaluation criteria for the improvement efforts or intervention that is being implemented and tested. It is necessary to provide an analytical assessment of an improvement effort to demonstrate measurable results. Defined, measurable criteria are articulated by operationally defining the metrics that will be used to achieve baseline measurements and postintervention or postimplementation measurements. Operational definitions are necessary to clearly define a numerical measure, as well as the tools or methods used to perform that measurement. For example, when defining a rate for "patient falls," it is necessary to define the term *fall* as well as how the rate will be measured. What are the numerator and the denominator for the rate, and are there specific inclusion and exclusion criteria that should be used? Evaluation of an improvement will guide the process of either disseminating the intervention established or changing the plan and revising the implementation if the goals and objectives set for the improvement are not met (Langley et al., 2009).

The final question in the MFI seeks to define the intervention that will be used to improve the process being evaluated. In this step, the team envisions a change that will lead to an improvement in the outcome defined by the measure or evaluation in the second guiding question. For example, if the team intended to improve the patient fall rate, then an intervention specific to falls would be developed. This may include processes such as developing and implementing a more accurate, evidence-based "falls risk assessment" tool on a nursing unit. The intervention is first defined and operationalized and then implemented and evaluated (Langley et al., 2009).

The three guiding questions of the MFI "set the stage" or provide the foundation for "testing" change that may lead to improving a process. Small tests of change are often accomplished with a plan–do–study–act (PDSA) cycle. The PDSA cycle is the engine for change that one would use to *plan* an improvement effort; *do,* or implement the plan; *study* the results of the implemented plan; and *act* upon the results by either disseminating the project or changing the plan and repeating in an iterative fashion. Small test-of-change, PDSA cycles are a method for testing improvement interventions in a systematic and focused manner.

Use of the MFI and PDSA approach may provide standardization of improvement efforts within a project plan and should be included in the written charter. The articulation and definition of these elements provide clarity for project efforts and may assist in focusing a project or improvement team on the project goals and objectives (Langley et al., 2009).

The project manager leads the team in conducting a SWOT analysis, in which the team identifies strengths and weaknesses (internal forces) as well as opportunities and threats (external forces). The strengths and opportunities are positive forces that can be exploited to efficiently implement a project. Weaknesses and threats may hamper project implementation if they are not considered regarding the overall aims and context of the project. Many organizations simultaneously conduct a needs assessment and a SWOT analysis and then compare findings. The needs assessment focuses on a summary of the following areas:

- Descriptions of the qualitative and quantitative data that support the need for the project
- The costs, resources, stakeholder buy-in, and work requirements necessary for a successful and meaningful project outcome before implementation
- Determination of whether needs are strategically aligned with the organization's mission and overall goals

The information gleaned from the needs assessment is pivotal and requires comprehensive consideration before planning and implementing a project. In this step, the role of the implementation project manager transitions into that of risk anticipator, assisting project stakeholders in devising a strategy means of overcoming potential barriers. It is best to begin with the end in mind. That is, what is the expectation for quality outcomes when undertaking a project initiative? Lighter (2011), for example, identified the need for stakeholders to consider the value proposition when implementing a project. More specifically, he proposed the following formula to calculate value:

$$\text{Value} = \text{quality/cost}$$

According to Skor (2013), establishing a substantive value proposition is critical to successful companies and projects undertaken to meet operational goals. This step starts the journey from the inception of an idea to completion of the project. Skor defines a value proposition as a positioning statement that outlines the benefits provided for the agent or company and explains how those benefits uniquely address the need. The target market, the problem to be solved, and why this solution is better than the alternatives are other information included in a well-stated value proposition. The creation of a compelling value proposition includes four steps: (1) defining, (2) evaluating, (3) measuring, and (4) building.

In the *defining* step, the team provides the information that determines if the problem is worth solving. Skor (2013) describes the four U's as being significant to defining the value proposition. If the answers are "yes" to most of these questions, it is likely that the project planners are moving in the right direction toward a compelling value proposition:

1. *Is the concern Unworkable?* If there were inaction regarding a real problem, perhaps someone gets fired without addressing the issue, or you lose a major customer, this would likely direct the need to finding a solution. For example, the person who may be fired would likely be an excellent internal champion of the project.
2. *Is fixing the problem Unavoidable?* If regulatory or accreditation issues are on the table, that factor drives fundamental requirements for compliance and accountability issues. Answering "yes" to this question would likely identify the group that should serve as a champion for the project.
3. *Is the concern Urgent?* Is this concern a top priority to the system? Without attention to the issue, would you likely lose market share or other major resources? If the answer is "yes," the corporate suite's attention will likely be drawn to the concern.
4. *Is the problem Underserved?* If there appears to be no (or limited) solution to the problem you want to address, you may be identifying a segment of the market (or white space) that would increase your organization's value. If you answer "yes" to this question, then your company may be primed to increase its market share.

Another tool that Skor (2013) recommends is qualifying the problem as "BLAC and White." BLAC is an acronym standing for Blatant, Latent, Aspirational, and Critical; White refers to the "white space" that the projects capitalize on as an opportunity for growth. Skor notes that concerns or problems that are blatant and critical are more likely to attract attention because they tend to stand in the way of doing business and are more acute than latent or aspirational problems. When a problem is latent, it is generally unacknowledged; aspirational problems are considered optional and are often the most difficult to consider in a fast-paced, frenetic market.

The second step, *evaluating*, seeks to determine whether the solution is unique or compelling enough to continue the effort in the planning. Once the problem is defined as critical for pursuing, the team must identify what is unique and compelling about a solution to this problem. Skor (2013) offers a useful approach in the context of the three D's. The three D's provide a thoughtful approach to considering the unique combination of *D*iscontinuous innovation, *D*efensible technology, and a *D*isruptive business model that makes a solution compelling to the team and its target—a possibly skeptical market. A *discontinuous* innovation provides transformative benefits over the status quo by viewing the problem through different lenses. *Defensible* technology encompasses intellectual property that can be protected to develop a barrier to entry and an unfair competitive advantage. *Disruptive* business models can catalyze the growth of the venture by enabling its employees to understand the value and cost rewards. Although "faster, cheaper, and better" may also be a useful metric, evaluating the three D's can expand thinking about a potential breakthrough.

Skor's (2013) third step, *measure*, considers the gain/pain ratio of potential adoption of a solution to a problem. This ratio compares the gain that the solution will deliver to the target market versus the pain and cost required for the solution's adoption. Skor reports that he looks for nondisruptive innovations—that is, those technologies that offer game-changing benefits yet require only minimal modifications to current processes and systems. Nondisruptive introduction is essential to new projects because the gains they deliver will be discounted by the risks associated with altering the current system. A successful venture delivers an order-of-magnitude improvement over the status quo. According to Skor, if you are not able to deliver a 10-fold gain/pain promise, stakeholders and the target market will typically default to "do nothing" rather than bearing the risk of working with you. To overcome this reluctance to change, you will need to assure that your innovation is measurable to a degree that change is notable.

Skor's (2013) final step, *build*, involves moving from defining, evaluating, and measuring to creating the value proposition. Skor recommends the following framework for the *building* step:

1. Who are your stakeholders? Your target customers?
2. Who and what are dissatisfied with your current performance?
3. What will this new strategy (product) be?
4. What will be provided? What provides key problem-solving capability?
5. What is unlike your product? What is the product (intervention) alternative?

According to Skor (2013), the most important consideration is the individual (*you*) that creates the value proposition and carries out the strategies. You, the project planner, are core to *your* value proposition. How do *you* understand and deliver uniquely? Which kind of disruptive business model can *you* bring? Skor describes being true to *yourself* as a thought leader to ensure that *you* will go far.

Inherent in the planning process is the development of an implementation strategy. The implementation strategy is meant to focus on the process from a stakeholder perspective and should be approved before execution. The most common implementation strategy is the phased approach for a project (Glaser, 2009). This approach is relatively safe for the organization because it allows the project team members to reassess their progress after each project phase is operationalized. For example, in a project to reduce catheter-acquired urinary tract infections (CAUTIs), phases may include determination of the extent of the problem, use of data to drive the urgency to act (magnitude of the problem), outcomes to be measured, implementation strategies, and evaluation protocols.

A key document in the implementation phase is the project charter. The project charter is an agreement between the organization providing the service and the stakeholder requesting the service and receiving the deliverables (Lewis, 2005).

It includes a comprehensive description of the project, a list of anticipated project team members, and those members' specific roles and responsibilities in the project. Also included in the charter is the level of authority for the project manager and the project outcomes. The project charter outlines the scope and measures of success and includes formal signatures for project authorization and approval. This process is critical to building consensus on project goals and documents communication between project stakeholders.

For example, a project aimed at reducing CAUTIs on an acute surgical unit might involve the clinical nurse leader (CNL), the infection control nurse, a patient representative, and staff nurses. The CNL may take the lead as project manager, outlining roles of each member (e.g., observing how patients' urinary catheters are handled during transport, monitoring the number of catheters inserted and discontinued). Tasks related to setting up communication channels, meeting times, and reviewing tools may also be established and delegated by the CNL. Although other team members are intimately involved in the implementation of the project and have an active voice in all project-related measures, the CNL is the project manager, but they cannot and should not be expected to produce the project outcomes alone.

Another phase of the project implementation may revolve around the action plan (based on the best available evidence) that delineates strategies. The action plan includes the following elements:

- How evidence-based interventions will be used to improve the system (system change) and practice
- The *how* to accomplish the stated purpose
- The collaboration and teamwork required to implement the project, its sustainability, and its relevance to an existing program or mission
- Information flow processes (informatics and technology)
- Interventions that will focus on educating others about the project and means by which the information provided will guide stakeholders throughout the implementation phase and result in the stated project goal/aim
- Descriptions of the theoretical or conceptual underpinnings and their relevance to the overall project and program mission
- How organizational and cultural dynamics will be addressed
- Anticipated impacts that the project will have and explanation of how findings will close gaps identified by the SWOT analysis and needs assessment
- Time-specific milestones

An evaluation phase to measure the success of actions taken is important to determine the efficacy of the plan. An evaluation plan includes the following elements:

- Methods and metrics for evaluating the project
- Timelines and data milestones
- Measurement types that include structure, process, and outcome
- Metrics that gather evidence relevant to stakeholders and the system, are scientifically sound, and are associated with processes that can be modified through reasonable methods and procedures
- Lessons learned, barriers that were overcome during the implementation phase, and strategies used to overcome the barriers that could further inform the project

Micro-, Meso-, and Macro-Collaboration

Collaboration across organizational stakeholders requires communication, commitment, accountability, and continuity (McElmurry et al., 2009). To ensure that a new initiative is realized to its full potential, stakeholders must see the strategic alignment. Administrative support for a project may enhance successful implementation and sustainability. For example, a project for reducing CAUTIs aimed at reducing patients' discomfort and costs of care serves to advance the mission of the organization. It addresses the overall mission of quality—that is, safe care. The implementation project manager translates to stakeholders how existing business processes would be improved with project implementation. Project stakeholders (project sponsors, decision-makers, and leaders) in a healthcare organization publicly endorsing the project may underscore the importance of the project's purpose.

In terms of the implementation of a project, collaboration with stakeholders is priceless. It is important to involve organizational stakeholders from the beginning, perform intermittent progress checks, be responsive to concerns, and address risks throughout implementation. At the point of implementation, the project manager ensures resource needs are clear and project risks are reviewed and validated. Stakeholder expectations must be managed during implementation through continued focus on the strategic goals of the project (McElmurry et al., 2009). Structure, process, and outcome indicators are continually evaluated to assure that resources are being used efficiently and effectively. Meetings to share progress and lessons learned—for example, actual reductions in CAUTI rates—will further enhance the credibility of the project team's work.

Communicate, Communicate, and Communicate

In addition to planning and collaboration, the other fundamental element of implementation is communication. The purpose of communications management is to share the right information, at the right time, with the right people, and in the right format. Good communications management requires expending effort on sharing information, which contributes to project success; conversely, lack of information can lead to failure. Most importantly, the project manager must identify the correct target audience for different categories of communications.

Strong communication must be accompanied by mutual trust. Both formal and informal methods can be used to disseminate information. Formal communication methods follow well-defined, systematic procedures, whereas informal communications are casual and more extemporaneous. Weekly status reports containing information about progress and issues are examples of a formal communication tool. Examples of informal communication include voice mail, email, and text messages. An effective and perhaps an efficient method of conveying information within a team is face-to-face conversation.

The implementation plan should be circulated to all stakeholders involved in the project. The implementation project manager must communicate continually to reinforce the messages related to that plan and make sure everyone is ready when implementation begins.

The management of communication is implemented through three essential processes:

- *Identification:* The process of identifying information to be shared, when it should be distributed, who should receive it, and how it should be prepared.
- *Reporting:* The process of collecting and preparing the information.
- *Distribution:* The process of disseminating the information and, for formal communications, storing the information in the project archive.

Change Management

Change management is possibly the most important factor in the implementation process. For example, when a healthcare organization is adopting a new clinical or financial information system, its business processes will undergo significant changes, so there will be a definite learning curve. The change process must be actively managed. Change management may be led by someone external to the organization, possibly a consultant, and begins at the same time as implementation. The individual or group of individuals charged with handling this task should collaborate with the implementation project manager and project stakeholders to craft a change management blueprint tailored for the organization.

An effective change management technique is for one department to test the new approach before it is rolled out more broadly. In other words, rather than a big-bang start, it is often more productive to begin with one unit or department trying out the project initiative. A staged approach allows the implementation project manager and stakeholders to monitor the initiative at work on a small scale and react to any resulting issues. This steady progression generates confidence and understanding throughout the organization, building buy-in for the project. This gradual process of integration can be replicated with employees as well. They are encouraged to start off slowly and build their knowledge and confidence related to the project initiative.

Faculty members from the University of South Alabama College of Nursing developed a model that visually illustrates the intersecting aspects of a system change project that can assist organizations and students when planning and implementing a project (**Figure 6-1**). Questions are posed for each intersecting aspect that can guide the implementation of the system change project. The intersecting aspects and accompanying questions are presented here.

Evidence-Based Practice: Incorporates Institute of Medicine (IOM) Aims, Models, Levels, Guidelines, and Critical Appraisal

- Is there a model or framework of how evidence is managed?
- Are level(s) identified?
- Is there a critical appraisal mechanism?

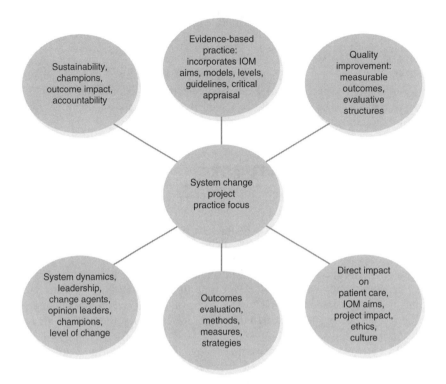

Figure 6-1 System Change Project Intersecting Aspects

Quality Improvement: Measurable Outcomes and Evaluative Structures

- Is a model/framework plan in place?
- What is the quality improvement process?

Direct Impact on Patient Care, IOM Aims, Project Impact, Ethics, and Culture

- Are the aims clearly defined?
- What is the direct impact on patient care?

Outcomes Evaluation, Methods, Measures, and Strategies

- Are outcomes defined?
- Are measures to be evaluated identified?
- Are methods to evaluate outcomes defined?

System Dynamics, Leadership, Change Agents, Opinion Leaders, Champions, and Level of Change

- Is there a conceptual/theoretical framework identified?
- Is it integrated into the project plan?
- Which system(s) are to be changed?
- Who are the change agents? Opinion leaders? Change champions?
- Is this an incremental change? Transformational change? How do you know?

Sustainability, Champions, Outcome Impact, and Accountability

- Do long-term plans exist?
- Which plans are in place to maintain sustainability?

Resistance to Change Is a Reality—Embrace It

Training and education play an important role in overcoming resistance in the adoption of new organizational initiatives. Research has revealed that adult learners have the capability to grasp new information early in the implementation phase of a project (Bond, 2006). The implementation project manager must collaborate with educational resources within the organization to develop training materials in the planning process of this project. Equally important is the support of decision-makers and leadership in providing these resources to support project efforts.

Post-Project Monitoring and Evaluation

Projects should be continuously evaluated for quality and appropriateness. Adjustments can then be made at the time of discovery, instead of waiting until the end of the project's implementation (Kitzmiller et al., 2006). With such an approach, the project may have more minor, smaller adjustments instead of larger, costlier swings in project scope and direction.

Postimplementation reviews can be conducted to identify value achievement progress and the steps still needed to achieve maximum gain. It is extremely rare for healthcare organizations to revisit their investments to determine whether promised value was achieved (Glaser, 2009). Some organizations believe that once the implementation is over and the change settles in, value will automatically be achieved (Glaser, 2009). It is wise for healthcare organizations to conduct reviews of projects periodically to evaluate progress.

Postimplementation reviews support the achievement of value by signaling leadership interest in ensuring the delivery of results, identifying the steps to ensure value, and reinforcing accountability for results. The reviews also answer questions such as the following:

- Which goals were expected to be met at the time the project was approved?
- How close has the organization come to achieving those project goals?
- How much has the organization invested in the project, and how does it compare with the original budget?
- If the organization had to implement the project again, what would it do differently?

Monitoring is an important component of the implementation phase to ensure that the project is implemented per the schedule. It is a continuous process that should be put in place before project implementation starts. Monitoring activities should be executed by all individuals and institutions that have an interest (stakeholders) in the project. To efficiently implement a project, the people planning and implementing it should plan for all the interrelated stages from the beginning. Metrics are also important to ensure that activities are implemented as planned. They help the implementation project manager measure how well project milestones and goals are being achieved. As such, the monitoring activities should appear on the work plan and should involve all stakeholders. If project activities are not going well, arrangements should be made to identify the problems as early as possible so that they can be corrected.

Organizations should benchmark their performance in achieving value against the performance of similar organizations (Glaser, 2009). These benchmarks may focus on process performance, using data to inform activities ranging from resource allocation to instructional practice. Stakeholders, especially project sponsors, should understand the accountability they have for the successful completion of the project. There should be an agreed-upon set of metrics that will be used to track value delivery. These metrics should complement the metrics used to evaluate project implementation.

Project Implementation Challenges and Risks

Project implementation can be improved by asking a series of questions, including seeking to know the activities that produce expected project outputs, inquiring about the sequencing and time frames for the planned activities, and determining who will be responsible for carrying out each activity. Several tools can be used to monitor these activities such as a Gantt chart, Critical Path Method (CPM) or Network analysis, and Project Evaluation and Review Techniques (PERT). For example, the Gantt chart is also referred to as the progress chart showing the timing of project activities using horizontal bars. The Gantt chart is one of the techniques of project scheduling that illustrates the frequency of activities and outlines the period for implementation. Using a Gantt chart can assist with determining the parts or implementation phases of the project, the sequencing of associated activities to be carried out, the estimated time required for each activity, and listing activities carried out at the same time and identifying those to be carried out sequentially. Constructing a Gantt chart involves a horizontal axis (time) and a vertical axis (activities). Specifically, bars are entered to determine the time designated for each activity and progression at any point in time (Bañuls et al., 2017).

Tools for implementation can facilitate successful projects. Other considerations for successful projects include political commitment, simplicity of design, careful preparation, good management, and involvement of beneficiaries/community. Conversely, factors and problems that lead to failure of projects may be financial problems, management problems, technical problems, and political problems. Other factors include poor scheduling of projects leading to delays in implementation, misallocation of funds, delay and sometimes lack of counterpart funding, lack of accountability and transparency, bureaucracy in decision-making, and selfishness/nepotism/favoritism by some project managers. Additional implementation problems may be weak monitoring systems, policy changes, migration of beneficiaries, lack of teamwork, and lack of incentives for implementers (Thompson & Cox, 2017).

Many potential challenges and risks may arise in the development, planning, and implementation of projects. Some of the common ones include funding and the management of stakeholders. If numerous stakeholders will be directly involved in the project, at least some political challenges will undoubtedly be encountered. Another frequent implementation challenge is the lack of communication among stakeholders, leadership, and the implementation project manager. Such miscommunication creates divergence in perceptions of critical initiatives that have great potential to benefit a healthcare organization, which in turn could lead to quality and safety risks.

Some common reasons for project implementation failure are poor communication with leadership and stakeholders, organizational resistance to change, scope creep, lack of project ownership and champion, and shifts in organizational priorities. It is important to consider leverage and capacity, describing their relationship in maintaining project and program efficacy. The recommended approach for achieving implementation success is the incorporation of agility into the project process (Kitzmiller et al., 2006). Agility is a concept that encourages flexibility, adaptation, and continuous learning as a part of the implementation process. The agility process accepts the complexity of a problem and addresses it through frequent inspection, responding with a flexible approach of constant adaptation (Kitzmiller et al., 2006). Agility considers the complexity of the problems faced in the current healthcare environment and enhances traditional implementation techniques.

Summary

- Implementation is the final process of moving the solution from development to production status.
- Successful implementation begins with an executable plan.
- SWOT analysis and needs assessment are critical to successful project implementation.
- Organizational and community assessments are essential to identifying the need to focus project planning and management.
- Project charters identify outcomes that can be tracked.
- Collaboration requires communication among and between all stakeholders.
- A system change project considers several aspects that impact practice outcomes.

Reflection Questions

1. What are two aspects of project planning that will ensure success? Compare them with situations in daily practice.
2. Which factors should be considered when dealing with external forces and barriers that can impede project implementation?
3. Consider a project that you have implemented. Which strengths, weaknesses, threats, and opportunities did you identify when implementing the project?

References

American Society for Quality. (n.d.). *The seven basic quality tools for process improvement.* https://asq
.org/quality-resources/seven-basic-quality-tools

Baldrige Excellence Builder. (2019–2020). *Key questions to improve your organization's performance.*
https://www.nist.gov/system/files/documents/2019/02/06/2019-2020-baldrige-excellence
-builder.pdf

Bañuls, V. A., López, C., Turoff, M., & Tejedor, F. (2017). Predicting the impact of multiple risks on
project performance: A scenario-based approach. *Project Management Journal, 48*(5), 95–114.
https://doi.org/10.1177%2F875697281704800507

Bond, G. E. (2006). Lessons learned from the implementation of web-based nursing intervention.
Computers in Nursing, 24(2), 66–74. https://doi.org/10.1097/00024665-200603000-00004

Centers for Disease Control and Prevention. (n.d.). *Community health assessments and health improvement plans.* https://www.cdc.gov/publichealthgateway/cha/plan.html

Gido, J., & Clements, J. P. (2015). *Successful project management* (6th ed.). Cengage Learning.

Glaser, J. (2009, July). Strategies for ensuring an IT project delivers value. *Healthcare Financial Management, 63*(7), 28–31. https://link.gale.com/apps/doc/A207643696/AONEu=anon~c940d87
f&rsid=googleScholar&xid=f9b21a84

Institute for Healthcare Improvement. (2017). *IHI Improvement Capability Self-Assessment Tool.*
http://www.ihi.org/resources/Pages/Tools/IHIImprovementCapabilitySelfAssessmentTool.aspx

Kitzmiller, R., Hunt, E., & Sproat, S. (2006). Adopting best practices: Agility moves from software
development to healthcare project management. *Computers in Nursing, 24*(2), 75–82. https://
doi.org/10.1097/00024665-200603000-00005

Langley, G. J., Moen, R. D., Nolan, K. M., Nolan, T. W., Norman, C. L., & Provost, L. P. (2009).
The improvement guide: A practical approach to enhancing organizational performance (2nd ed.).
Jossey-Bass.

Lewis, J. (2005). *Project planning, scheduling, and control.* McGraw-Hill.

Lighter, D. E. (2011). *Advanced performance improvement in health care.* Jones & Bartlett Learning.

McElmurry, B. J., McCreary, L. L., Park, C. G., Ramos, L., Martinez, E., Parikh, R., Kozik, K., &
Fogelfeld, L. (2009). Implementation, outcomes, and lessons learned from a collaborative pri-
mary health care program to improve diabetes care among urban Latino populations. *Health
Promotion Practice, 10*(2), 293–302. https://doi.org/10.1177/1524839907306406

Phelan, B., & Stockwell, C. (2014). Are your projects delivering business value? *Bright Hub
Project Management.* http://www.brighthubpm.com/project-planning/128738-are-your-projects
-delivering-business-value

Project Management Institute. (2020). Ahead of the curve: Forging a future-focused culture. *Pulse
of the Profession.* https://www.pmi.org/learning/library/forging-future-focused-culture-11908

Richter, L., & Scudder, R. (2014). What is a project charter? *Bright Hub Project Management.* http://
www.brighthubpm.com/project-planning/5161-what-is-a-project-charter

Roussel, L., & Dearman, C. (2009). *DNP project plan model.* Unpublished work documents in DNP
program development.

Skor, M. (2013, June 14). Four steps to building a compelling value proposition. *Forbes.* http://www
.forbes.com/sites/michaelskok/2013/06/14/4-steps-to-building-a-compelling-value-proposition

Thompson, S., & Cox, E. (2017). How coaching is used and understood by project managers in organizations. *Project Management Journal, 48*(5), 64–77. http://dx.doi.org/10.1177
/875697281704800505

Case Exemplar

Managing Patients with Diabetes Distress

Swapna Thomas

The burdensome chronic disease of diabetes mellitus causes a significant emotional impact called "diabetes distress" leading to poor outcomes in patients. The importance of identifying and managing diabetes distress is being increasingly recognized, and guidelines from agencies like the American Diabetes Association (ADA) recommend routine screening for diabetes distress using valid screening tools. A SWOT (Strengths, Weaknesses, Opportunities, and Threats) analysis was done to assess current practice, understand what will and will not work for the organization, and to identify the specific steps needed to be undertaken (MindTools, n.d.). In their article, Li et al. (2018) identified six interrelated organizational contextual features that influence the implementation of evidence-based practices within organizations; they are the culture of an organization, its leadership, communication and networks, available resources, evaluation systems, monitoring and feedback processes, and champions. Interventions to address the issue were also recommended, one of them being Cognitive Behavioral Therapy (CBT), which was found to be beneficial in managing diabetes distress in several studies. The project was designed to reduce diabetes distress and to improve outcomes in Type 2 Diabetes Mellitus (T2DM) using the framework of the health promotion model. The goal was to augment the comprehensive care of T2DM patients by the addition of the Problem Areas in Diabetes-5 (PAID-5) screening tool for diabetes distress, referral for and participation in CBT, and follow-up. The project employed multidisciplinary collaboration to deliver the intervention, and the feedback from the two-week follow-up call and the analysis of outcomes data indicated that the screening and intervention were beneficial. There was a significant reduction in diabetes distress and improvement in glycemic control in the patients. This project added to the knowledge base about the feasibility of screening and intervention in diabetes distress.

Reflection Questions

1. Describe the reasons why a SWOT analysis is important to developing a project idea, and identifying strategies for successful project implementation.
2. Select two of the six interrelated organizational contextual features that have influenced your own project planning, implementation, and evaluation.

References

American Diabetes Association. (2020). Standards of Medical Care in Diabetes—2020 abridged for primary care providers. *Clinical Diabetes, 38*(1), 10–38. https://doi.org/10.2337/cd20-as01

Li, S. A., Jeffs, L., Barwick, M., & Stevens, B. (2018). Organizational contextual features that influence the implementation of evidence-based practices across healthcare settings: A systematic integrative review. *Systematic reviews, 7*(1), 72. https://doi.org/10.1186/s13643-018-0734-5

Mind Tools. (n.d.). *SWOT analysis: How to develop a strategy for success.* https://www.mindtools.com/pages/article/newTMC_05.htm

Synthesizing, Leveling, and Assessing the Fidelity of Evidence in Support of Project Implementation and Proposed Interventions

Catherine Dearman
Lolita Chappel-Aiken

CHAPTER OBJECTIVES

1. Examine the process for synthesizing and leveling literature findings to form the basis for project implementation and evaluation.
2. Design a matrix to facilitate synthesis of literature and establish fidelity of evidence in support of improvement projects.
3. Use the synthesis matrix to seamlessly align the literature and evidence with project objectives.
4. Promote fidelity of evidence in support of improvement projects and proposed interventions.
5. Review levels of evidence to assure the highest levels are available to support the project.

KEY TERMS

Evidence
Fidelity
Levels of evidence
Organization and alignment

Project interventions
Synthesis matrix

ROLES

Faculty	Practitioner
Leader	Project leader
Manager	Reviewer

PROFESSIONAL VALUES

Ethics	Quality and safety
Evidence evaluation and grading	Synthesis, writing, and organization

CORE COMPETENCIES

Alignment	Fidelity of evidence
Analysis	Project evaluation
Design	Project implementation
Development	Synthesis

Introduction

Synthesizing, organizing, and sharing relevant literature that is aligned or can be aligned to your project objectives and implementation plan are essential components of translating evidence into practice and designing quality improvement projects. *Synthesis* is defined as "a process of combining ideas, concepts, and/or constructs to advance knowledge" (Synthesis, n.d.). Ultimately, the result of synthesis is the development of a new, higher level of knowledge regarding a subject of interest. The compelling attributes of synthesis are that it involves higher-order thinking skills and focuses on the production of something new and unique—something that has not occurred before—such as a quality improvement project. Individuals synthesize information on a daily basis. New parents review multiple daycare agencies, synthesize the evidence, and choose the best one for them and their child. Students synthesize information from peers and relevant sources to determine which professor's course they will take. Busy parents synthesize information about their work schedules and their children's activities so that they can assure they have constructed an appropriate plan to include all essential aspects. One may not have fully developed a synthesis writing skill set; continuing development, however, is integral to the combination of critical thinking and creative reasoning in the development of a unique project.

Assuring the fidelity of evidence is essential to the development of a high-quality improvement project that can drive decision-making and promote improved patient care. Fidelity of evidence includes assessing the level of the evidence, the relevance of the evidence to the project at hand, and the impact on implementation of the project. Each of these components will be discussed later in the chapter.

The skill of synthesis thinking and writing is essential to the development of new ideas and forms the basis of quality improvement projects such as those conducted by doctor of nursing practice (DNP), clinical nurse leader (CNL), and nurse executive students. Synthesis thinking and writing seek to address a gap in evidence or clinical practice and propose solutions to that gap (Hain & Kear, 2015).

The aspects of analyzing and categorizing evidence into relevant structures; the synthesis of available evidence into new, unique projects; and the alignment of the evidence to the project objectives/implementation plan will be discussed. Such evidence includes "best research evidence, clinical expertise, and values of the patient or subject" (Roberts, 2013, p. 5). Tools, guidelines, and techniques for categorizing and synthesizing evidence that aligns with your project will be presented.

Literature Synthesis and Establishing the Fidelity of Evidence

The primary aspect of literature synthesis begins with the supporting evidence. Writers must search for and critically appraise all available evidence in order to clearly identify what is known and not known about the topic, to establish a reliable knowledge base, and to highlight opportunities for the new project (Briner & Denyer, 2012). Leveling the evidence and establishing the fidelity of the evidence is foundational to synthesis. According to Glasgow et al. (2012), "translation of . . . evidence to . . . practice has been conceptualized as a linear process—a pipeline or roadmap which is slow and inconsistent" (p. 646). These authors propose a different way to conceptualize translation processes, an evidence integration triangle to align science with practice. Similarly, Kilbourne et al. (2007) proposed a replicating-effective-programs framework to facilitate the implementation of evidence-based interventions proposed through research or quality improvement projects. All of these mechanisms were predicated on effective collection and critical appraisal of the evidence.

Assessing the Fidelity of Evidence

The first step in establishing the fidelity of evidence is leveling or grading the evidence. According to Burns et al. (2011), the Canadian Task Force on the Periodic Health Examination established a three-level hierarchial system of rating evidence on the probability of bias. Sackett (1989) further expanded the levels of evidence to four levels, a system which formed the basis for the individualization evident today:

Level 1: Randomized controlled trials (RCT) using randomization or quasi-randomization

Level 2: Nonrandomized controlled trials that predict eligibility criteria and outcome measures

Level 3: Observational studies with controls; case-controlled studies, and cohort studies

Level 4: Observational studies without controls; expert opinions

Progressively, the available evidence and the strength of that evidence within different specialties and subspecialties has advanced at exponentially different rates, leading to modifications in the levels of evidence. These modifications have added to the specificity of the levels of evidence and include meta-analyses, systematic reviews, critically appraised topics, and critically appraised individual articles. However, the strength of evidence varies widely among professions and within professions.

According to Murad et al. (2016), evidence-based medicine currently uses the pyramid that follows, which includes systematic reviews and meta-analyses.

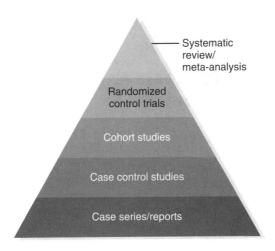

Nursing, similar to medicine, has a significant number of meta-analyses and systematic reviews that form the basis for new inquiry. However, the argument exists that not all worthy evidence-based projects or even research will be based on these higher levels of evidence. In some specialties and subspecialties, the level of evidence simply does not rise to this standard. In many areas, beginning-level researchers are beginning to establish case control studies and cohort studies.

Some may question, then, if the project based on these lower levels of evidence has sufficient foundation to move forward. Can the project have merit if based on lower levels of evidence? Yes, they should move forward and can have merit! In the not-so-distant past, trial and error was the basis for new knowledge development. Evidence-based practice projects are designed to directly affect practice and create a significant difference in patient care. Eliminating them simply because the foundation is a cohort study rather than a meta-analysis is short sighted and ultimately will have a negative impact on health care.

The mantra for evidence-based practice projects becomes "use the best available evidence, whatever the level." Continuous quality improvement is vital to the nursing profession and patients; therefore, all efforts to develop new practices or impact practice changes should be at the forefront in the development, implementation, and evaluation of projects.

Organization of Evidence

The guiding principle in organizing evidence is to lead the reader to the realization that the project is the only logical conclusion to the gap in evidence. Several tools and teaching methods exist in the literature that propose strategies for synthesis writing. Synthesize eLecture and Lippincott's NursingCenter.com, as well as several university writing centers provide writing advice and tools to help writers organize and effectively present evidence.

Most of the articles and websites propose beginning with a thesis statement worded similarly to this example: This project is going to address (*topic/issue/problem*) through (*strategy*). Writers can use this basic template and fill in the blanks with specifics related to their project.

Developing outlines is an effective way of organizing thoughts and events and provides an effective guide to writing the literature review. Some outlines are chronological; however, in the case of synthesis writing, the outline is based on the primary topics associated with the project or idea being proposed. Outlines may be more effective after content is organized using a synthesis matrix such as the one proposed in the Tools, Guidelines, and Techniques for Literature Synthesis and Project Alignment section in this chapter.

Aligning Evidence with Project Interventions and Implementation

Aligning supporting evidence with project interventions and implementation requires that the writer be knowledgeable regarding the subject matter and all aspects of the project. The writer should locate all available resources, published and unpublished, that are linked to the project ideas and appraise the quality and relevance of the evidence to inform the project (Gough, 2007). The intent is to clearly establish that the writer is fully conversant with what is known and not known about the topic. Therefore, negative and contradictory evidence must be discovered and reviewed carefully to gauge the impact on the project. The writer should assure that all information in the review of the literature is supported by existing evidence. Evidence is broader than research findings alone and encompasses current clinical practices, the strategies that have worked in the individual agency or institution in prior projects, and the writer's personal experiences (Glasgow et al., 2012). Ultimately, the object of aligning any existing evidence to the project objectives and implementation plan is to clearly highlight a "gap" in the knowledge base, which presents an opportunity for the project being proposed (Briner & Denyer, 2012).

Synthesis involves assembling ideas into a new or unique product or plan that presents a solution to a previously unanswered problem (Kelly, 2017). Glasgow et al. (2012) promote the use of a "straightforward and systematic" path from new idea to integration into practice (p. 646). Typical action verbs associated with synthesis thinking include the following: *create* new ideas; *predict*, *modify*, or *change* a mechanism; and *organize*, *adapt*, *elaborate*, and *draw conclusions* regarding a topic or set of topics.

Establishing and Maintaining Fidelity of Implementation

"Tracking progress, monitoring, and maintaining fidelity determine if outcomes can be attributed to the evidence-based practice or program" (Iris Center, n.d., p. 8). A quality improvement project is virtually unusable if the outcomes cannot be directly or indirectly attributed to the project. Attributing the outcomes directly to a project is highly dependent on establishing implementation measures and monitoring the extent to which the intervention and the delivery of the intervention adhere to established project protocols or models—in other words, establishing the fidelity or the internal validity of the project.

Establishing the model and the methods designed to achieve the desired outcomes is foundational to measuring the effectiveness of an intervention (Mowbray et al., 2003). Consistent measuring of program aspects is an effective way to prevent program deviations from the intended model. Loss of program fidelity or variations in interventions can account for a significant amount of variance in outcomes (Bond et al., 2009). One effective way of assuring program consistency or validity is the use of a fidelity scale (Bond et al., 2009). Fidelity scales are tools to assess the quality and consistency of implementation in a program or clinical unit (Ruud et al., 2020).

A fidelity review process is critical to successful implementation and is a powerful influence on change. Fidelity is "best measured through the use of observational data" (Iris Center, n.d., p. 6); in other words, having colleagues observe or perform self-assessment of videotaped interventions. These direct observations provide assistance in establishing a pattern of interventions over time. Other methods for assessing fidelity of implementation include structured supervision, program audits, and strict adherence to data-driven continuous quality improvement principles that are focused on improvement (Bond et al., 2009). The outcomes of maintaining fidelity of implementation have driven the development and use of valid fidelity criteria to the extent that it is now an expected component of evidence-based practice evaluation protocols (Mowbray et al., 2003).

Successfully translating evidence-based projects into practice is predicated on maintenance of treatment fidelity (Bleijenberg et al., 2016). There is considerable discussion in the literature about the efficacy of persistently maintaining rigid control of all aspects versus adapting the protocols and program as the project matures. There is strong evidence for either strategy. Strict adherence to protocols provides a clear linkage between the intervention and the outcomes. However, adaptive strategies can be more effective if the innovation involves unstructured interventions or when the data support tailoring the project to specific circumstances through establishing the importance of context to the intervention or the treatment group (Mowbray et al., 2003). However, one must monitor adaptive practices to assure that the basic underlying premise of the project is not compromised. There is an ever-present chance of program and/or treatment "drift" when adaptations are not closely monitored (Mowbray et al., 2003).

Tools, Guidelines, and Techniques for Literature Synthesis and Project Alignment

In order to provide context for tools, guidelines, and literature synthesis techniques, an overview and examples are provided. The following content provides an explanation of each.

Cognitive Maps

According to wisegeek.com, cognitive mapping is the "means through which people process with environment, solve problems and use memory." Although cognitive maps are generally used to help learners connect new information to that previously learned, they can also be useful for writers trying to express a disparate data set. Synthesis writing uses topics and subtopics to organize a literature review. The cognitive map that follows (**Figure 7-1**) can also be used to diagram topics and subtopics before writing about them.

Synthesis Matrix

Table 7-1, adapted from a chart created by the North Carolina State University Writing and Speaking Tutorial Service (2006) (https://tutorial.dasa.ncsu.edu/wp-content/uploads/sites/29/2015/06/synthesis-matrix.pdf), provides a tabular view of the same information. To use the chart, enter comprehensive information as you review each article/reference. Once all the references are entered into the chart, you can develop an outline or write directly from the chart.

As one examines the evidence that has been collected, the matrix may be modified as needed. The matrix, upon completion, provides a guideline for writing. As one enters the information into the matrix, data relatedness is evident, or not. Not all sources will have information that fits into the matrix completely. Some may have

Figure 7-1 Cognitive Map

Table 7-1 Synthesis Matrix for Literature Review

Author/ Title	Purpose of Project	Framework	Similarities/ Controversies to Your Project	Results	Implications for Practice, Research, and Theory

more information; some may have less. If the completed matrix has gaps or areas where little or no information is included, these areas may guide one's consideration of what is known and what is not known about the topic. Patterns of information may become readily visible within the matrix. All of this information will guide the synthesis of the evidence.

Synthesis Writing

A clear, comprehensive review of the literature is based on synthesis writing. Drew University has an online resource for writers regarding synthesis writing and describes the process as "combining two or more summaries in a meaningful way" (Drew University, n.d.) that supports the writer's thesis. Synthesis involves integrating themes or ideas from the literature into one's thinking/writing and allows the creation of new, unique outcomes. Synthesis is dependent on analysis of concepts, classifications, and categorizations but does not stop at this point. Synthesis involves the "search for links between materials for the purpose of constructing a thesis or theory" (Drew University, n.d.), which assimilates the disparate ideas and concepts into harmony, creating a meaningful new structure.

Synthesis writing can be achieved using an "explanatory" or an "argumentative" approach (Kelly, 2017). In the explanatory synthesis option, the writer is simply describing objectively without presenting a position or opinion. Argumentative synthesis writing involves the writer selecting a position and providing justification for that position. The argumentative option is more suitable for quality improvement or innovation projects because they require the writer to propose a new idea that is supported by existing literature but does not duplicate that literature. The idea is new and unique but is well founded in current evidence (Drew University, n.d.).

In either type of synthesis writing, the writer first proposes a one-sentence thesis statement, not a question, that is the focus of the project (Drew University, n.d.). The thesis statement reflects the synthesis of supporting literature while identifying the innovation or improvement. The remainder of the paper is composed of paragraphs that provide detail from the literature and other evidence to assist the reader in viewing the information in a new way. Each paragraph reflects a blending of reference material, not a summary of each source, and is linked to one or more key elements or subtopics associated with the idea or project. The paper culminates in a conclusion that addresses the "so what" and links back to the thesis (Kelly, 2017).

Synthesis writing is accurate, organized, and helps the reader make sense of information in order to identify the overlaps and gaps in the available data. To accomplish these aspects of synthesis writing, the writer must locate all studies, positive, negative, supportive, and contradictory, creating a clear path forward that is fully supported by existing evidence (Briner & Denyer, 2012). The paragraphs in a synthesized document are organized by topic or subtopic rather than by source and present a coherent assessment of the subject. Synthesis writing answers the question, "What do we know about . . . (the topic)?" The ultimate goal is to demonstrate that the writer is highly knowledgeable about the topic, has developed a perspective and/or interpretation of the evidence, and can assert that "no one has addressed XX," which will, in turn, become this writer's project.

Summary

- This chapter discusses a literature synthesis, methods of organizing the evidence, purposeful synthesis writing, and aligning evidence with the project interventions and implementation.
- Tools, guidelines, and techniques to assist the writer are provided to give a new perspective and interpretation of the evidence surrounding the project.
- When implementing an evidence-based project, leveling or grading and fidelity are paramount to project implementation and outcomes.
- Fidelity of evidence can be demonstrated by providing a systematic approach to individualize the evidence or data.
- Merit-based research employs meta-analyses and systematic reviews; however, relevance or practice change can occur with each level of evidence. It is always best to use the best evidence available when developing new methods or strategies, or when implementing practice changes.

Reflection Questions

1. Why is it essential for the writer to identify, read, and synthesize data that both support and do not support the project?
2. What action verbs associated with synthesis writing provide the writer with a way to design an appropriate quality improvement project?
3. How is synthesis writing different from other types of writing? How does that difference impact aligning the evidence with project interventions and implementations?

References

Bleijenberg, N., TenDam, V. H., Drubbel, I., Numans, M. E., deWit, N. J., & Schurrmans, M. J. (2016). Treatment fidelity of evidence-based nurse-led intervention in a proactive primary care program for older people. *Worldviews Evidence Based Nursing, 13*(1), 75–84. https://doi.org/10.1111/wvn.12151

Bond, G. R., Drake, R. E., McHugo, G. J., Rapp, C. A., & Whitley, R (2009). *Strategies for improving fidelity in the National Evidence-Based Practice Project. Research on social work practice.* https://doi.org/10.1177/1049731509335531

Briner, R. B., & Denyer, D. (2012). Systematic review and evidence synthesis as a practice and scholarship tool. In D. M. Rousseau (Ed.), *Handbook of evidence-based management: Companies, classrooms and research* (pp. 112–119). Oxford University Press.

Burns, P. B., Rohrich, R. J., & Chung, K. C. (2011). The levels of evidence and their roles in evidence-based medicine. *Plastic Reconstructive Surgery, 128*(1), 305–310. https://dx.doi.org/10.1097%2FPRS.0b013e318219c171

Canadian Task Force ON Preventive Healthcare (1979) The Periodic Health Examination. *Can Med Assoc J.* Pub Med PMID115569

Drew University. (n.d.). *Synthesis writing.* https://users.drew.edu/sjamieso/Webresources.html

Glasgow, R. E., Green, L. W., Taylor, M. V., & Stange, K. C. (2012). An evidence integration triangle for aligning science with policy and practice. *American Journal of Preventive Medicine, 42*(6), 646–654. https://doi.org/10.1016/j.amepre.2012.02.016

Gough, D. (2007). Weight of evidence: A framework for the appraisal of the quality and relevance of evidence. *Research Papers in Education, 22*(2), 213–228. https://doi.org/10.1080/0267 1520701296189

Hain, D. J., & Kear, T. M. (2015). Using evidence-based practice to move beyond doing things the way we have always done them. *Nephrology Nursing Journal*, 42(1), 11–21. http://152.12.30.4:2048/login?url=https://search.proquest.com/docview/1655480007?accountid=15070

IRIS Center. (n.d.). *Evidence based practices: Evaluating learner outcomes and fidelity*. Iris.peabody.vanderbilt.edu/module/ebp_03, pp. 6–8.

Kelly, M. (2017). *Higher level thinking: Synthesis in Bloom's taxonomy: Putting the parts together to create new meaning*. http://www1.center.k12.mo.us/edtech/Blooms/Synthesis.htm

Kilbourne, A. M., Neumann, M. S., Pincus, H. A., Bauer, M. S., & Stall, R. (2007). Implementing evidence-based interventions in healthcare: Application of the replicating effective programs framework. *Implementation Science*, 2(42). https://doi.org/10.1186/1748-5908-2-42

Mowbray, C. T., Holder, M. C., Teague, G. B., & Bybee, D. (2003). Fidelity criteria: Development, measurement and validation. *American Journal of Evaluation*, 24(3), 315–340. https://doi.org/10.1177/109821400302400303

North Carolina State University Writing and Speaking Tutorial Service. (2006). *Writing a literature review and using a synthesis matrix*. https://tutorial.dasa.ncsu.edu/wp-content/uploads/sites/29/2015/06/synthesis-matrix.pdf

Murad, M.H., Noor, A., Alsawas, M., & Alahdab, F. (2016). New evidence pyramid. *BMJ Evidence-Based Medicine 21*, 125–127. https://doi.org/10.1136/ebmed-2016-110401

Roberts, B. (2013). Doctor of nursing practice: Integrating theory, research, and evidence-based practice. *Clinical Scholars Review*, 6(1), 4–8. http://152.12.30.4:2048/login?url=https://search.proquest.com/docview/1348259634?accountid=15070

Ruud, T., Drake, R. E., & Bond, G. R. (2020). Measuring fidelity to evidence-based practices: Psychometrics. *Administration and Policy in Mental Health and Mental Health Services Research*, 47(6), 871–873. https://doi.org/10.1007/s10488-020-01074-7

Sackett, D. L. (1989). Rules of evidence and clinical recommendataions on the use of antithrombotic agents. Chest 95: 2S-4S.

Synthesis. (n.d.). In *Merriam-Webster's online dictionary*. https://www.merriam-webster.com/dictionary/synthesis?src=search-dict-box

U.S. Department of Health and Human Services. http:www.ahrq.gov

Case Exemplars

Synthesis Writing (Hand Hygiene)

The DNP student has identified a rise in hospital-acquired infections that is limited to the medical–surgical units. Hand-hygiene protocols are in place on all units throughout the facility. The DNP student wishes to compare the protocol to actual practice and identify a gap for project development. The first step is to identify and synthesize the literature and evidence from practice.

Sample of Synthesis Writing Related to Hand Hygiene

Hand hygiene is one of the most effective methods for preventing infection (Aziz, 2013; Mortell, 2012; Spruce, 2013). In the mid-1800s, Dr. Semmelweis was one of the first physicians to recognize the importance of hand hygiene for preventing infection (Aziz, 2013; Molinari, 2017; Mortell, 2012). There is a lack of adherence to hand-hygiene protocols among healthcare workers (Aziz, 2013; Mortell, 2012). This can lead to an increase in healthcare-associated infections, spreading drug-resistant microorganisms (Molinari, 2017; Mortell, 2012). Some reasons for nonadherence to hand hygiene include a lack of priority, allergy to or intolerance of antiseptics, and a lack of leadership (Mortell, 2012; Spruce, 2013). It is important to increase hand-hygiene compliance because it can improve patient outcomes (Molinari, 2017; Mortell, 2012).

Identification of Gap

The standard hand-hygiene protocols currently in place need to be assessed to determine compliance and to improve health outcomes.

Thesis Statement for Project Development

This project will compare current standard hand-hygiene protocol to clinical practice on three specific medical–surgical units to determine compliance.

References

Aziz, A. (2013). How better availability of materials improved hand-hygiene compliance. *British Journal of Nursing*, 22(8), 458–463. https://doi.org/10.12968/bjon.2013.22.8.458

Molinari, J. A. (2017). Effective, sensible, and safe hand hygiene: Poor compliance among clinicians still leads to associated infections. *RDH*, 37(10), 62–65.

Mortell, M. (2012). Hand hygiene compliance: Is there a theory-practice-ethics gap? *British Journal of Nursing, 21*(17), 1011–1014. https://doi.org/10.12968/bjon.2012.21.17.1011

Spruce, L. (2013). Back to basics: Hand hygiene and surgical hand antisepsis. *AORN Journal, 98*(5), 449–460. https://doi.org/10.1016/j.aorn.2013.08.017

Case Exemplar

A community-based, nurse-led, family-centered practice is experiencing increased numbers of patients exhibiting hypertensive issues. The vulnerable, low-income, and predominantly African American patient population has been provided with literature on best practices with regard to management of hypertension. Nutritionists have provided evidence-based meal plans for each of the patients. Pharmacological treatments have been prescribed for all.

Yet, the majority of patients are not experiencing a decrease in their blood pressure. The CNL student is interested in this issue and has devised a protocol to identify causes, relational factors, and patient views as a basis for a clinical innovation project.

Reflection Questions

1. What process should she follow?
2. What literature does she need to review?
3. What practice policies does she need to review?
4. What practice standards exist that may or may not be used in this practice?
5. What steps does the CNL student need to take to assure comprehensiveness of the project?

CHAPTER 8

Building the Improvement Project Budget: Quantifying the Cost and Quality Equation

Patricia L. Thomas
James L. Harris

CHAPTER OBJECTIVES

1. Explore the concept of cost and quality as drivers of decision-making in project management.
2. Examine elements of a project budget.
3. Explore key financial considerations in the design of improvement projects.
4. Review ways return on investment is established in project budgets.
5. Propose communication plans that communicate budgetary and financial considerations.

KEY TERMS

Management	Stakeholders
Project budget	Stewardship
Project management	Sustainability
Project plan	Teams
Return on investment	Value

ROLES

Communicator	Leader
Designer	Manager

PROFESSIONAL VALUES

Accountability	Integrity
Fiscal stewardship	Patient-centeredness

CORE COMPETENCIES

Analysis	Integration
Assessment	Leadership
Communication	Risk anticipation and mitigation
Critical thinking	Systems thinking

Introduction

In the last decade, decision-making attention has shifted from a singular focus on care quality and outcomes to include the cost of care. Organizations and leaders now expect proposed projects to include financial, clinical, and operational improvement to prioritize resources and projects within any approval process.

As providers, organizations, and systems shift attention toward defining "value" within the context of value-based purchasing payment models and patient satisfaction, a crucial consideration has evolved. Demonstration of value directed toward innovation and responsiveness to patient/family feedback is an expectation. This awareness requires that implementation and sustainability have a cost. Regardless of the industry, transformation is central to future success in a local, national, and global economy. What was once viewed as desired, but not essential, in terms of cost has been replaced with a survival instinct within market distinction and a competitive alternative. Sustainable project plans and value-based programs have become the cornerstone for prioritization of organizational resources and fiscal investment.

Quality metrics and indicators have also become measures of value with resultant reimbursement or financial penalty from third-party payors. Leaders have become focused on the costs of work, projects, and programs.

Recent attention regarding the cost of continual change on employees has also been articulated in the Quadruple Aim. Initially articulated by the Institute for Healthcare Improvement (IHI), the Triple Aim focuses on improvement in the patient experience, health of a population, and reduction in care costs (IHI, 2014). The addition of the Quadruple Aim adds the dimension of employee experience recognizing burnout and exhaustion of providers, caregivers, and how staff may hinder attainment of the other elements in the Triple Aim (Bodenheimer & Sinsky, 2014; Previs Health, 2019).

Innovation and patient-centeredness, enabled by technology, have facilitated a silent revolution of individuals and global leaders dedicated to seamless integration, coordination, and expectation that benefit the health and economic well-being of society. A review of 10 years of contributions by the Robert Wood Johnson Foundation (2014) established an array of improvements directed toward health that are achieved by expanding its definition to include social determinants of health such as education, income, communities, job opportunities, and the environment outside health systems. An approach guided by strength-based focus, rather than gap or deficit drivers, has gained prominence in strategic project planning and evaluation as catalysts for organizational change (Sankaran et al., 2017; Stratton-Berkessel, 2010).

Successful planning and implementation that recognizes social determinants of health and health equity now strengthen the focus of system thinking. Pending universal agreement, achievement of social justice and health equity will require attention to health determinants that extend beyond the location of care and services. This represents a distinct modification in how projects are planned, requiring consideration and incorporation of known social determinants that influence outcomes. As knowledge is gained, knowledge transfer becomes an imperative. Evidence is spread and systems of care are strengthened and sustained. This is relevant in the current environment, where the focus of work is on obtaining the right outcomes, as opposed to past decades, where performing the right processes was emphasized (Porter-O'Grady & Malloch, 2015) as previously addressed. The relevance is increasingly predominant in a market-driven economy by value-based versus volume-based care delivery and reimbursement (Frist, 2016). Effective system strengthening, inherent in project management, requires systems thinking and attention to how the parts work together to create a seamless whole.

This chapter focuses on the financial components of project planning and management, building on content from Chapters 1, 2, 4, and 6. Definitions and strategies to articulate cost, quality, and sustainability are guided by tangible and visible financial metrics established in the project plan initially and evaluated at the termination of project work. General principles of budget development and monitoring will be provided with an understanding that the organizational complexities and unique attributes of budget planning are outside the scope of this chapter. Collaboration with finance departments, organizational leaders, and operational managers is essential for effective budget planning; however, all project team members need to have an appreciation for the alignment of the project plan elements, articulation of the cost–quality goals, and areas of focus related to cost in the implementation of any project. This assists the team to communicate consistently toward strategies that the project is fiscally responsible to those not on the project team, and benefits the initiation of a common language that defines and describes impact.

As the evolving era of healthcare reform has highlighted, ignoring costs is both outdated and detrimental. Team composition must demonstrate a positive impact toward the financial landscape within an organization. This distinguishes activities directed toward continuous work or workstreams from those identified for elimination. Gone are the days when quality reigned as the single driver of clinical success; today, efficiency, effectiveness, and awareness of cost support improvement in quality and clinical outcomes (Marquis & Huston, 2017; Thomas & Collins, 2021).

Although this is not new work, it actually represents decades of extensive work that has been persistent and only moderately successful. In 1999, the Institute of Medicine (IOM) report, *Crossing the Quality Chasm: A New Health System for the 21st Century*, recommended sweeping healthcare systems changes to address quality and safety. The 2003 IOM report, *Health Professions Education: A Bridge to Quality*, addressed a radical redesign of health professional education in support of quality and safety centered on competencies of patient-centeredness, teamwork, collaboration, evidence-based practices, and informatics. What followed was the publication of IOM landmark reports to address the contemporary issues and complexity of care delivery in the United States, noting healthcare errors and mistakes cost between

$17 and $29 billion annually. Additionally, payment and reimbursement modifications by the Centers for Medicare and Medicaid Services (CMS) and third-party payors have linked cost and quality in value-based purchasing reimbursement models and innovative expectations for reporting clinical quality and patient satisfaction indicators to reimbursement incentives or penalty payments (Sherwood & Barnsteiner, 2017).

Several terms related to costs are regularly used. It is important for project managers and team members to establish where the project exists in relation to the cost–quality equation. Caution must be used when discussing cost because spending money or having a higher cost can be advantageous if the clinical care outcomes are improved and consistent. Significant healthcare expenditures occur on duplicative care, readmissions, and incomplete care. Therefore, consultation with financial analysts and individuals with a systems lens to examine upstream and downstream impacts is key.

Key Definitions and Budgeting Principles

It is not within the scope of this chapter to offer all the possibilities and options related to budgeting, but rather the intent is to offer key attributes and considerations for project budgets. As pressures and expectations rise in regard to fiscal stewardship, the importance of having a detailed and comprehensive view of costs and anticipated expenses, including supply, personnel, and information management required in order for a realistic set of expectations, is presented to the leadership team, sponsors, stakeholders, and project team members. Transparency in this information builds trust and achievable results whereby a lack of information or transparency leads to disappointment absent of a shared vision and goals not established initially.

The link of cost in a project, both what will be saved and what will be spent, has become the norm and often a primary consideration in decision-making related to allocation of resources and project approval. A return on investment, sustainable improvement in a financial reimbursement metric, or cost–benefit related to competitive market advantage or patient/consumer satisfaction motivates the deliberations and prioritization for project approval (Hampton, 2018; Thomas & Collins, 2021). Cost analysis and evaluation need to be established during project design, allowing for the articulation of how the cost (or cost savings) aligns with the project goals toward value. Clear and specific definitions in project charters, executive summaries, and project updates need to reiterate the terms and definitions and provide a direction about whether targets are met or undefined/unexpected costs or revenue loss have ensued. This is of paramount importance for project team credibility and organizational decision-making related to replication or elimination of a project.

Context and Definitions for Projects, Project Plans, and Project Management

A project plan captures essential components that culminate into a realistic, clear, and well-planned sequence of actions and processes. It extends beyond goals and scope to include details that put structure and meaning to how a particular project warrants implementation based on the value it offers to the organization. As described in Chapter 1, project plans include a budget, scheduled work activities, and a schedule with supporting documents for deliverable outcomes that are communicated. Success of all project management includes a specific and detailed budget that aligns activities, actions, and individuals to specific measures and expected cost or expense.

The Project Budget

A well-developed project budget is based on objectives and a detailed estimate of all costs required from inception to completion. Project budgets should be flexible, have standards, and use available sources to avoid unnecessary costs. A typical project budget includes costs for staff labor, materials and their procurement, on-going operation costs, other direct costs such as travel and education, and indirect costs that support the project such as building expenses. The proposed budget provides information to develop a cost–benefit analysis and a return on investment expressed in a ratio as net profit divided by total investment times 100 (Finkler et al., 2014).

Harrin (2015) identified four sequential steps to a well-planned project budget. First, break down the tasks. Breaking down the work and listing what is needed for the project's completion is important from the onset. Second, estimate the tasks based on expert knowledge and past experiences. Third, total the estimates in order to create the total for the planned budget. Fourth, include extras that may arise unexpectedly as the project proceeds. A 10% contingency is common in most cases where costs are poorly estimated. An example of a project budget template is provided in **Table 8-1**.

Attributes of a Well-Constructed Project Budget

A thoughtfully constructed project budget is a roadmap to ensure adequate startup funding, cost controls, and a concise depiction of fiscal stewardship (Viter, 2021). The budget outlines expected costs and forecasted revenue or savings, is visible to those involved in the project, and indicates what is anticipated and expected. A

Table 8-1 Project Budget Template

Line Item	FY 20XX–20XX			
	Labor	Material	Other	FY Total
Total				

Total Project Budget: $_____   **Return on Investment:** _____%

FY, fiscal year.

budget should be developed with input from stakeholders, leaders, sponsors, and financial analysts to ensure a wide set of perspectives.

A common technique to generate a budget is from the bottom up, using the project charter and milestones with each task, activity, and phase to project costs (Viter, 2021). This granular level of detail may be tedious, but it is precisely the specificity needed to prevent surprises or disappointment. Once budget costs are totaled, it is important to align costs with tasks and/or milestones germane for the project outcomes.

Many project teams struggle with the creation of a budget because there is a desire to look at "best case" performance or "worst case" performance. Therefore, it is prudent to consider the best case, worst case, and likely case (Viter, 2021). Often benchmarks from other units, departments, or organizations are available, and at other times one can rely upon the expertise of the project team. Understanding what leads to best and worst cases in terms of individuals, equipment, and supplies influence project design decisions.

Often Overlooked Cost

Quality and process improvement initiatives include descriptions readily identified as cost found in supplies, staffing levels, and reduced processing steps. Irrespective of the quality or process framework utilized, reducing waste, simplifying processes, or initiating a new supply makes cost visible and, by extension, quantifiable (Thomas et al., 2020).

When costs associated with making change are overlooked, it often leads to disappointment when the financial metrics in a project are not achieved. As an example, many projects related to reductions in length of stay or readmission have been undertaken with inconsistent cost improvements. Likewise, the purchase and integration of technology, notably electronic health records, have not yielded the anticipated improvements in efficiency or sustainability. In deconstructing project plans to evaluate disappointing outcomes, several key costs or expenses were excluded when the project budget or return on investment calculations were established at the onset of program design or implementation.

- Training and development costs (conferences, seminars) and cost to train staff
- Professional services (legal advice, consultants, market research)
- Material resources (software, equipment, supplies)
- Equipment or technical upgrades
- Travel (Viter, 2021)

Language and Definitions in the Budget Process

Attention to terms and definitions commonly used as part of the project budget follows with key terms and definitions that offer clear wording and language. This benefits the entire project team. Many organizations have definitions and application points, so it is important to verify and validate the way a term is used to ensure a shared meaning. **Table 8-2** provides examples and language definitions associated with the budget process.

Table 8-2 Types of Costs

Types	Definition	Example
Fixed costs	Costs that remain the same regardless of activity	Rent, insurance, taxes, depreciation, utilities (Marquette et al., 2015)
Variable costs	Costs that change dependent on level of volume	Overtime labor, materials, staffing, med–surg supplies, linen (Marquette et al., 2015)
Direct costs	Costs readily assigned to a project	Supplies charged to a patient, a specific clinical procedure, labor costs per produced unit (Barton & Jones, 2020)
Indirect costs	Costs that cannot be attributed to a specific patient or process	Depreciation, utilities, taxes, floor space, administration (Barton & Jones, 2020)

Types of Budgets

Generally speaking, there are two types of budgets commonly discussed in project planning: the operating budget and the capital budget. An operating budget includes revenue and expenses (both fixed and variable) for the year. It includes items relevant to day-to-day operations such as wages, office supplies, repair and maintenance costs, travel, and subscriptions as well as clinical supplies such as thermometers, otoscopes, and sphygmomanometers (Finkler et al., 2014; Marquette et al., 2015; Thomas & Roussel, 2020). Supply and equipment are typically found in the operating budget unless the dollar threshold established by the organization moves it to a capital expense.

The capital budget reflects major expenditures that typically undergo separate review and approval. Items in a capital budget may include equipment, land acquisition, or buildings. Unique to this budgeting process are the deliberate review of strategic initiatives and consideration about services offered that are related to competitive market advantage. There is a formal process to consider regarding how the expenditure would impact service lines, quality and safety, personnel, facility renovation including depreciation, maintenance, payment methods, and replacement. Capital budgets are used in renovations, remodeling, and costly equipment; for example, purchase of an MRI and CT scan machines, operating room autoclaves, and electronic health records. Purchase of land to build a new facility to address market share and purchase of hospital beds or a medication distribution system throughout an organization are other examples (Marquette et al., 2015; Thomas & Roussel, 2020).

Cost Avoidance, Cost-Effectiveness, and Cost–Benefit

When establishing the financial impact of any project, defining terms for both team members and stakeholders is needed. When engaged in change work, it is common to assume that the leader for the project remains in cost-reduction mode, often translated as job loss. Project managers have an important leadership responsibility in reducing the stress and fear of a team so that creative and innovative solutions can be formulated. Cost avoidance is defined as costs in the future that will not be incurred because of a change in practice or process. Think of this the same way as you would think of preventative maintenance on your car. Often you have a cost in the short run (such as an oil change), but you avoid blowing your head gasket. The same holds true in health care. If we spend money on this now, we could avoid expenses (and potentially negative health outcomes). Some view this kind of savings as a "soft saving" because you have not spent the money yet, and other factors could arise that negate the savings. The downside to cost avoidance as rationale to implement a project is that the baseline costs or expenses may not represent future costs. Consider, for example, the cost of a loaf of bread 3 years ago versus the cost today. This may be avoided by using cost savings as tangible dollars that are related within a financial report including items such as avoided overtime or reduced supply use, often elements that are accomplished through quality and process improvement initiatives (Thomas & Collins, 2021).

Cost-effectiveness analysis is often used to highlight areas where resources are used differently to achieve a desired effect. It captures opportunities to employ inexpensive interventions that have the potential to reduce disease burden, achieve outcomes, and reduce expense. An example of this could include oral rehydration for children with diarrhea. One million children die from dehydration annually. Although oral rehydration does not decrease the incidence of diarrhea in children, it can reduce the severity and mortality. The cost of the oral rehydration diminishes in comparison to the hospitalization costs and critical care expenses associated with childhood diarrhea. Cost–benefit analysis assigns a dollar value on both the cost and the effectiveness of an intervention, recognizing individual and societal benefits that often influence policy- and decision-makers. An example of this is purchasing lift equipment to avoid employee injuries, recognizing it will take time to pay for the equipment, but that will be offset by having fewer employees injured during lift or transfer. The equipment will accrue benefits to include the money saved on lost time from work, workers' compensation costs, and overtime. A project manager would need to keep the potential or desired financial impact in view for the teams they lead. Often, a member of the finance department will be a member of the project team or will serve as a consultant to the team so that financial analysis is based on the design and development of each specific project.

Thomas et al. (2018) highlighted the utility of applying a business model to immersive improvement projects, which includes value proposition resources and processes, as well as a profit formula. The value proposition assists teams in accomplishing the goals for a project. Resources represent human, supply, and fiscal resources and encompass the knowledge, skills, and abilities necessary to accomplish the desired outcomes so executive leaders and sponsors can appreciate the complexity of the work and what will be needed to sustain it. The final element is the profit formula, whereby cost, benefit, reimbursement models, value-based purchasing incentives, bundled payment, and cross continuum impacts are considered as part of the system lens for decision-making.

Common Pitfalls in the Establishment of Project Budgets or Expected Financial Outcomes

The thoughtful planning and review may result in a gap in budget planning. For example, in the design phase of a project, tasks and work may not be apparent or new tasks are added during implementation (Viter, 2021). Technology upgrades may not have been apparent in the design phase, but are required to move forward in a project. Wiring in a facility, internet signals, and accreditation requirements can sometimes add unexpected costs.

Detailing a budget with input from stakeholders and financial analysts is an advantage because the detail generated in the task list and milestones generate an agreed upon baseline that allows the project manager and sponsors to validate where the gap occurred and provide the means to adjust expectations.

Summary

- Planning successful projects requires a series of deliberate and purposeful activities and a well-developed budget that results in an attainable goal.
- Budgets must be inclusive of anticipated, avoidable, and identified cost.
- Involvement of stakeholders during and throughout the project is essential for success.

Reflection Questions

1. You are tasked with developing a project budget. What are the primary components to include in the budget?
2. Sustainability of practice change has been difficult in the department. Staff are weary from repeated change where cost savings are not achieved despite significant attention during implementation. Given what you have learned about a project budget, what elements were missed or underrepresented in the planning?
3. You have been asked to lead a project team for an important organization-wide project. There is enthusiasm in the stakeholder and sponsor groups. Although improved clinical outcomes are anticipated, it is likely that supply, information technology, and staff time costs will be high. How will you document and visualize the cost analysis to highlight cost–benefit and cost avoidance to ensure realistic expectations?

References

Barton, A., & Jones, P. (2020). Cost analysis in DNP projects. In G. Armstrong & S. Sables-Baus (Eds.), *Leadership and systems improvement for the DNP*, 295–308. Springer Publishing.

Bodenheimer, T., & Sinsky, C. (2014). From Triple to Quadruple Aim: Care of the patient requires care of the provider. *Annals of Family Medicine*, 12(6), 573–576. https://doi.org/10.1370/afm.1713

Finkler, S. A., Jones, C. B., & Kovner, C. T. (2014). *Financial management or nurse managers and executives* (4th ed.). Elsevier.

Frist, B. (2016). From volume to value: Achieving bold change in our healthcare payment systems. *Forbes.* https://www.forbes.com/sites/billfrist/2016/06/30/from-volume-to-value-achieving-bold-change-in-our-healthcare-payment-systems/?sh=1a4afd4a9c82

Greiner, A., Knebel, E. (Eds.); Institute of Medicine Committee on the Health Professions Education. (2003). *Health professions education: A bridge to quality.* National Academies Press. https://www.ncbi.nlm.nih.gov/books/NBK221528/

Hampton, D. (2018). Cost analysis and nurse leadership: Implementing projects and purchases requires an understanding of costs and benefits. *American Nurse Today, 13*(10), 53–55.

Harrin, E. (2015). *How to plan a project budget.* https://www.projectmanager.com/blog/how-to-plan-a-project-budget

Institute for Healthcare Improvement. (2014). *The IHI Triple Aim.* http://www.ihi.org.Engage/Initiatives/TripleAIM/Pages/default.aspx

Institute of Medicine Committee on Quality of Health Care in America. (1999). *Crossing the quality chasm: A new health system for the 21st century.* National Academies Press (US). PMID: 25057539.

Lighter, D. M. (2011). *Advanced performance improvement in health care.* Jones & Bartlett Learning.

Marquette, R., Dunham-Taylor, J., & Pinczuk, J. (2015). Budgeting. In J. Dunham-Taylor & J. Pinczuk, *Financial management for nurse managers* (3rd ed.), 445–524. Jones & Bartlett Learning.

Marquis, B., & Huston, C. (2017). *Leadership roles and management functions in nursing: Theory and application* (9th ed). Wolters Kluwer.

Porter-O'Grady, T., & Malloch, K. (2015). *Quantum leadership: Building better partnerships for sustainable health.* Jones & Bartlett Learning.

Previs Health. (2019). *What is the Quadruple Aim and what role does it play in healthcare?* https://www.privishealth.com/what-is-the-quadruple-aim-and-what-role-does-it-play-in-healthcare/

Robert Wood Johnson Foundation. (2014). *Time to act: Investing in the health of our children and communities. Recommendations from the Robert Wood Johnson Foundation Commission to Build a Healthier America executive summary.* https://www.rwjf.org/en/library/research/2014/01/recommendations-from-the-rwjf-commission-to-build-a-healthier-am.html

Sankaran, S., Müller, R., & Drouin, N. (2017). *Cambridge handbook of organizational project management.* Cambridge University Press.

Sherwood, G., & Barnsteiner, J. (2017). *Quality and safety in nursing: A competency approach to improving outcomes* (2nd ed.). John Wiley & Sons, Inc.

Stratton-Berkessel, R. (2010). *Appreciative inquiry for collaboration skills: 21-system-based workshop.* John Wiley & Sons, Inc.

Thomas, P., & Collins, B. (2021). Selecting the right tools for the job: From idea to execution. In P. Thomas, J. Harris, & B. Collins (Eds.), *Data-driven quality improvement and sustainability in health care: An interprofessional approach.* Springer Publishing.

Thomas, P., Harris, J., & Collins, B. (2020). *Data driven quality improvement and sustainability in health care: An interprofessional approach.* Springer Publishing.

Thomas, P., Harris, J., & Roussel, L. (2018). Creative and meaningful clinical immersions. In J. Harris, L. Roussel, & P. Thomas, *Initiating and sustaining the clinical nurse leader role: A practical guide* (3rd ed.). Jones & Bartlett Learning.

Thomas, P., & Roussel, L. (2020). Procuring and sustaining resources: The budgeting process, in L. Roussel, P. Thomas, & J. Harris *Management and Leadership for Nurse Administrators*, (8th eds.) pp. 155–188. Jones & Bartlett Learning.

Viter, I. (2021). *Creating a project budget – A complete guide for 2021.* https://www.forecast.app/blog/how-to-create-a-project-budget#what-is-project-budgeting

Case Exemplar

The Value of Project Improvement Budgets

James L. Harris and Patricia L. Thomas

Project budgets are pivotal to selling any projected improvement plan. Void of a budget, administrators, stakeholders, and team members easily question the value of any improvement project. Throughout any improvement planning process is the requirement to include all informed parties. Inclusivity and collective engagement and thought offer opportunities for a well-developed budget and plan. As others are involved in a project, new ideas emerge and a comprehensive budget is developed. As discussed in this chapter, budgets are drivers that provide a roadmap useful for expenditures, measurement, and dissemination of any improvement. Although there are no specific templates or models for budget development noted in the chapter, many exist within the literature. An outline is provided in this chapter that focuses on how including others during the budget process must be linked to quality, safety, and value acknowledged by a larger community of interest.

CHAPTER 9

Information Management in Clinical Projects: Technology, Metrics, and Measurement

Patricia L. Thomas

CHAPTER OBJECTIVES

1. Describe the role of information management as an enabler of effective projects.
2. Explain the value of linking projects to information systems for enhanced functionality, data conversion, and data utility.
3. Recognize the importance of organizational culture and evidence-based practice improvement for successful project planning and management.
4. Examine process and outcome measures as cornerstones in project management supported by appropriate selection and project design.
5. Identify methods and tools to capture project milestones and management that ascribe meaning and value in sustainment.

KEY TERMS

Big data
Information management
Information technology
Metrics

Small data
Stakeholder
Value

ROLES

Communicator
Decision-maker
Information manager
Integrator

Leader
Partner
Team member

PROFESSIONAL VALUES

Efficiency	Performance
Integrity	Quality

CORE COMPETENCIES

Analyzing	Data management
Communication	Design
Coordination	Interpersonal influence
Critical thinking	Systems thinking

Introduction

The Patient Protection and Affordable Care Act, known more simply as the Affordable Care Act (ACA), represents the largest change to the U.S. healthcare system since the genesis of the Medicare and Medicaid programs in 1965 (Institute of Medicine [IOM], 2001, 2011). The U.S. healthcare system has experienced numerous changes, and how the healthcare industry responds to changes in technology, care mandates, reimbursement models, and the information age are influenced by knowledgeable decision-makers represented by consumers and leaders. The momentum needed for competitive advantage and organizational survival will largely be shaped by how well and how accurately needs are assessed and technology is leveraged, as well as the ways innovation and implementation generate sustainable outcomes. Quantum leaps in efficiency and effectiveness will be realized as the diffusion of technology drives projects and determines the role that the information specialists will play in the process (Geibert, 2017). However, such projects will only be as effective as the partnership that is built between transformative clinical project managers and interprofessional teams. Clinical project managers, in partnership with clinical stakeholders and informaticists, guide project activities with necessary tools, issue management, and coordination for success (Davies et al., 2020; Gallagher, 2012; Kudyba, 2021). The transformation of action to quantifiable results and communication of improvements that appeal to patients, families, administrators, regulators, and payors serves as the springboard to articulate value.

At its core, the act of "measurement" is fundamentally about communicating change. The more structured and clear the communication, the more likely the change will be accepted, supported, sustained, and replicated (Datsenko & Schenk, 2013; Meyer, 2019). Communication can take many forms, ranging from large national impact through academic, peer-reviewed journal publications to local demonstrations within single inpatient units using dashboards, posted charts, and/or graphs. Regardless of scale and audience, the important story to tell is that of performance optimization and, more broadly, quality improvement. A clear value proposition statement for leaders and stakeholders brings a direct line of sight between fragmented and inefficient care delivery systems and improvement (Petersilge, 2020; Radnor et al., 2012).

Information Technology as an Enabler for Clinical Project Success

The availability of electronic networks 24/7 provides access across points of care. Equally, evidence-based data are readily available as clinical projects are envisioned and initiated. But what enables a clinical project's success and its management? Although there is no single formula that guarantees project aims are met, the use of informatics represents a valuable tool in today's evolving technological healthcare environment. Investing in new ways to mix technology with project ideas by engaging information management and clinical informaticists has expanded based on the realization that a knowledge gap exists when only clinical team members guide change. The potential to enhance practice, solve clinical problems, and improve care has been expedited through the inclusion of informatics, contributions of professionals outside the healthcare sector, and deliberate project management processes to articulate results that appeal to diverse stakeholders (Kelly, 2012; Kudyba, 2021). Engaging clinicians with experts in information management and technology fills a knowledge void and serves as a catalyst in effective and efficient project design that promotes the likelihood of positive project results. Leveraging the skills of informatics specialists and utilizing appropriate measurement tools can optimize the iterative and address areas that lend themselves to workarounds. Informatics and technological advances provide clinical applications that can process transactions with tools for productivity, business strategies, collaboration, and innovations by exploiting unique technological advances, consistency, and standardization (Deloitte Insights, 2020; Shane, 2014).

To answer the earlier question of what enables a project's success and its ongoing management, numerous individuals and organizations have identified enablers to support projects, programs, and organizational efficacy to improve care (California HealthCare Foundation and First Consulting Group, 2002; Davies et al., 2020, DeLaune & Ladner, 2009; Fox, 2011; Stevens & Staley, 2006):

- Computerized order entry
- Electronic health records
- Peer-to-peer health care
- Mobile communication devices
- Secure messaging and email
- Automated documentation templates and clinical reminders
- Medication administration and management systems
- Evidence-based knowledge and information retrieval systems with remote library, smartphone, and internet resources
- Quality improvement data collection and data summary systems
- Data mining techniques for sorting large data batches
- Webpages for personalizing information
- Disease surveillance systems
- Computerized data encounter archives

To maximize these enablers and information technology (IT) systems when planning a project, many considerations and data points must be taken into account. The benefits can range from the needs assessment phase to completion of the project and dissemination of results.

Big and small data are valuable data sets and are analyzed and integrated into a project design (Austin & LaFlamme, 2021; Beal, 2014). Big data is generated from multiple sources and provides a snapshot of what is happening without answering why. It is used to describe, interpret, and predict (Henly, 2014). Small data provides information to answer a specific question or address an identified problem. Small data feeds big data by creating new knowledge and care advances (McCartney, 2015). Big and small data analysis are key to improvement initiatives (Austin & LaFlamme, 2021, Thomas et al., 2021; Welton et al., 2020).

Stakeholder and Partner Roles in Information Technology

Identifying and engaging stakeholders continuously during a clinical project is pivotal to project success. Similarly, IT is integral in data retrieval and meaningful use as discussed in Chapter 11. As stakeholders participate in a project, whether by engaging in the approval process or by offering encouragement in keeping with representation of interests, the clinical enterprise is the centerpiece. When stakeholders participate, partnerships emerge, ownership is reinforced, and support for the project takes center stage.

Informatics Core Competencies and Skill Sets

In today's global environment and economy, IT has become a thread woven throughout all types of organizations. Whether an individual is directly or indirectly involved in patient care or beginning a clinical project, that person must be armed with a general knowledge of informatics. The need for organizational and care efficiency, for example, requires healthcare team members to review and mine data so that they can design or redesign care delivery models and productivity. Such activities require competency and skills in informatics, both general and advanced. For those individuals with limited informatics knowledge, knowing where to seek assistance is essential if goals are to be attained. This need resonates with one of the IOM's healthcare professional core competencies (utilize informatics); indeed, its fifth healthcare professional core competency is delineated as the ability to "communicate, manage knowledge, mitigate error, and support decision-making using information technology" (IOM, 2003, p. 4). Likewise, the Robert Wood Johnson/IOM report *The Future of Nursing* (2010); the National Academies of Sciences, Engineering, and Medicine (2021); and the position statement from the Healthcare Information and Management Systems Society (2011) echo the need for nurses to possess informatics competency and skills (Matney et al., 2021).

Recognition of the significance of IT core competencies and skills for successful projects and management dates to early work at the University of Maryland that identified three levels of competencies (technical, professional, and advanced) for its multidisciplinary student body (Ball & Douglas, 1989). Grobe's (1988, 1989) seminal work describes informatics competencies for medical students that was later modified to create seven levels of informatics competencies for nursing

---

Box 9-1 Grobe's Nursing Informatics Competencies for Basic and Graduate Nursing Education

---

1. Use basic information-handling tools.
2. Independently learn about computers and information management.
3. Use computer systems and access databases.
4. Knowledgeably use systems and specialized databases.
5. Perceive new applications.
6. Build systems for personal applications.
7. Utilize tool building.

---

students and other allied health disciplines. **Box 9-1** identifies these seven levels of competencies.

Grobe's work was an initial step in establishing a comprehensive taxonomy of competencies on a continuum ranging from user to modifier to innovator. For decades, healthcare professionals have advanced their care delivery as new competencies have emerged, including those related to informatics. This work continues today and no single system has been established for electronic medical records to record nursing care (Cipriano, 2014). Clark and Lang (1992) identified the key shortcoming associated with this practice: "If we cannot name it, we cannot control it, finance it, teach it, research it, or put [it] into public policy" (p. 109). Although advancing clinical competencies is necessary to meet care demands, the ongoing development of informatics competencies will be required for successful data management. This persistent need is apparent in the review of baccalaureate, master's, and doctor of nursing practice (DNP) end-of-program competencies (American Association of Colleges of Nursing [AACN], 2006, 2008, 2011) and the recent revisions to the AACN *Essentials* (2021) document approved for competence-guided nursing education in the future.

The Value of Linking Projects to Information Systems

From the inception to dissemination of any project, its value must be considered. Value must be attainable and measured to ensure that the resources allotted to a project did, in fact, advance the mission and vision of the organization. Likewise, the value to stakeholders must be measurable and attainable, as they are the end recipients of a clinical project.

Measuring value can be complex and requires the use of data from various sources. The data must be informative, relevant, and sensitive to the intent of a project so that a difference is evident in desired outcomes. Meeting this standard requires one to link the project to information systems; otherwise, changing inefficient processes will be more difficult, and the value produced may be questionable (Harris & Thomas, 2021; Nelson et al., 2007; Thomas & Bleich, 2020).

Information systems are the "nervous system" for meaningful projects and can provide the context for how a project benefits practice, education, quality improvement, management, and policy. When planning the project, one must select those

Table 9-1 Clinical Success Metric

Success Metric	Attainable, Measurable Outcomes from Information System
Improved quality, safe, and efficient patient care processes	■ Medication order entry errors (pharmacy, medical, and nursing services) ■ Timely signing and verification of emergency verbal orders (medical and nursing services, health information management, pharmacy, and quality improvement)

metrics that will measure specific outcomes based on the project's aim. Aligning the metrics to the correct information system will isolate the effect of the project based on desired outcomes and allows for greater functionality, conversion, and utility of the data gathered. Conversely, failure to ensure such alignment is a common flaw in the design process. Metrics that effectively measure success extend beyond business and strategic goals and are linked to stakeholders who have a vested interest in the success of any project. Those metrics must be specific and quantifiable (A. Lewis, 2011; Thomas et al., 2021). To further illustrate this point, consider the example of a clinical success metric identified in **Table 9-1**.

If quality, safety, efficiency, and continuous improvement are to be achieved with the initiation of any project and its subsequent sustainment, ongoing measurement is pivotal to success. Donabedian (1978) provided an excellent way to characterize medical quality, based on structure, process, and outcome measures. Using Donabedian's model, quality improvement teams consistently use these measures to guide the development of metrics that are linked to data warehouses for easy retrieval. Specifically, structure measures describe the facilities, staff, and culture of an organization (e.g., number of licensed beds). Process measures relate to the interface between the patient and the provider (e.g., patient satisfaction). Finally, outcome measures are associated with the efficiency and effectiveness of processes, both clinical and business. Accrediting agencies such as The Joint Commission and the Centers for Medicare and Medicaid Services have developed standards and measures using Donabedian's model that demonstrate desirable characteristics to showcase relevance, scientific soundness, and feasibility.

Organizational Culture and Project Management

Although the discipline of project management framed by data is critical to project or program success, the culture within an organization or unit cannot be ignored. In recent years, recognition for both the "soft" and "hard" sides of leadership and project management have been recognized, in large part because projects or programs failed (Radnor et al., 2012; Sheppy et al., 2012; Thomas, 2020). Malloch and Porter-O'Grady (2010); Melnyk and Fineout-Overholt (2015); and Nelson et al. (2007) address organizational culture and change leadership as foundational to implementation of evidence-based practices and quality improvement, emphasizing the need to honestly assess the environment to leverage strengths (and champions) and prepare for resistance or compliance proactively. The challenges of the digital age call on each of us to perceive work and roles openly so different perspectives inform transformational thinking and action that spans disciplines and care settings to fit in a sociotechnical culture (Porter-O'Grady & Malloch, 2015).

Common barriers to successful implementation of projects or their replication are lack of leader champions, insufficient human and fiscal resources, and unrealistic expectations regarding the time necessary for design and achieving desired outcomes. Schein (2004) describes organizational culture and leadership as two sides of the same coin with both having the significant influence within organizations, particularly when instituting change. Inclusive of the spoken and unspoken values, norms, and espoused beliefs, awareness of the culture is essential to success but is often overlooked at the start of a program or project. Setting project goals and developing a charter for the work team that outlines expectations, timelines, and lines of accountability and authority structure expectations is an initial step. What is often missed is the discussion and planning directed toward perceptions, change leadership strategies, and methods to address the team activities that will be undertaken if the agreed-upon changes start to backslide to the previous state. Each of these has distinct strategies for management and requires acknowledgment of the power that culture has in influencing them (Andre & Sjovold, 2017; Shirley, 2011).

The link to organizational readiness and assessment of this readiness, including data availability, administrative support, and outcome analyst support, provide organizational information to determine how poised a team is to accept change. The rationale for a change readiness assessment or evaluation of the culture provides important information to leaders that can reduce or eliminate impacts on staffing and caregivers who will be affected by a project (B. Brown & Hough-Falk, 2014; Miake-Lye et al., 2020), which is described more fully in Chapters 5 and 6.

Use of Evidence-Based Practice: An Intertwined Element

Evidence-based practice and evidence-based medicine are established "buzzwords" that get affirmative nods from many practitioners across disciplinary lines. Despite this affirmation, many disciplines have been slow to adopt evidence-based practices and often identify solutions to problems or new changes to implement without the benefit of evidence. For discussions related to the selection of metrics, project development, and the ensuing evaluation and alignment to evidence in the design of the program or project aims and in the development of activities or interventions, is essential (Malloch & Porter-O'Grady, 2010; Nelson et al., 2007; Thomas et al., 2021). Without clarity derived from definitions and reputable evidence found in the literature, selection of interventions, replication, and credibility of outcomes is questioned (Hall & Roussel, 2022; Melnyk & Fineout-Overholt, 2015). Although outside the focus of this chapter (but detailed in Chapter 7), understanding levels of evidence is key to project success and an important consideration for project managers.

Selecting the Right Variables to Tell Your Story

Selecting variables to establish measures of progress and success can be daunting. Members of the project team often come from different disciplines, educational programs, and job or role expectations, bringing diversity and a wide space for misunderstandings. As the project manager, one of the roles will be to simplify the process and bring a sense of confidence and inclusion to those completing work. To that end, using metaphors that bring common meaning and understanding offers a space for shared learning. When discussing metrics, measures, and variables, a helpful metaphor for groups that will implement change is that of "telling a story through data." People can envision their home library and the varied genres of books. Applying this to health care, they can appreciate how each person involved in a project has unique interests (and unique home library genres) that bring distinct perspectives. Team participants will have unique stories and different ways to share them. The unifier will be the data and the shared lens of "data telling the story" in support of measurement. Each chart, graph, and dashboard represents a chapter in the story being told. Each measure or variable represents a different character in the story with a specific role and perspective.

Fundamental Types of Measures

Process Measures

Measures of clinical process describe "activities carried out by healthcare workers to deliver services" (Agency for Healthcare Research and Quality [AHRQ], 2014; Thomas & Collins, 2021). Measures of this type reflect specific and observable aspects of clinical practice. A prominent example comes from emergency cardiac care. For patients presenting to the emergency department (ED) with STEMI (ST-segment elevation myocardial infarction), door-to-balloon time measures a process that starts with the patient's arrival and ends with intervention in the cardiac catheterization laboratory. This is a process measure that describes the total time necessary to complete a series of processes associated with treating a patient with STEMI, performed by multiple care team members. A key feature of process measures is that they can be easily and clearly defined. As a result, when properly defined, process measures are generally not case-mix or risk-adjusted.

Information about completed processes emerges from two sources. First, the process can be directly observed. Staff with a stopwatch can time how long it takes to complete a specific task or shadow clinicians to ensure a specific task is completed or not. This is referred to as upstream measurement—the measurement is taken *as the action is being completed*. One example is the observational audit of staff to ensure that the proper handwashing procedure is followed.

On the other hand, downstream measurement is generated from information on processes that *have already been completed*. Here, data are often extracted from administrative sources such as patient charts or the electronic medical record. Door-to-balloon time for STEMI patients is an example of downstream measurement because the measure is reported as the sum of the time it takes to complete multiple processes and therefore is typically extracted from the medical record after the sample population of patients has been discharged. Another example is the examination of a patient's chart to see if fall prevention education was delivered. The chart review takes place after the process of delivering fall prevention education has been completed.

Downstream measures have two important limitations that cannot be overlooked. First, downstream measures typically only indicate whether or not a process was completed; they are binary indicators, lacking any qualifiers. They do not clearly indicate *how* the process was completed. Expanding on the example of fall prevention education, using a downstream measure for this process would not reveal any information about how much time was taken to speak to the patient and gives no indication that the patient fully comprehended the information provided, two pieces of information that could be captured if the process had been directly observed. Second, downstream measurement introduces recall bias by relying on staff to record information after the task has been completed, sometimes several hours later. For these reasons, upstream measurement is the preferred option where available but should be balanced against the greater demands placed on the cost of gathering this data (such as staff time and expense).

Outcome Measures

Although representing different viewpoints, both measures of process and measures of outcomes must be included to tell the complete story of any project or program. Outcome measures are the cornerstone of quality improvement. For many projects and programs, improving patient outcomes is the final goal. Outcomes capture a variety of health states such as mortality, physiologic measures (blood pressure, laboratory test results), and patient-reported health status (functional status and symptoms) (AHRQ, 2014; Thomas & Collins, 2021). These variables represent final goals of clinical interventions and processes—improved health status for patients or populations.

Process and outcomes measures are intrinsically linked. One of the most common mistakes made in measurement strategy is the conflation of the two. Evaluating a care management training program on medication reconciliation in primary care practices represents two things. First, are the process measures derived from the training process? Second, are the outcomes or results of this training on medication reconciliation? It is not uncommon for these distinct measures to be described as one entity. In developing a project or program, calling out the distinctions between process and outcomes is essential so that measurement and clarity around accountability and results can be determined.

Qualitative Measures

Although quantitative measurement is most commonly used based on specificity and ease in data gathering and analysis, qualitative measurement offers a different perspective. Measures that tell the story of a stakeholder's opinion about a process are called qualitative measures because they convey deeper meaning regarding quality, or how *well* a given process was fulfilled. A plethora of qualitative measures can be found on the Hospital Consumer Assessment of Healthcare Providers and Systems, or HCAHPS, survey (also known as the HCAHPS Hospital Survey). HCAHPS is a national, standardized, publicly reported survey of patient perceptions of care received during a hospitalization (Centers for Medicare and Medicaid Services [CMS], 2020).

It is a 29-question survey about a patient's recent hospital stay, taken from a random, monthly sample of all eligible discharges. One example qualitative measure from this survey tool is the percentage of patients who report that their nurses "always" communicated well during their stay (H-COMP-1-A-P). This measure is considered to be qualitative because it reflects a person's opinion about nurse communication—what is considered to be "good" or "effective" communication varies from person to person. Similar surveys exist for home and hospice care (HHCAPS).

Selecting the Right Data

When possible, measure sets are best focused on the patient or individual, commonly referred to as "patient-centric." This means that when read together, the measures show how a patient or population of patients progresses through a given process or disease state. This simplifies understanding and provides a platform for replication.

Matching Populations

When selecting sets of variables, care should be taken to represent the same time frame and the same target population across the entire set. Mismatches of this type are common. Using **Table 9-2** as a reference, there would be little insight to be

Table 9-2 Sample Inpatient Heart Failure Measure Set

Variable Description	Data Source	Measure Type
Heart Failure & Shock with Major Complications (MS-DRG 291)	CMS (ICD-10-CM)	Outcome; quantitative
Heart Failure & Shock with Complications (MS-DRG 292)	CMS (ICD-10-CM)	Outcome; quantitative
Heart Failure and Shock Without Complications or Major Complications (MS-DRG 293)	CMS (ICD-10-CM)	Outcome; quantitative
Average Length of Stay (ALOS)	Administrative clinical data; EMR	Process; quantitative
30-Day, All-Cause Mortality Rate	Administrative clinical data; EMR	Outcome; quantitative
Patients Discharged to Ambulatory Care or Home Health Care	Administrative clinical data; EMR	Process; quantitative
30-Day, All-Cause Unplanned Readmission Rate	Administrative clinical data; EMR	Outcome; quantitative
Patients Who Received Heart Failure Education	Administrative clinical data; EMR	Process; quantitative

CMS, Centers for Medicare and Medicaid Services; EMR, electronic medical record.

gained by reporting the average length of stay for a population of patients discharged between the months of January to June at the same time as 30-day all-cause mortality rate for patients discharged between the months of July and December. By definition, these are two different populations with two different stories to tell. This noise makes interpreting any trend, change, or intervention outcome difficult or even impossible to discern. In addition to reporting time frames, other mismatches can arise in the underlying population (different groups of patients) and processes without connection or causal relationship. Drawing conclusions about the impact a change has when the "noise" is not accounted for can lead to attribution that is distorted or inaccurate.

Common Data Sources

- CMS
- Press Ganey
- National Database of Nursing Quality Indicators (NDNQI)
- AHRQ National Quality Measures Clearinghouse
- Healthcare Effectiveness Data and Information Set (HEDIS)
- Organizational administrative and claims data

Benefits of Using Established Measures

Many individuals are tempted to write or establish individual data definitions as a means to highlight the uniqueness of an organization or a patient population. This can be initiated because individuals recognize that the current available data are valued by those engaged in the project or data that are readily available. Oftentimes, individuals look for ways to stimulate "buy-in," particularly when the "charge" or expectation to make meaningful change originates outside the work team expected to generate the change. Although tempting, this undertaking requires knowledge and analysis not generally found in healthcare organizations and should be avoided if established national or specialty-specific data definitions exist. Over the last decade, significant progress has been made in establishing evidence-based, validated, credible data definitions that promote comparability within a single facility or to other organizations, especially when participating in regional or national quality improvement collaboratives.

Eliminating Unnecessary Measures

In Lean and Project Management Book of Knowledge (PMBOK) methodology, any work that adds cost or time, or expands the scope of this work without also adding value, is considered to be wasteful. One specific type of waste that is applicable to measurement strategy is called overprocessing. Overprocessing can take many forms, including requesting and processing more information than is necessary or information that will never be used, or reporting duplicative information (Hadfield et al., 2012; Thomas & Collins, 2021). A central tenet of Lean is to only measure that which one intends to impact through a project or program. Eliminating waste from your dashboard—in the form of vestigial or unnecessary variables—will increase the clarity and impact of the story being told therein. Additionally, and perhaps more importantly, it will increase the ability to glean new knowledge such as trends from the data, which could otherwise be hidden behind the noise of unnecessary measures. For example, if the goal of a program is to establish a process for complex care coordination in the emergency department (ED), the measurement of ED median arrival-to-discharge time adds no valuable information.

To eliminate waste from an established dashboard of measures, begin by clarifying the reporting and communication needs of involved stakeholders. Look for measures that do not include information which is being expressly requested. This step is also a centerpiece of change management—if stakeholders are not involved early in the process of making changes, there is a higher risk that disruptions could arise further on.

Data Management Plan

No matter what program or project is going to be evaluated, a data management plan should be developed to help guide the process of selecting the correct metrics. Using a structured approach provides a proactive guide to ensure the best measurement is initially identified and that all of the information needed for evaluation is obtained. There are six basic steps to follow, which are: (1) define data needs, (2) identify data sources, (3) identify performance measures, (4) design the study, (5) retrieve the data, and (6) analyze the data.

Step One: Define Data Needs

Defining necessary data depends upon the questions to be answered. There are two general types of questions. First are quantitative questions such as "Who?" "What?" and "How many?" These questions generate numerical data that can be counted, ranked, and statistically analyzed, such as volume and frequency data. Quantitative questions are generally asked to verify something or make a prediction (Shank, 2006; Thomas et al., 2021). Calculated means or averages can be trended over time. Medians, or the middle point of data sets, are better to use for data sets with extreme values (D. Brown et al., 2008; Geary & Clanton, 2011; Thomas, 2020).

The second type of question, qualitative, seeks to answer "Why?" "Why not?" and "How?" These questions are open ended to generate lots of information and gain a deeper understanding of the issue being studied. Analysis of qualitative responses is done by reviewing the responses and identifying any common themes. Qualitative questions are not as frequently used in hospitals but can often give you more timely data and be less expensive to generate (Geary & Clanton, 2011; Hoff & Sutcliffe, 2006; Thomas, 2020).

Using both quantitative and qualitative questions can result in a measurement set that more thoroughly evaluates a process or program. The patient satisfaction surveys used by most hospitals include both quantitative and qualitative questions. Quantitative questions ask patients to rank their response on some sort of numerical scale and address items such as level of satisfaction with nursing care, discharge planning, pain management, environmental cleanliness, and quality of food. These data can be compared and trended over time to include previous information. Most surveys also have open-ended questions that assess patients' opinions or comments.

When specific comments are recurrent, then trends can be identified. Qualitative information can direct how an aspect of care might be improved or identify processes that can be replicated. Using both quantitative and qualitative data provides a holistic approach to any type of evaluation and should be used whenever possible (Geary & Clanton, 2011; Thomas, 2020).

Two quality-control tools that are useful in determining specific types of questions and measurements needed for program evaluation are process flowcharts and cause-and-effect diagrams. Process flow diagrams provide a visualization of all of the steps and decision points involved in a process. The first step in creating a flow diagram is to identify the beginning and the end point of the process. An oval shape is used to represent these points. Hospital processes are usually very complex, so it is important to establish exactly what part of the process is being reviewed. The different steps within a process are represented by rectangles and appear in the order as they occur in the process. All processes have decision points that are represented in a flow diagram as diamonds. The different answers at these decision points will either lead to the next step in the process or outside the process where some other step or decision must be made before the process can continue. The number of decision points contained in a process is an indication of the process complexity. The more complex the process is, the greater the chance for breakdown or undesired outcomes (Geary & Clanton, 2011; Thomas et al., 2021).

Key measurements for analysis can be identified by reviewing the flowchart key process steps and decision points (Geary & Clanton, 2011; Okes & Westcott, 2001; Thomas & Collins, 2021; Westcott, 2013). For example, flow diagrams can identify missing, redundant, or erroneous steps and point to improvement actions. An example of a flow diagram is shown in **Figure 9-1**.

A cause-and-effect diagram is useful in demonstrating the many different contributing causes of a particular problem. To construct this type of diagram, the problem (effect) is noted in the box at the right side of the chart, and then major categories and subcategories that identify possible different causes are listed. Typical categories when discussing patient care problems are patient factors, staff factors, physician factors, administrative factors (policies and procedures), environmental factors, and equipment factors. A benefit of creating a cause-and-effect diagram is the brainstorming of all possible factors, which yields a broad range of possible measurements, ensuring a thorough review. The cause-and-effect diagram shown in **Figure 9-2** is a continuation of Figure 9-1 (Geary & Clanton, 2011, p. 129; Thomas & Collins, 2021). After reviewing the process flow, the step of cross-matching the patient's blood specimen was identified as being a common cause for the delay. A cause-and-effect diagram was constructed to illustrate all of the possible reasons why a problem with blood cross-matching might occur (Geary & Clanton, 2011; Thomas & Collins, 2021).

Step Two: Identify Data Sources

Healthcare facilities today, more than ever, collect a large amount of data. Much of what hospitals measure is required by the CMS to receive reimbursement for services or by The Joint Commission to demonstrate compliance with accreditation standards. The Joint Commission Hospital Standards require hospitals to collect data to monitor performance pertaining to restraint use, moderate sedation, adverse drug reactions, medication errors, results of resuscitation, use of blood

Operating room blood process

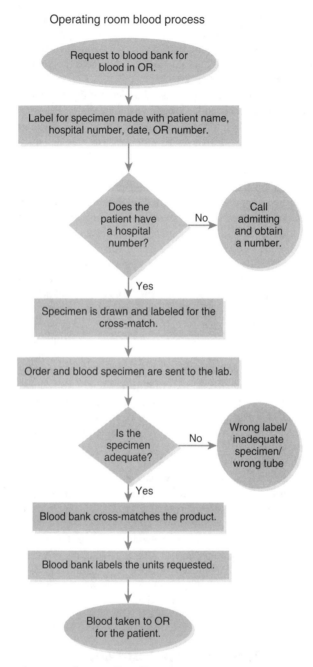

Figure 9-1 Process Flow Diagram

products, procedure complications, and preoperative and postoperative diagnosis discrepancies (The Joint Commission, 2017). Hospitals also have ongoing measurements/counts of infection rates, patient falls, mortality, length of patient stay, and other metrics designed to analyze processes of care and productivity of

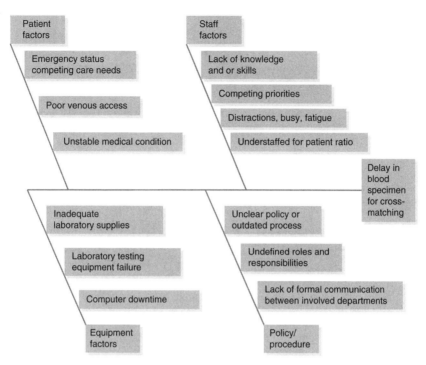

Figure 9-2 Cause-and-Effect Diagram

services. In addition to acute care metrics, HEDIS data for population health metrics and community-based care services are gaining prominence.

Many hospitals participate in disease-specific registries such as the Society of Thoracic Surgeons, the American College of Cardiology, and the National Surgical Quality Improvement Program. These national databases have validated measures of risk-adjusted patient outcomes for specific procedures such as coronary artery bypass surgery, percutaneous coronary interventions, and surgical care. The metrics are designed to measure evidence-based physician practices.

The most common direct measure of nursing is the NDNQI. This metric set was developed in 1998 by the American Nurses Association; it became part of Press Ganey in 2014 and is used by more than 40,000 organizations in the United States (Press Ganey, 2014, 2021). The NDNQI based on the National Quality Forum endorsed safe practices. The National Quality Forum's *Safe Practices for Better Healthcare* was originally released in 2003 and has been updated four times since then to incorporate current evidence and new measures (National Quality Forum, 2010). Of these measures, those most closely linked to nursing practice are referred to as nursing-sensitive measures and include nursing workforce (staffing plan and resource allocation), patient care information, order read-back and abbreviations, labeling of diagnostic studies, discharge systems, medication reconciliation, hand hygiene, surgical site infection prevention, multidrug-resistant organism prevention, venous thrombosis prevention, glycemic control, wrong-site-surgery prevention, pressure ulcer prevalence, patient falls, urinary catheter-associated infections, central line catheter-associated bloodstream infections, and ventilator-associated pneumonia (Geary & Clanton, 2011; National Quality Forum, 2010).

Caution is needed when using the CMS core measures, Hospital Acquired Condition (HAC) data, or any data derived from administrative or coded data for analysis or conclusions. Administrative data are generated from patient classification and billing codes. Diagnostic, procedural, and complication codes are determined by medical record reviewers based on what is documented in the medical record according to established coding criteria. Thus, only what is documented in the record and interpreted by the coders will be part of the administrative database. Administrative data is not risk-adjusted for patient condition and does not include information on how care delivery is organized in a facility. Examples of structural measures such as staffing ratios, patient skill mix, and procedure volumes are commonly found in administrative databases. Structural measures can be indirectly related to both process and outcome measures but recognizing limitations is key (**Table 9-3**).

Step Three: Identify Performance Measures

Process measures typically evaluate whether processes are being followed as designed. They can measure specific steps of a process or an entire process and usually fall into categories of financial, utilization, compliance, disease-specific, and satisfaction with care (Missel & Thomas, 2015; Thomas, 2020). The CMS core measures are all process measures designed to determine the frequency of specific evidence-based practices. The CMS requires measuring processes to facilitate optimal patient outcomes that should occur. The underlying assumption is that if the core measure practices for pneumonia patients, for example, are instituted, then a patient with pneumonia will have a greater chance of having a positive outcome. However, many factors and processes can influence patients' outcomes, so inferences regarding any causal relationships should be made with caution. The patient's other health risks may affect their recovery, infection prevention practices of the patient's caregivers could cause the patient to develop a nosocomial infection, and the skill of the cardiologist can determine the success of any cardiac interventions. Therefore, measuring outcomes such as complications, infections, and mortality is also important in the overall evaluation of a program or project (Geary & Clanton, 2011; Thomas, 2020; Thomas & Collins, 2021).

Outcome measures are used to determine the effectiveness of processes. Two types of outcomes are common in health care—operational and clinical outcomes. Both are important in program evaluation. Operational outcomes measure how well a nonclinical process is performing and includes financial data, environmental inspection data, patient satisfaction with food, and cleanliness. Clinical outcome measures are specific to a clinical condition or the result of specific treatment and care. Many national registries such as the National Surgical Quality Improvement Program provide clinical outcome data that is risk adjusted for each patient according to comorbidities and other identified related factors (Ko, 2009; Missel & Thomas, 2015; Thomas, 2020). Risk-adjusted outcome data are a more accurate measure of how well a treatment or process is working.

There are many valid and reliable assessment tools that can be used to define concepts to be measured. For example, when measuring patients' risk for skin breakdown, using the Braden Scale to define high risk gives a specific definition and ensures an objective, consistent measurement. One should not assume to know the meaning, as many concepts can be subjectively defined. For example, measuring a patient's level of pain will vary from patient to patient and could vary based on

Table 9-3 Structure, Process, and Outcome Measures for Cardiac Catheterization

Measure	Jan	Feb	Mar	Apr	May	June	July	Aug	Sept	Oct	Nov	Dec	Total
Volume (structural measures)													
No. of catheters													
No. of diagnostic													
No. of interventional													
Process measures													
Closure device used (Y/N)													
Fluoro time													
No. of stents													
Complications (outcome measures)													
No. of hematomas													
No. of required transfusions													

(continues)

Table 9-3 Structure, Process, and Outcome Measures for Cardiac Catheterization

(continued)

Measure	Jan	Feb	Mar	Apr	May	June	July	Aug	Sept	Oct	Nov	Dec	Total
No. requiring surgery													
No. requiring unplanned intervention													
No. of acute closures													
No. of closures w/in 6 mos													
No. of codes E—expired; S—survived													
No. of balloon pumps used													
No. of AMI* following catheterization													
No. of deaths													

*AMI, acute myocardial infarction.

what specific type of pain measurement scale is used to quantify the pain. A level-5 pain may be the most severe pain on a 1 to 5 scale but moderate pain on a 1 to 10 scale. Another example is the different definitions of fall rates; some include patient and visitor falls whereas others include only patients. Performance measures must be defined before measuring and preferably using definitions that have already been validated and used in the nursing literature (Geary & Clanton, 2011; Thomas, 2020).

Performance measures need to be reliable and valid. Reliability is defined as the extent to which the data generated are consistent with what is being measured and the variable of interest is measured the same way in each participant (Missel & Thomas, 2015; Polit & Beck, 2020). Performance measures are said to be valid when they measure what is intended to be studied. Poor validity can occur if the measure is indirectly linked to a concept or if the variables are not clearly defined.

Step Four: Design the Study

The study design is determined by the focus of the project or program and the specific aspects being evaluated. However, some basic concepts are defining the population of interest and determining the sample size. For example, if the project focuses on preventing urinary tract infections in hospitalized patients, the population of interest would be all patients who have an indwelling catheter. In a large hospital, it may not be possible to include all patients, so a representative sample would be needed. The current minimum sample size is 5% or 30 items, whichever is greater (Williams & Geary, 1997). If the population is less than 30, every case needs to be reviewed (Geary & Clanton, 2011; Thomas, 2020).

Step Five: Retrieve the Data

Many projects fail because data retrieval is not systematically planned, resulting in wrong or incomplete data being obtained, leading to an inability to analyze or measure the concept of interest (Lighter, 2011; Missel & Thomas, 2015; Thomas et al., 2021). Systematically planning the retrieval of data includes deciding where and how to access data that are already being collected, or, if data are not already available, deciding who will collect the data, how data will be gathered, and the specific time period for the collection. This is especially critical to do if more than one person is doing the data retrieval to ensure consistent methods. Data collection tools, such as the one shown in **Table 9-4** (Geary & Clanton, 2011, pp. 136–138), are helpful in ensuring consistency in data retrieval.

Data can come from a variety of sources and retrieval methods and can include observation, medical record review, surveys, and interviews. The information needed will determine the best source of the data; the more direct measure of a concept, the stronger the analysis. For example, observing a practice is a more accurate measure than reviewing a chart for documentation of the practice. The ease of obtaining data is also an important factor and can sometimes cause one to use a more indirect measure of the concept (Geary & Clanton, 2011; Thomas et al., 2021).

It is also necessary to decide on the time period for measurement. Most administrative data, such as core measures, are retrospective measurements. Advantages of retrospective data collection include convenience and use of administrative databases, which allow for quick and large-scale evaluations to be done. Examples

Table 9-4 Patient Safety Liaisons Data Collection Form

Patient Safety Unit-Based Rounds Unit: _____ Month/Year _____ Completed by: _____					
Issue—Mark Each as Yes, No, or n/a	MR No.	MR No.	MR No.	MR No.	MR No.
Patient Interview and Observation Items					
1. The patient was encouraged not to leave their clinical area and, if they do, to have a signed release in the chart.					
2. The correct armband is on the patient.					
3. Ask the patient if new caregivers are asking them to state their full name and checking their armband before giving them medications or blood.					
4. Patients at a high risk for falling have on a yellow armband and a fall leaf placed on the door.					
Medications/IV Solutions					
5. IV medications are labeled with correct patient name, time IV hung, and ordered drug/dose if not already labeled.					
6. The IV site is dated, timed, and changed every 72 hours.					
7. The IV pump library is in use for heparin, insulin, and chemotherapy agents.					
8. A medication reconciliation form is completed on admission.					
9. PCA pumps have a booklet and a warning label for the patient to push only.					
Patient Safety Unit-Based Rounds Unit: _____ Month/Year _____ Completed by: _____					
Issue—Mark Each as Yes, No, or n/a	MR No.	MR No.	MR No.	MR No.	MR No.

Chart Review					
10. Documentation of read-back of orders has been done.					
11. Documentation of read-back of critical values, tests, and procedure results has been done.					
12. Allergies are documented on all required forms.					
13. Signature indicating informed consent has been obtained for any surgical or invasive bed-side procedure and matches the procedure on the order or postprocedure note.					
14. All invasive procedures have a final time out entered.					
15. No "do not use" abbreviations are found in the progress notes or orders. If they are, list which ones (write "none" or the specific abbreviations used).					
16. The Morse Fall Scale is re-corded on the graphics ac-cording to the patient's risk level.					
17. The Braden Scale is recorded on the initial assessment sheet according to the pa-tient's risk level.					

Patient Safety Unit-Based Rounds
Unit: _____ Month/Year _____ Completed by: _____

Issue—Mark Each as Yes, No, or n/a	MR No.	MR No.	MR No.	MR No.	MR No.

Observation Measure (Actual Number of Behaviors Observed/Total Number of Behaviors Possible)

18. The number of times hand hygiene was done/number of times hand hygiene should have been done (before and after patient care, staff breaks, eating, etc.).	/	/	/	/	/

(continues)

Table 9-4 Patient Safety Liaisons Data Collection Form   *(continued)*

19. Ask the nurse whether patient transporters are initiating the "ticket to ride."					
20. Refrigerator logs are being completed to document temperature checks.					
21. Code carts are being checked and documented daily.					

MR, medical record.

of retrospective data retrieval include using administrative data based on specific codes, medical record abstractions from previous hospitalizations, and posthospital/ procedure surveys. A disadvantage of retrospective data is that there is a delay of sometimes several months between when a process change or improvement action is implemented and when the retrospective data will be available to analyze for any effects. Therefore, retrospective data are not best for projects of an urgent nature needing immediate review.

Concurrent measurement refers to real-time data collection; the length of time for data collection depends on the amount of data needed to reach the appropriate sample size. The disadvantage of concurrent measurement is that it takes more time and effort to collect the data. The advantages, however, are that data can be trended (Geary & Clanton, 2011; Missel & Thomas, 2015; Thomas, 2020). During this collection time, any issues can be promptly identified and addressed. With retrospective data, any issues have already occurred, and there is no opportunity to intervene at the time of occurrence.

Step Six: Analyze the Data

The last step of the data management plan is to analyze the measurement data to determine any necessary changes. Data analysis is often the weakest step and is frequently inadequately performed. There are some simple statistical tools that can assist in analyzing the effect of an action or the success of a project. Several different types of charts can easily be constructed using standard computer programs. The type of chart needed will depend on the measures and the information needing analysis.

One of the most basic charts designed to identify trends in the variables is a run chart. Run charts are line graphs that display data over time and can show whether there has been a change in the performance after an intervention is implemented. One process or several can be shown on the same chart if the data are being analyzed for comparisons in trends. This type of chart is shown in **Figure 9-3**. This line (or run) in the chart depicts the process variation. All processes have variation that is either part of the process itself (common cause variation) or caused by external influences (special cause variation) (Geary & Clanton, 2011; Lighter, 2011; Missel & Thomas, 2015; Thomas, 2020). Being able to recognize the special cause variation is important, especially when analyzing for effects from an intervention.

Figure 9-3 Run Chart Comparing Two Processes: Rapid Response Team Calls and Codes

Run charts typically have the time interval on the horizontal axis and the variable being measured on the vertical axis. The data are plotted over time, and variation is evaluated. Two special cause trends are runs and shifts. Runs mean there is a continual increase or decrease seen for six data points in a row, and shifts cause data points to all fall above or below the average or centerline. Runs and shifts need to be analyzed further in order to determine the cause of the variation.

   Control charts are run charts that include the process parameters of mean and standard deviation calculated from the process data. These parameters make the centerline (mean) and the upper and lower control limits. The control limits are determined by adding or subtracting the standard deviation to or from the mean. Control limits can be set as one, two, or three standard deviations above and below the process mean depending on what is being measured and how much variance is acceptable. The more standard deviations are used, the larger the control limits and the more variation is accepted before the process is said to need additional analysis. So, if the control chart is trending serious patient issues (mortalities, infections, etc.), the control limits would best be set at one or two standard deviations so that only minimum occurrences would be tolerated. Both the run chart and control chart are useful tools to use when analyzing data over time to determine if a process is performing as designed or if a change has occurred—whether intentional, unintentional, positive, or negative. If data stay within the control limits, the process is stable. The process is unstable when data points are found to be outside of the control limits, and further investigation is needed to determine the special cause(s) of the variation. In the control chart example shown in **Figure 9-4**, there are 3 months when the number of patients leaving the ED before they are seen were outside the control limits. All three of these months should be further reviewed to determine any specific causes or common factors (Geary & Clanton, 2011; Thomas, 2020).

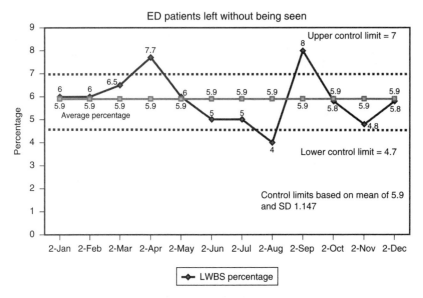

Figure 9-4 Control Chart with Mean, Standard Deviations

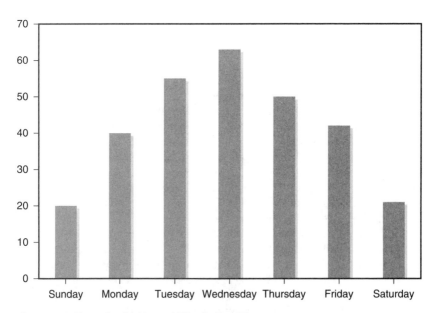

Figure 9-5 Example of a Normal Distribution Histogram

Two types of bar charts that are useful for analyzing the frequency or pattern of the data over a time period are histograms and Pareto charts. A histogram, as shown in **Figure 9-5**, is used to determine if the process has a normal distribution. Data are said to be bell shaped or normally distributed when the most frequent data appear within the center of the graph, with equal data points appearing on either side (Geary & Clanton, 2011; Missel & Thomas, 2015; Okes & Westcott, 2001;

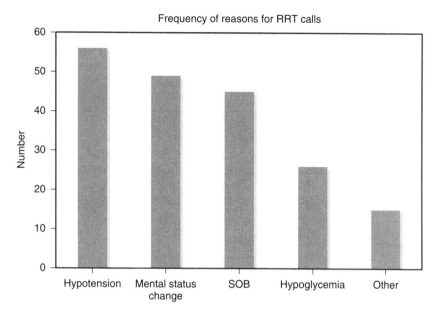

RRT, rapid response team; SOB, shortness of breath.

Figure 9-6 Pareto Chart Showing Most Frequent to Least Frequent Reason for Rapid Response Team Calls

Thomas, 2020; Westcott, 2013). An abnormal distribution or shape indicates that the process is not performing as designed and additional review is needed.

A Pareto chart is a bar chart that shows the frequency of measures. This type of graph is based upon the Pareto principle, which states that 80% of the process variation, or cause of a problem, is based on 20% of the variables (Geary & Clanton, 2011; Missel & Thomas, 2015; Okes & Westcott, 2001; Thomas, 2020; Westcott, 2013). The bars in the Pareto chart are ranked in descending frequency with the variables listed on the horizontal axis and frequency on the vertical axis. In **Figure 9-6**, the most frequent cause identified for calling the rapid response team is patients having hypotension. Being able to make this analysis helps direct any additional information needed to identify any common factors contributing to these patients developing hypotension.

The last chart that is helpful in analyzing data is a scatter diagram. Scatter diagrams are useful in determining if there is a correlation between two variables. A positive correlation is indicated when there is an upward slope found among the data points. A negative correlation is seen when the pattern slopes downward, which occurs when one variable's increase correlates with the other variable's decrease. When an identifiable pattern is not found, the scatter diagram is interpreted as showing there is no correlation between the two variables. A positive or negative correlation does not necessarily mean there is a direct cause-and-effect relationship between the two variables. There is also no way to determine the strength of the correlation from a scatter diagram. Additional measurement would be needed for that type of analysis. The first step involved in constructing a scatter diagram is to determine the variables and the type of relationship being investigated

■ Interpreting scatter diagram patterns

- Positive correlation: an increase in y may depend on an increase in x.

- Negative correlation: an increase in x may cause a decrease in y.

- No correlation: Y may be dependent on another variable.

Figure 9-7 Different Correlations Found in Scatter Diagrams

(cause/cause; cause/effect). Next, obtain paired data for the two variables and place the cause on the horizontal axis and the effect on the vertical axis. Finally, plot the data and check for any patterns. Patterns are interpreted as positive correlations, no correlations, or negative correlations, as shown in **Figure 9-7** (Geary & Clanton, 2011; Missel & Thomas, 2015; Thomas, 2020).

It is important to have a data management plan to determine the measures needed to support and evaluate any project or new program. Many different hospital departments perform ongoing measurement to evaluate different processes and outcomes. Some of these measures are suitable to use to evaluate and analyze new aspects of care, but often additional data are needed to be able to do a true analysis of an issue. If additional measures are needed, then the most direct measurement of the concept should be considered. Also, there are always new questions raised when analyzing a project or program. Using the appropriate statistical process tools will contribute to a comprehensive analysis and guide decision-making (Geary & Clanton, 2011; Missel & Thomas, 2015; Thomas, 2020).

Summary

- Today's more knowledgeable consumers are demanding accurate and timely data that are easily retrievable and understandable.
- Big data provides a snapshot of what is happening without answering why.
- Small data provides information to answer a specific question and feeds big data by creating knowledge and advancing care.
- Involving IT specialists in projects can lead to more successful projects.
- Interprofessional participation in clinical environments is key to success given the complexity and interconnectedness of care activities.
- The health professionals of the 21st century require information technology knowledge and competence for success.

- Quality, safety, and continuous improvement will be driven by data, processes, and tools to extract data and spread evidence.
- As the healthcare delivery system is reformed, an essential lever will be measuring meaningful elements of our practice to improve outcomes. This will include a thoughtful data plan as well as appropriate metrics.
- Building from research and evidence-based practice implementation, the disciplines of project management and quality improvement serve as guardrails for selection of meaningful metrics.

Reflection Questions and Learning Activities

1. What is the role of nurses, project planners, and interprofessional team members in ensuring projects align health care with trends?
2. Consider the definitions of process and outcome indicators. Select an area of practice you believe a project could be developed for. What are some of the process metrics you might consider to demonstrate progress or improvements in care? What are some of the outcome measures you would consider? What key big and small data would you consider?
3. Reflect on your current practice. Where would you go to get information about data available in your organization? Data in the electronic medical record? Administrative data? Claims data? Data sets or data warehouse? Who are the people (or roles and departments) to help you develop knowledge and understanding of the available data?
4. How might a project planner outline the steps needed to add value-based project outcomes? What are ways you could engage stakeholders in moving toward meaningful outcomes?

References

Agency for Healthcare Research and Quality (AHRQ) National Quality Measures Clearinghouse. (2014). *Uses of quality measures*. http://www.qualitymeasures.ahrq.gov /tutorial/using.aspx

American Association of Colleges of Nursing. (2006). *The essentials of doctor of nursing educator for professional nursing practice*. Author.

American Association of Colleges of Nursing. (2008). *The essentials of baccalaureate education for professional nursing practice*. Author.

American Association of Colleges of Nursing. (2011). *The essentials of masters education for professional nursing practice*. Author.

American Association of Colleges of Nursing. (2021). *The essentials: Core competencies for professional nursing education*. Author.

Andre, B., & Sjovold, E. (2017). What characterizes the work culture at a hospital unit that successfully implements change—a correlation study. *BMC Health Services Research, 17*(486). https://doi .org/10.1186/s12913-017-2436-4

Austin, R., & LaFlamme, A. (2021). Information systems/technology and patient care technology for the improvement and transformation of healthcare. In M. Zaccagnini & M. Pechacek (Eds.), *The doctor of nursing practice essentials: A new model for advanced practice nursing* (4th ed.), 111–130. Jones & Bartlett Learning.

Ball, M. J., & Douglas, J. V. (1989). Informatics in professional education. *Methods of Information in Medicine, 28*(4), 250–254. https://doi.org/10.1055/s-0038-1636794

Beal, V. (2014). *Big data*. https://www.webopedia.com/TERM/B/big_data.html

Brown, B., & Hough-Falk, L. (2014). Embarking on performance improvement. *Healthcare Financial Management, 68*(6), 98–103.

Brown, D., Aydin, C., & Donaldson, N. (2008). Quartile dashboards: Translating large data sets into performance improvement priorities. *Journal for Healthcare Quality, 30*(6), 18–30. https://doi .org/10.1111/j.1945-1474.2008.tb01166.x

California HealthCare Foundation and First Consulting Group. (2002). *Report identifies positive impact technology can have on nurse productivity and satisfaction.* https://www.chcf.org/press-release /report-identifies-positive-impact-technology-can-have-on-nurse-productivity-and-satisfaction

Centers for Medicare and Medicaid Services. (2020). *HCAHPS: Patients' perspectives of care survey.* https://www.cms.gov/Medicare/Quality-Initiatives-Patient-Assessment-Instruments/Hospital QualityInits/HospitalHCAHPS

Cipriano, P. F. (2014). What we measure, we can improve. *The American Nurse.* http://www .theamericannurse.org/2015/01/05/what-we-measure-we-can-improve

Clark, J., & Lang, N. (1992). Nursing's next advance: An internal classification for nursing practice. *International Nursing Review, 39*(4), 109–111, 128. PMID: 1517047.

Datsenko, Y., & Schenk, J. (2013). Leading clinical projects. *Applied Clinical Trials Online, 22*(1), 22–28. http://pph-plus.com/sites/pph-plus.com/files/pictures/2013-01-28_act_leading_clinical _projects.pdf

Davies, A., Mueller, J., & Moulton, G. (2020). *Core competencies for clinical informaticians: A systematic review.* Elsevier. https://doi.org/10.1016/j.ijmedinf.2020.104237

DeLaune, S. C., & Ladner, P. K. (2009). *Fundamentals of nursing standards and practice* (3rd ed.). Delmar Cengage Learning.

Deloitte Insights. (2020). *Tech Trends 2020.* https://www2.deloitte.com/content/dam/Deloitte/cz /Documents/technology/DI_TechTrends2020.pdf

Donabedian, A. (1978). The quality of medical care. *Science, 4344,* 856–864. https://doi .org/10.1126/science.417400

Fox, S. (2011, February 28). Peer-to-peer health care. *Pew Research Center.* http://www.pewinternet .org/2011/02/28/peer-to-peer-health-care-2

Gallagher, T. (2012, October 8). The role of informatics in project management. *HIMSS Clinical Informatics Insights.* http://s3.amazonaws.com/rdcms-himss/files/production/public/newsletters /ClinicalInformatics/201210_CII.pdf

Geary, M., & Clanton, C. (2011). Developing metrics that support projects and programs. In J. Harris, L. Roussel, S. Walters, & C. Dearman, *Project planning and management: A guide for CNLs, DNPs, and nurse executives,* 119–145. Jones & Bartlett Learning.

Geibert, R. C. (2017). The information revolution: Using data and technology to support patient care. In S. Davidson, D. Weberg, T. Porter-O'Grady, & K. Malloch (Eds.), *Leadership for evidence-based innovation in nursing and health professions* (pp. 241–262). Jones & Bartlett Learning.

Grobe, S. J. (1988). Nursing informatics competencies for nurse educators and researchers. In H. Peterson & U. Gerdin-Jelger (Eds.), *Preparing nurses for using information systems: Recommended informatics competencies* (pp. 25–40, 117–138). National League for Nursing.

Grobe, S. J. (1989). Nursing informatics competencies. *Methods of Information in Medicine, 28*(4), 267–269. https://doi.org/10.1055/s-0038-1636804

Hadfield, D., Holmes, S., Kozlowski, S., Sperl, T., & Tapping, D. (2012). *The new lean healthcare pocket guide: Tools for the elimination of waste in hospitals, clinics, and other healthcare facilities.* MCS Media, Inc.

Hall, H., & Roussel, L. (2022). *Evidence-based practice: An integrative approach to research, administration, and practice* (3rd ed.). Jones & Bartlett Learning.

Harris, J., & Thomas, P. (2021). Data as the centerpiece for administrative and clinical decisions. In P. Thomas, J. Harris, & B. Collins, *Data-driven quality improvement and sustainability in healthcare.* Springer Publishing.

Healthcare Information and Management Systems Society. (2011, June 17). *Position statement on transforming nursing practice through technology and informatics.* http://www.himss.org/news /transforming-nursing-practice-through-technology-informatics-0

Henly, S. J. (2014). Mother load and mining tools: Big data for science. *Nursing Research, 63*(3), 155. https://doi.org/10.1097/NNR.0000000000000041

Hoff, T., & Sutcliffe, K. (2006). Studying patient safety in health care organizations: Accentuate the qualitative. *The Joint Commission Journal on Quality and Patient Safety*, 32(1), 5–15. https://doi .org/10.1016/s1553-7250(06)32002-8

Institute of Medicine. (2001). *Crossing the quality chasm: A new health system for the 21st century*. National Academy Press.

Institute of Medicine. (2003). *Health professions education: A bridge to quality*. National Academies Press.

Institute of Medicine. (2011). *The future of nursing: Leading change, advancing health*. National Academies Press.

Kelly, P. (2012). *Nursing leadership and management* (3rd ed.). Delmar.

Ko, C. Y. (2009, November/December). Measuring and improving surgical quality. *Patient Safety and Quality Healthcare*. https://www.psqh.com/analysis/measuring -and-improving-surgical-quality

Kudyba, S. (2021). *Healthcare informatics: Strategies for the digital era*. Auerbach Publishers, Incorporated.

Lewis, A. (2011, November 8). Project management. Part II: What works in nursing informatics? *Advance Web*. http://community.advanceweb.com/blogs/nurses_18/archive/2011/11/08 /project-management-part-ii-what-works-in-nursing-informatics.aspx

Lighter, D. M. (2011). *Advanced performance improvement in health care*. Jones & Bartlett Learning.

Malloch, K., & Porter-O'Grady, T. (2010). *Introduction to evidence-based practice in nursing and health care* (2nd ed.). Jones & Bartlett Learning.

Matney, S., Langford, L., & Staggers, N. (2021). Are nursing informatics competencies good enough? *JBI Evidence Synthesis*, 19(4), 747–748. https://doi.org/10.11124/JBIES-21-00092

McCartney, P. R. (2015). Big data science. *The American Journal of Maternal/Child Nursing*, 40(2), 130. https://doi.org/10.1097/NMC.0000000000000118

Melnyk, B. M., & Fineout-Overholt, E. (2015). *Evidence-based practice in nursing & healthcare: A guide to best practice* (3rd ed.). Wolters Kluwer.

Meyer, M. (2019). Competencies required for healthcare improvement ositions. *International Journal of Health Care Quality Assurance*, 33(1), 281–295. https://doi.org/10.1108/ijhcqa-12-2017-0236

Miake-Lye, I., Delevan, D., Ganz, D., Mittman, B., & Finley, E. (2020). Unpacking organizational readiness for change: An updated systematic review and content analysis of assessments. *BMC Health Services Research*, 20, 1. https://doi.org/10.1186/s12913-020-4926-z

Missel, A., & Thomas, P. (2015). Developing metrics that support projects and programs. In J. Harris, L. Roussel, C. Dearman, & P. Thomas, *Project planning and management: A guide for nurses and interprofessional teams* (2nd ed.). Jones & Bartlett Learning.

National Academies of Sciences, Engineering, and Medicine. (2021). *The future of nursing 2020–2030: Charting a path to achieve health equity*. The National Academies Press. https://doi .org/10.17226/25982

National Quality Forum. (2010). *Safe practices for better care*. https://www.qualityforum.org/News _And_Resources/Press_Kits/Safe_Practices_for_Better_Healthcare.aspx

Nelson, E. C., Batalden, P. B., & Godfrey, M. M. (2007). *Quality by design: A clinical microsystems approach*. Jossey-Bass.

Okes, D., & Westcott, R. (2001). *The certified quality manager handbook*. American Society for Quality Press Publications.

Petersilge, C. (2020). The enterprise imaging value proposition. *Journal of Digital Imaging*, 33(1), 37–48. https://doi.org/10.1007/s10278-019-00293-1

Polit, D., & Beck, C. (2020). *Nursing research: Generating and accessing evidence for nursing practice* (11th ed.). Lippincott Williams & Wilkins.

Porter-O'Grady, T., & Malloch, K. (2015). *Quantum leadership: Building better partnerships for sustainable health*. Jones & Bartlett Learning.

Press Ganey. (2014, June 10). Press Ganey acquires national database of nursing quality indicators (NDNQI®). *PR Newswire*. https://www.prnewswire.com/news-releases/press-ganey -acquires-national-database-of-nursing-quality-indicators-ndnqi-262538811.html

Press Ganey. (2021). About. https://www.pressganey.com/about-us

Radnor, Z., Holweg, M., & Waring, J. (2012). Lean in healthcare: The unfilled promise? *Social Science & Medicine*, 74, 364–371. https://doi.org/10.1016/j.socscimed.2011.02.011

Robert Wood Johnson Foundation & The Institute of Medicine. (2010). *The future of nursing: Leading change, advancing health.* http://www.nationalacademies.org/hmd/Reports/2010/The-Future-of-Nursing-Leading-Change-Advancing-Health.aspx

Schein, E. (2004). *Organizational culture and leadership* (3rd ed.). Jossey-Bass.

Shane, B. (2014). *Informatics planning model essential to maximize the effectiveness of IT in supporting program goals.* https://www.bpcgallery.com/publications/informatics-planning-model/

Shank, G. (2006). *Qualitative research* (2nd ed.). Pearson.

Sheppy, B., Zuliani, J., & McIntosh, B. (2012). Science or art: Risk and project management in healthcare. *British Journal of Healthcare Management, 18*(11), 586–590. http://dx.doi.org/10.12968/bjhc.2012.18.11.586

Shirley, D. (2011). *Project management for healthcare.* CRC Press.

Stevens, K. R., & Staley, J. M. (2006). The quality chasm reports, evidence-based practice, and nursing response to improve healthcare. *Nursing Outlook, 54*(2), 94–101. https://doi.org/10.1016/j.outlook.2005.11.007

The Joint Commission. (2017). *Hospital standards CAMH.* https://www.jointcommission.org/standards_information/hap_requirements.aspx

Thomas, P. (2020). Developing metrics that support projects and programs, interventions, and programs. In J. Harris, L. Roussel, C. Dearman, & P. Thomas, *Project planning and management: A guide for nurses and interprofessional teams* (3rd ed.). Jones & Bartlett Learning.

Thomas, P., & Bleich, M. (2020). Measuring the value of projects within organizations, healthcare systems, and globally. In J. Harris, L. Roussel, C. Dearman, & P. Thomas, *Project planning and management: A guide for nurses and interprofessional teams* (3rd ed.). Jones & Bartlett Learning.

Thomas, P., & Collins, B. (2021). Selecting the right tools for the job: From idea to execution. In P. Thomas, J. Harris, & B. Collins, *Data-driven quality improvement and sustainability in healthcare: An interprofessional approach,* 171–188. Springer Publishing.

Thomas, P., Harris, J., & Collins, B. (2021). *Data-driven quality improvement and sustainability in healthcare: An interprofessional approach.* Springer Publishing.

Welton, J., Sables-Baus, S., & Kleiner, C. (2020). Improvement and big data. I G. Armstrong & S. Sables-Baus, *Leadership and systems improvement for the DNP.* Springer Publishing.

Westcott, R. (2013). *The certified manager of quality: Organizational excellence handbook* (4th ed.). American Society for Quality Press Publications.

Williams, T., & Geary, M. (1997). *Improving nursing performance.* Precept Press.

CHAPTER 10

The Institutional Review Board Process

Catherine Dearman
Dionne Roberts
Lolita Chappel-Aiken

CHAPTER OBJECTIVES

1. Examine the process for initiating and completing the institutional review board (IRB) process—the when, why, and how to navigate the process.
2. Formulate a methodology featuring initiating and completing the IRB process.
3. Differentiate the IRB process and outcomes for quality improvement projects and research.
4. Propose the strategies involved in implementation and evaluation of the project once IRB and institutional review processes are complete.

KEY TERMS

Human-subject protection
Human subjects
Implementation and evaluation of
   projects

Informed consent
Institutional review board (IRB)
Quality improvement projects versus
   research

ROLES

Participant
Researcher

Reviewer

PROFESSIONAL VALUES

Beneficence
Quality

Respect for persons
Social justice

CORE COMPETENCIES

Analysis	Development
Communication	Evaluation
Design	Implementation

Introduction

This chapter reviews the role of the institutional review board (IRB) in an organization and describes the basic process used in the review of a study or quality improvement project. The IRB is integral to the protection of human subjects and connecting those subjects to the protocols and safeguards included in completing an IRB application. Organizations sponsoring research and other scholarly work must consider the impact of that work on human subjects and be able to determine whether information gleaned from the work can be generalized to the public. Therefore, IRB approval should be secured before any data collection for research and quality improvement projects. Following the approval from the IRB and the internal institutional requirements, the next essential step is the implementation and evaluation of the processes and outcomes.

The IRB is composed of a representative group of faculty and staff within an institution who are experienced in research processes and thoroughly understand how the rights of subjects in the research are protected. The IRB reviews all research and many quality improvement protocols involving human subjects before their implementation, to assure that subjects' human rights are protected. In many cases, IRB approval is a basic requirement to publication of the findings, including those from quality improvement projects. In addition to an IRB review, many institutions have internal quality controls that must be addressed before data collection and ongoing throughout the implementation and evaluation. Those internal controls are individual to the organization and are consistent with the inherent institutional goals and values. Completing the IRB does not preclude these institutional requirements.

Inherent in the IRB review is the independent nature of the review and the reviewers—that is, researchers do not review their own work; instead, independent members of the IRB review each submission. In some cases, more than one IRB will need to be involved in the review of the research, especially if the university is not connected to the clinical facility where the research will occur.

Regardless of the project that is identified, the initial step is to complete a needs assessment, analyze the data, and assimilate data as background support when building the business case. However, one cannot dismiss the need to obtain IRB approval if the data or outcomes of a project will be disseminated beyond the immediate organization or system. Securing IRB approval at the beginning of the project limits future issues.

Historical Perspective Related to Protection of Human Subjects

The Federal Policy for the Protection of Human Subjects requires universities or other institutions that receive federal funds and conduct biomedical or behavioral research involving human subjects to establish an institutional review process.

The "Common Rule," as the policy is widely known, requires a research institution to assure the protection of the human rights of human subjects who participate in research. The institution is bound by law, then, to assure that all researchers follow this rule with regard to selecting subjects and obtaining informed consent from them (U.S. Department of Health and Human Services [DHHS], 2016a).

IRBs emerged based on principles included in the Nuremberg Code (U.S. GPO, 1949), the Declaration of Helsinki (World Medical Association, 2008), and the Belmont Report (National Commission for the Protection of Human Subjects of Biomedical and Behavioral Research, 1979). These documents define the minimum codes for conducting research with human beings, as well as the ethical principles of beneficence, respect, and justice, which form the basis for all human research endeavors. The concept of beneficence assures that the study is structured in such a way that it will benefit—and not harm—the subjects. Researchers must then address the risks and benefits inherent in the research for all participants. Respect for persons and their right to choose to participate or not, as well as their right to cease participation at any point, is addressed through the informed consent process. Justice addresses the potential for all persons to be included in the study; no single person or group—and particularly not a vulnerable person or group—can be singled out to receive benefits or harm from the research (National Commission for the Protection of Human Subjects of Biomedical and Behavioral Research, 1979).

What is a human subject? Human subjects are living participants who are working with one or more researchers who are studying a phenomenon to acquire data by involvement (can be via distance; not required to be face-to-face) or data that can be used to distinguish one phenomenon from another.

The History of the Human-Subjects' Protection System

Human-subject protection began with the Nuremberg Code, which was developed for the Nuremberg Military Tribunal as a standard against which to judge the human experimentation conducted by the Nazis during World War II. The Nuremberg Code captures many of what are now taken to be the basic principles governing the ethical conduct of research involving human subjects. Its first provision states that "the voluntary consent of the human subject is absolutely essential" (U.S. GPO, 1949). Freely given consent to participate in research is the cornerstone of ethical experimentation involving human subjects. The Nuremberg Code also provides the details implied by such a requirement—namely, capacity to consent, freedom from coercion, and comprehension of the risks and benefits involved. Other provisions require that risk and harm be minimized, that the risk/benefit ratio be determined and shared with the potential subjects of the research, that qualified investigators use appropriate research designs, and that subjects have the freedom to withdraw at any time.

Similar recommendations were made by the World Medical Association in its *Declaration of Helsinki: Recommendations Guiding Medical Doctors in Biomedical Research Involving Human Subjects*, first adopted by the 18th World Medical Assembly in Helsinki, Finland, in 1964 and subsequently revised by the 29th World Medical Assembly, Tokyo, Japan, 1975, and by the 41st World Medical Assembly, Hong Kong, 1989 (World Medical Association, 2008). The Declaration of Helsinki further distinguishes therapeutic from nontherapeutic research (Steneck, 2007).

In the United States, regulations protecting human subjects first became effective on May 30, 1974. These regulations were promulgated by the Department of Health, Education and Welfare (DHEW) and raised to regulatory status in 1966 as the National Institutes of Health's (NIH) Policies for the Protection of Human Subjects. The regulations established the IRB as one mechanism through which human subjects could be protected.

In July 1974, the National Commission for the Protection of Human Subjects of Biomedical and Behavioral Research was established. The Commission met from 1974 to 1978 and issued reports identifying the basic ethical principles that should underlie the conduct of biomedical and behavioral research involving human subjects and recommending guidelines to ensure that research is conducted in accordance with those principles. Its report setting forth the basic ethical principles that should underlie the conduct of biomedical and behavioral research involving human subjects is titled *The Belmont Report: Ethical Principles and Guidelines for the Protection of Human Subjects of Research*. The Belmont Report, which is named after the Belmont Conference Center at the Smithsonian Institution, sets forth the basic ethical principles underlying the acceptable conduct of research involving human subjects. Those principles—respect for persons, beneficence, and justice—are now accepted as the three quintessential requirements for the ethical conduct of research involving human subjects and are discussed in the text that follows:

- *Respect for persons* involves a researcher and their team recognizing the personal dignity and autonomy of individuals and providing for special protection of those persons with diminished autonomy.
- *Beneficence* entails an obligation to protect persons from harm by maximizing anticipated benefits and minimizing possible risks of harm.
- *Justice* requires that the benefits and burdens of research be distributed fairly (National Commission for the Protection of Human Subjects of Biomedical and Behavioral Research, 1979).

The Belmont Report also describes how these principles apply to the conduct of research. Specifically, the principle of respect for persons underlies the need to obtain informed consent, the principle of beneficence underlies the need to engage in a risk/benefit analysis and to minimize risks, and the principle of justice requires that subjects be fairly selected. As was mandated by the congressional charge to the National Commission, the Belmont Report also provides a distinction between "practice" and "research." The text of the Belmont Report is thus divided into two sections: (1) boundaries between practice and research and (2) basic ethical principles (DHHS, 2010).

The DHHS regulations are codified at Title 45 Part 46 of the Code of Federal Regulations and became final on January 16, 1981; these regulations were revised effective March 4, 1983, and June 18, 1991. The 1991 revision involved the adoption of the Federal Policy for the Protection of Human Subjects. The Federal Policy ("Common Rule") was promulgated by the 16 federal agencies that conduct, support, or otherwise regulate human-subjects research; the Food and Drug Administration (FDA) also adopted certain provisions. The Federal Policy is designed to make the human-subjects protection system uniform in all relevant federal agencies and departments. Additional protections for various vulnerable populations have been adopted by the DHHS reflecting vulnerable populations such as pregnant women (August 8, 1975; revised January 11, 1978, and November 3, 1978), prisoners (November 16, 1978), and children (March 8, 1983, and revised June 18, 1991) (DHHS, 2010).

An account of the history of human-subjects research and the human-subjects protection system in the United States can be found in Rothman's *Strangers at the Bedside: A History of How Law and Bioethics Transformed Medical Decision Making* and in Maloney's *Protection of Human Research Subjects*. Rothman details the abuses to which human subjects were exposed, culminating in Beecher's 1966 article, "Ethics and Clinical Research," published in the *New England Journal of Medicine*, and ultimately contributing to the impetus for the first NIH and FDA regulations (Fain, 2009).

Definition of Research

Research is a "diligent and systematic inquiry or investigation into a subject in order to discover or revise facts, theories, applications . . ." (Research, n.d.). The intent to publish findings is generally considered as contributing to generalizable knowledge. An investigation, then, must meet certain criteria to be classified as research. Research studies are designed in an organized, logical process that can support a range of goals, from basic scientific inquiry to a qualitative research study of a specified group. Research processes, measurement, assessment, and data collection are required elements of the study itself. Essentially, research is completed in a manner that will allow findings, experiences, or understandings gleaned from the work to be generalized to the broader population. Some research involves rodents, larger animals, or even primates. These studies are evaluated differently than research involving human subjects. When humans are involved, the research processes and procedures that include consent forms and the issue of informed consent must be evaluated by an IRB (DHHS, 2010).

The research project is usually described in a formal protocol that sets forth an objective and a set of procedures designed to reach that objective. The Belmont Report recognizes that "experimental" procedures do not necessarily constitute research, and that research and practice may occur simultaneously. It suggests that the safety and effectiveness of such "experimental" procedures should be investigated early, and that institutional oversight mechanisms, such as medical practice committees, can ensure that this need is met by requiring that "major innovation[s] be incorporated into a formal research project" (National Commission for the Protection of Human Subjects of Biomedical and Behavioral Research, 1979).

Boundaries Between Practice and Research

Why discuss IRBs when quality improvement processes and quality assessments are the foci for most clinical nurse leaders (CNLs), nurse executives, doctor of nursing practice (DNP) candidates, and other clinical doctorate students? If the IRB is predominantly focused on the ethical conduct of research, then why should quality improvement projects be reviewed by the IRB? After all, quality improvement is not research, is it? Although recognizing that the distinction between research and therapy is often blurred, practice is described as interventions that are designed solely to enhance the well-being of an individual patient or client and that have a reasonable expectation of success. The purpose of medical or behavioral practice, then, is to provide diagnosis, preventive treatment, or therapy to particular individuals.

Ultimately, patients are the focus of quality improvement/process improvement projects, and their rights must be protected (Speers, 2008); the IRB process offers that protection. Similarly, community needs assessments can impact individuals and populations; thus, their protection is also warranted.

Quality improvement activities are widely regarded as critical to the effort to reduce healthcare errors and improve patient outcomes. Most can be readily distinguished from research; however, some cannot (Speers, 2008). The issue for students in nurse executive, CNL, and DNP programs is that they are not generating new knowledge; instead, they are testing and translating research findings into practice and the care of patients. To share with colleagues a project's success in improving quality of care, results are published, which brings quality improvement projects into the realm of review by the IRB.

In 2007, national attention was brought to the impact of quality improvement studies on patient care. In turn, many healthcare professionals became involved in heated arguments about the differences between research and quality improvement. For example, a major care provider implemented a checklist for insertion of large intravenous (IV) lines in patients. As a part of this checklist, providers were reminded to wash their hands before the procedure and to wear sterile gloves and a gown. Within 3 months, IV line infection rates fell precipitously, resulting in a simultaneous reduction in costs for the provider. However, because the checklist was determined to be an intervention that impacted patients and no consent had been obtained from those patients, the Office of Human Research Protection closed down the program. This was done despite the benign nature of the intervention and the significantly positive outcomes realized for patients.

As a result of these events, more attention is now being paid to process and quality improvement projects, which drive the review of projects by IRBs. The problem that most students and project managers face with regard to completion of the application to the IRB for projects is that the application uses research language, not quality improvement language. Students frequently attempt, in error, to reconcile quality improvement projects with research language, such as describing an experimental design when presenting an intervention.

The information that IRB members need with regard to quality improvement projects is generally confined to the "W" questions and answers: What will be done? Who will do it? Who will be involved in it? When will it be done (include stages)? Where will it be done, and how will it impact processes in the location(s)? Why is it necessary (include the potential impact on practice and improving health care)? In addition to these questions, the researcher/project manager needs to answer the "How" questions: How will the project unfold? How long will it take? How will the impact be measured? Clarity is essential in the application process; students and faculty should seek help on an as-needed basis.

Applying the Ethical Principles to Both Research and Quality Improvement

The responsible conduct of research (RCR) requires investigators involved in any level of the research to complete basic training in the protection of human subjects. Scholarship in the health sciences requires a clear understanding of the ethics involved in conducting research. This basic training can be obtained through the NIH or the Collaborative Institutional Training Initiative (CITI) modules (NIH, 2018).

Respect for Persons

RCR training addresses the ethical principles of respect for persons. Informed consent to participate in research or a quality improvement project is required by the ethical principle of "respect for persons." It includes three elements: information, comprehension, and voluntariness.

First, potential subjects must be given sufficient information to be able to decide whether to participate, including the research procedures, their purposes, risks and anticipated benefits, alternative procedures (where therapy is involved), and a statement offering the subject the opportunity to ask questions and to withdraw at any time from the research. Incomplete disclosure is justified only if it is clear that: (1) the goals of the research cannot be accomplished if full disclosure is made; (2) the undisclosed risks are minimal; and (3) when appropriate, subjects will be debriefed and provided with the research results.

Second, subjects must be able to comprehend the information that is given to them. The presentation of information must be adapted to the subject's capacity to understand it; researchers may be required to test potential subjects to assure they understand. Where persons with limited ability to comprehend are involved, they should be given the opportunity to choose whether to participate (to the extent they are able to do so), and their objections should not be overridden. Each such class of persons should be considered on its own terms (e.g., minors, persons with impaired mental capacities, the terminally ill, and the comatose).

Third, consent to participate must be voluntarily given. The conditions under which an agreement to participate is made must be free from coercion and undue influence. IRBs are especially sensitive to these factors when particularly vulnerable subjects are involved.

Beneficence

The principle of beneficence addresses risk/benefit assessments and includes information on the probability and potential magnitude of possible harms and benefits. Researchers must define the nature and scope of the risks and benefits while systematically assessing them. All possible harms—not just physical or psychological pain or injury—should be considered. The principle of beneficence requires both protecting individual subjects against risk of harm and considering not only the benefits for the individual but also the societal benefits that might be gained from the research.

Justice

The principle of justice mandates that the process used to select research subjects must be fair and must result in fair selection outcomes. The "justness" of subject selection relates both to the subject as an individual and to the subject as a member of social, racial, sexual, or ethnic groups.

With respect to their status as individuals, researchers need to assure that certain persons (poor, racial or ethnic minorities, or those who are institutionalized) are not selected simply because they are available or their circumstances are easily manipulated (NIH, Office of Extramural Research, 2018).

Informed Consent

The process of assuring that the participants in research or quality improvement projects are aware of their rights and the three primary principles of respect for persons, beneficence, and justice is termed *informed consent*. Informed consent documents must present the information clearly and in readily understandable language without esoteric terms or convoluted sentence structure or word use.

The two primary elements to be addressed in the informed consent process are the provision of complete information about the study/project and the understanding of the participant regarding that information. Providing information alone is not sufficient to meet the standard of informed consent—the participant must also fully understand what they are agreeing to as a part of the study/project.

Some key elements of informed consent were discussed previously in relation to respect for persons, beneficence, and justice. However, some populations may be fully informed and voice understanding yet not truly understand. Such may be the case with individuals with low literacy, for example. Options for assisting those with low literacy skills include reading the consent form for the participant and allowing sufficient time for the participant to consult with another individual, such as a family member or clergy.

Another special case arises with children who participate in research/projects. Parents must provide consent for all minors participating in research. The children, too, must give permission (assent) to be involved in the study. In cases where higher risks are associated, the researcher may be required to obtain assent from the child as well as consent from both parents.

Typically, informed consent takes the form of a signed, written document. However, a waiver of written informed consent can be approved if the presence of a signed document could increase the risk associated with participation. It is significant to note that the waiver, if used, applies only to the signed written document; it does not apply to the actual process of informing the participants.

Informed consent is as essential in quality improvement projects as in research studies. Any participant in any organized project must be afforded their rights, including informed consent.

Institutional Review Board Processes and Procedures

Having to complete an IRB application can appear to be quite complicated and off-putting, but the process actually is straightforward and procedurally oriented. When one considers that the overall purpose of the IRB is to protect human subjects, the process becomes fairly benign.

IRB reviewers look for clear explanations of what will be done, who will do it, when it will be done, and how it will be done so that the board members can determine if the project requires full board review or is eligible for expedited or exempt status. A clear understanding of the intent of the project is critical to the IRB review process. The discussion that follows highlights some ways to respond to the nature of the question without categorizing the quality improvement project in research terms while assuring ready understanding by IRB review teams. Some of the areas of the application are readily discernable, and others take a bit more information.

The remainder of this section provides details on the information needed to complete an IRB application. The basic processes the application will follow during the staged review are also addressed.

Research Purpose

Typically, the researcher needs to provide a brief description of the intent of the project. This section is basically the same for research studies or quality improvement projects. The applicant needs to answer the question: What is the problem, and which impacts will the proposed research/project have?

Subject or Population

Who will be involved in the project and how? To which population will the results be generalizable? Again, this section is the same for research studies or for quality improvement projects, even though findings from quality improvement studies are not typically considered to be generalizable to larger populations because of agency variations. Basically, the information presented must allow investigators, institutions, or IRBs to determine if the proposed methods of selecting participants could result in unjust distributions of the burdens and benefits of research. For example, subjects should not be selected simply because they are readily available in settings where research is conducted or because they are "easy to manipulate as a result of their illness or socioeconomic condition" (DHHS, 2010).

Design of the Study

This section is very different for research studies and quality improvement projects. The applicant will need to provide enough information for reviewers to determine if the design fits the purpose and has the potential to yield the anticipated outcomes.

For research studies, the discussion of study design should address the overall nature of the study—experimental, quasi-experimental, descriptive, or mixed methods. Applicants must provide specific aims that the research will address and explain how the design will facilitate achieving those aims. Some indication of the underlying quantitative or qualitative focus is included.

For quality improvement studies, the quality improvement design must be linked to the project and to the project site as well as to the quantitative and/or qualitative nature of the project. Some typical quality improvement designs are the FADE model (focus, analyze, develop, and execute), PDSA (plan–do–study–act), and Six Sigma. Six Sigma actually encompasses two different models: DMAIC (define–measure–analyze–improve–control) and DMADV (define–measure–analyze–design–verify), which are used for existing and new processes, respectively. The basic premise is the same regardless of which design is specified: Reviewers must know how the project will be conducted.

Privacy and Confidentiality

How will the researcher protect the information collected? Will participants be recognizable? Will responses be linked to participants? How and where will the data be stored? Who will have access? This last issue is particularly relevant to staff or patient participants who may fear retribution if they answer questions truthfully. In quality improvement projects, participant pools are typically smaller and site-specific. The researcher must carefully assure that the privacy of all participants is protected.

Inclusion/Exclusion Criteria

How will the researcher determine the eligibility of participants? The applicant must describe the processes and procedures used in determining who is eligible to participate in the research/project versus who is not eligible. The researcher will also need to ensure that the issue of vulnerability is addressed. Frequently, quality improvement projects do not include children or other vulnerable populations, although that is not a hard-and-fast rule. Consequently, the researcher must describe inclusion and exclusion criteria comprehensively. If a population or subgroup is excluded for any reason, the application must clearly address those criteria. The researcher must be aware that the IRB application may require a stipulation whether or not any vulnerable population is included.

Risks and Benefits from Participation

Even if they are minimal, the researcher needs to address all risks and benefits to the participant, actual or potential, including physical and psychological risks and benefits, inconvenience, and loss of privacy. If subjects will be paid to participate in the research, the amount of payment and the restrictions on the payment need to be explained in detail. With regard to risks and benefits, more attention is generally paid to the risks than to the benefits. Therefore, the IRB members must independently assess the risk to the participants to determine if they agree with the risk assessment in the application. Additionally, the IRB must determine the type, probability, and extent of the risk as much as possible. It must determine if the researcher's estimates of harm or benefit to participants are reasonable, given the facts and results of other studies.

Five basic principles apply to risk/benefit assessment:

1. "Brutal or inhumane treatment of human subjects is never morally justified."
2. Risks should be minimized, including the avoidance of using human subjects if at all possible.
3. IRBs must be scrupulous in insisting on sufficient justification for research involving "significant risk of serious impairment" (direct benefit to the subject or "manifest voluntariness of the participation").

4. The appropriateness of involving vulnerable populations must be demonstrated.
5. The proposed informed consent process must thoroughly and completely disclose relevant risks and benefits (IRBNet, 2012).

If the researcher or project manager offers compensation to participants, the IRB must also be cognizant of the amount and impact of that compensation. Is the compensation commensurate with the participation? Could the amount of compensation affect an individual's participation to the extent that it affects the outcomes of the project/research?

Outcomes

The researcher must describe how the findings will be used. Are the findings sufficient to propose a change in policy or practice, or will more research be needed with different groups, under different circumstances, or some other criterion?

For quality improvement projects, will the project potentially change practice? How might that change occur? Whom will the change affect?

Informed Consent Form

A copy of the informed consent document is included in the packet provided to the IRB so that an assessment can be made with regard to the accuracy of information shared with participants and the reading level required to ensure true understanding.

Levels of Institutional Review Board Reviews

The IRB has the authority to approve or not approve research and/or quality improvement projects (Fain, 2009). IRB reviews occur on three distinct levels depending on the degree to which the study is considered to constitute potential harm or violation of one or more ethical principles. Those three levels are full review, expedited, and exempt (Polit & Beck, 2020). An applicant can request a specific level of review, but the final decision regarding that level rests with the IRB staff and committee.

The full review process requires that a full IRB committee, including scientific, nonscientific, and community members, evaluate the study. All members of the IRB read, consider, and evaluate each study. Primary and secondary reviewers are stipulated to present the salient facts of the study to the full board, including all components of human-subject protection. The researcher maintains responsibility for the RCR, even with a full board review. A full board review is typically reserved for studies with inherent risks to participants. Examples of studies that fit this criterion are those focused on sensitive topics such as race, ethnicity, and sexual behaviors; studies focused on vulnerable populations; and clinical trials, especially related to medication regimens.

Expedited reviews are reserved for studies in which "minimal" exposure to risk is projected. Minimal risk is defined as the participants being at no greater risk than they could encounter as a part of daily life. Expedited reviews are typically conducted by one or two members of the IRB committee and are reported at the IRB meeting but not discussed there. Many quality improvement projects qualify for an expedited review, as they constitute minimal risk to subjects.

An exempt review designation is typically reserved for studies where no human subjects are involved or for studies where there is no risk to humans. Typically, exempt studies include situations where subjects cannot be identified, secondary review of existing data, studies in which data are gathered through observation of public behavior, and anonymous surveys (DHHS, 2010).

Multiple Institutional Review Boards

In most research studies, a single IRB is responsible for assuring compliance with human-subject protection. Typically, this review board exists within the primary agency/institution that maintains responsibility for the project. Once approval is obtained from this review board, evidence of that approval is provided to other partner agencies.

In the case of quality improvement projects, however, multiple IRBs may be indicated. The primary agency/institution's IRB is typically approached first. Clinical agencies where the project will be implemented may assert the need to file a separate application through their on-site IRB. This practice is becoming more commonplace as more clinical agencies have established IRBs.

Implementation and Evaluation of Outcomes

Following the successful IRB review and approval of internal institutional requirements, the project or research can be implemented and evaluated. This process is critical to the nature of the research and/or project and the protocols described in the previous sections must be scrupulously followed. Sabatier (1986) described the state of the science related to implementation research. Curran et al. (2012) advanced the idea that strengthening implementation science can contribute to the integration of findings into practice, improve clinical effectiveness, and promote high-quality patient outcomes. Implementation facilitates generation of knowledge regarding the "what, why, and how" the intervention works in real-world settings and promotes an integrated approach to improve public health (Peters et al., 2013, p. 1).

Summary

- This chapter has provided an overview of the role of the institutional review board (IRB) in an organization, a review of the basic processes involved in the review of a study or project, and methods involved in the protection of human subjects.
- The IRB is the primary mechanism used by institutions to ensure the protection of human subjects through informed consent, justice, beneficence, and

respect for persons. The IRB also reviews quality improvement studies to ensure that human subjects are protected.

- Researchers must be aware of the IRB policies within their institutions and be prepared to complete the processes to ensure the protection of the persons involved in their research.
- Project implementation is integral to use of findings in practice and determining impact on health outcomes.

Reflection Questions

1. Which institutional criteria are used to review an IRB application?
2. What differentiates a quality improvement project from research?

References

Beecher, H. K. (1966). Ethics and clinical research. *New England Journal of Medicine* 274, 1354–1360.

Collaborative Institutional Training Initiative (CITI Program). CITIprogram.org.

Curran, G. M., Bauer, M., Mittman, B., Pyne, J., & Stetler, C. (2012). Effectiveness and implementation of hybrid designs: Combining elements of clinical effectiveness and implementation research to enhance public health impact. *Medical Care*, 50, 217–226. https://doi.org/10.1097/mlr.0b013e3182408812

Fain, J. A. (2009). *Reading, understanding, and applying nursing research* (3rd ed.). F. A. Davis.

IRBNet. (2012). *Innovative solutions for compliance and research management.* https://www.irbnet.org

Maloney, D. M. (1984). *Protection of human research subjects.* Springer.

National Commission for the Protection of Human Subjects of Biomedical and Behavioral Research. (1979). *The Belmont report: Ethical principles and guidelines for the protection of human subjects of research.* http://www.fda.gov/ohrms/dockets/ac/05/briefing/2005-4178b_09_02 _Belmont%20Report.pdf

National Institutes of Health, Office of Extramural Research. (2018). *Protecting human research participants.* http://phrp.nihtraining.cm/users/login.php

Peters, D. H., Adam, T., Alonge, O., Agyepong, I. A., & Tran, N. (2013). https://doi.org/10.1136/bmj

Polit, D. F., & Beck, C. T. (2020). *Nursing research: Generating and assessing evidence for nursing practice* (11th ed.). Lippincott Williams & Wilkins.

Research. (n.d.). *Dictionary.com.* http://www.dictionary.reference.com/browse/research?s=t

Rothman, D. J. (2017). A history of how law and bioethics transformed medical decision making. https://doi.org/10.4324/9781315130286

Sabatier, P. A. (1986). Top down and bottom-up approaches to implementation research. *Journal of Public Policy*, 6(1), 21–48. https://doi.org/ 10.1017/S0143814X00003846

Speers, M. A. (2008). Editorial: Quality improvement: Research or non-research? AAHRPP perspective. *Association for the Accreditation of Human Research Protection Programs, Advance*, 5(2), 1–2.

Steneck, N. H. (2007). *ORI: Introduction to the responsible conduct of research.* https://ori.hhs.gov/ori-introduction-responsible-conduct-research

U.S. Department of Health and Human Services. (2010). *Guidance on IRB continuing review of research.* http://www.hhs.gov/ohrp/policy/continuingreview2010.html

U.S. Department of Health and Human Services. (2016a). *Institutional review board written procedures: Guidance for institutions and IRBs.* https://www.hhs.gov/ohrp/regulations-and-policy

U.S. Department of Health and Human Services. (2016b). *The federal policy for human subject protections ('Common Rule').* http://www.hhs.gov/ohrp/regulations-and-policy/regulations/common-rule/index.html

U.S. Department of Health and Human Services. (2017). *ANPRM for revision to common rule.* https://www.hhs.gov/ohrp/regulations-and-policy/regulations/anprm-for-revision-to-common-rule/index.html

U.S. Food and Drug Administration. (2019). *Institutional review boards (IRBs) and protection of human subjects in clinical trials.* https://fda.gov/about-fda/center-drug-evaluation-and-research-cder /institutional-review-boards-irbs-and-protection-human-subjects-clinical-trials

U.S. Government Printing Office. (1949). *Trials of war criminals before the Nuremberg military tribunals under control council law, 10*(2), 181–182. https://history.nih.gov/research /downloads /nuremberg.pdf

World Medical Association. (2008). *World Medical Association Declaration of Helsinki: Ethical principles for medical research involving human subjects.* https://www.wma.net/policies-post /wma-declaration-of-helsinki-ethical-principles-for-medical-research-involving-human-subjects

Case Exemplars

Vulnerable Population

Dionne Roberts

A DNP student proposed implementing a practice change intervention to increase the vaccination of preteen/adolescent patients with the human papillomavirus (HPV) vaccination. The change will involve a deliberate discussion regarding HPV prevention at each office visit, including sick visits, and will involve the nursing staff, the preteen/adolescent patient, and a parent. The participant will be between 11 and 18 years of age. The DNP student will develop written and verbal information to be shared with all eligible patients and their parents and will be available to discuss options directly at the time of the visit. The nursing staff will inform the DNP student when eligible patients arrive and will notify the patients/parents that someone will come to discuss a potential study with them. The information sharing discussion will require the DNP student to discuss, briefly, the relationship of sexual activity and HPV with the possible participants. The intervention will require the revision of the Centers for Disease Control and Prevention (CDC) HPV fact sheet to be discussed in 5 minutes with allocated time for questions. An HPV knowledge instrument will be used before and after the intervention.

Reflection Questions

1. With this type of DNP project, would this proposal require an expedited or full IRB review?
2. Will this project require an assent from the preteen/adolescent as well as an informed consent from the parent?
3. Can the DNP student speak with the preteen/adolescent without the parent?
4. In reviewing this proposed project, would you offer any specific advice to the DNP student regarding the information to be shared or the approach to be used?

Institutional Review Board Application for Quality Improvement Project

Dionne Roberts

The IRB application for a research study and for a DNP/CNL/nurse executive project will have similarities and differences. Specifically, the project application will require information on the clinical mentor, stakeholders, resources, and quality improvement efforts. The application itself must remain intact; therefore, the student must incorporate the additional information into the existing format, which can be challenging. The use of a PICOT (population, intervention, comparison, outcome, and time) rather than a research question may also be challenging for the IRB member who is not familiar with the practice-focused quality improvement projects. Review the IRB template—the quality improvement project IRB application may not include the SWOT (strengths, weaknesses, opportunities, and threats) analysis as part of the literature review. However, the methodology is important, and the full description of the quality improvement project is critical to the review.

Reflection Questions

1. Why is an IRB needed for a quality improvement project if all the sections of the application do not apply?
2. How does the IRB application for a quality improvement project address the protection of human subjects?
3. What strategies can the DNP/CNL/nurse executive student use to assure the accurate completion of the IRB application for a quality improvement project?

The Capstone Project: An Experiential and Transformative Process

Theodora Ledford

Differentiating quality projects from research often challenges students to ensure that the objective of the project is met and any impact on human-subjects' protection is determined. Upon completing a microsystem needs assessment and engaging in dialogue with the IRB, it was established that the CNL project was needed to obtain information that supported nursing quality improvement data. Data gleaned from the project would be useful for detecting trends in and patterns of performance that affected more than the identified microsystem. Data collected would be utilized in the development of action plans in collaboration with other practice committees concerning nurse-sensitive indicators directed at quality, safe, and efficient patient outcomes. Additionally, data could engender interprofessional collaboration, opportunities to monitor and evaluate compliance with standards, recommendations to enhance continuous quality improvements, and the spread of safety initiatives throughout the healthcare system.

Although the capstone project started initially as an outcomes-based endeavor where differentiating quality improvement from research was of foremost importance, the transformative processes that followed were valuable. The experience culminated in thoughts of how unit-based quality nursing councils could use data to create more solid structures and processes. As a result, an innovative environment was envisioned where professional practice would flourish and the mission, vision, and values would come to life. This notion can become a reality. However, during dialogue with colleagues and quality improvement staff, a fundamental action was needed—namely, the development of a guide for other nurses to understand the differences between quality improvement projects and research and the steps necessary for accomplishing meaningful and value-added quality projects that are patient-centric and advance care delivery. Steps are in process for the action to become reality.

Reflection Questions

1. Which individual challenges do students confront when completing IRB applications for universities and clinical agencies?
2. How might students create opportunities from challenges associated with quality improvement and research endeavors?

CHAPTER 11

Big Data and Information Systems: Understanding the Value for Improvement Projects

James L. Harris
Todd Harlan
Lonnie K. Williams

CHAPTER OBJECTIVES

1. Define big data and information systems within the context of project improvement value.
2. Discuss how big data and information systems facilitate improvement and its sustainability.
3. Recognize the importance of stakeholder involvement and partnerships when developing information systems and the management of big data.
4. Justify the importance of the five Vs of big data to outcomes measurement and continuous improvement.
5. Examine the importance of data integrity, accuracy, and relevance of information systems for future improvement priorities.

KEY TERMS

Big data
Continuous improvement
Critical success factor (CSF)
Data accuracy and integrity
Facilitator
Five Vs of big data (volume, variety, velocity, veracity, value)
Improvement

Information systems and technology
Knowledge
Management
Outcomes
Partnership
Privacy
Relevance
Security

Small data   Sustainability
Stakeholder   Value

ROLES

Collaborator   Partner
Educator   Team member
Leader

PROFESSIONAL VALUES

Advocacy   Protection
Integrity   Quality
Privacy

CORE COMPETENCIES

Apply business principles using   Management of information systems
  information systems and data   and big data
Big data analysis   Understand value and its relation to big
Effective communication   data and information systems

Introduction

Health care remains at a crossroad with constant change imposed by competition, a pandemic, regulatory mandates, and consumers who are informed and technologically knowledgeable. Survival will depend on multiple factors. The use of big data will be a contributing factor for a healthcare organization's survival. This chapter builds upon the content in Chapter 9, defining big data and information systems within the context of their value to continuous improvement. The importance of stakeholders and partnerships will be briefly discussed as they relate to information system development, value, and management of big data. The importance of the five Vs of big data to measurement and improvement sustainability are addressed. The content will conclude with an overview of the relevance of data quality, integrity, and accuracy for future improvement priorities.

Big Data and Information Systems Defined and the Link to Value

To define big data and information systems within the context of healthcare value requires one to consider the human computer interaction and information systems. Further consideration that links decision support processes and workflow generated from discrete electronic clinical documentation inputs is required to define each term. An impactful advantage that adds value is realized as data are entered once and used multiple times and ways (Sensmeier, 2015).

Value must be attainable and measured to ensure that information is relevant and advances the mission and goals of an organization. Although measuring value is complex, using multiple sources will assist in the process. Complexity science supports this notion and can inform how value is determined and documented. Linking projects to the correct metrics are central for measuring value (Porter-O'Grady & Malloch, 2015). To measure the value of health-related improvement projects, Gallagher (2012) identified five phases that provide valuable information for personnel ranging from the novice to the expert: First, the initiation phase should involve an informaticist when developing project requirements, scope, and vendor contracts and requirements. This can eliminate incongruity between customer expectations and the product. Second, the planning phase includes the determination of tasks to ensure design, workflow, and barrier identification. Third, execution begins, and the end users of the project are involved as products are tested, adjustments are made, super users are identified, and education is continuous. The fourth stage involves monitoring to ensure all deliverables are met and issues are resolved. Otherwise, the progress of the project can be jeopardized, including the budget. In the final phase, closing, all open issues are resolved and any additional modifications are completed for a smooth and effective project that will have meaningful use to all involved.

As improvement projects are developed and implemented, considering the Donabedian (1978) model of structure, process, and outcome (discussed in Chapter 9) can assist team members to analyze the value of projects and link it to information systems. The publication of the Meaningful Use Final Rule (U.S. Department of Health and Human Services, 2014a) assists project developers as improvement processes are designed. This will contribute teams to measure the impact of enrolling patients in a clinical patient portal of many electronic medical record (EMR) systems. However, ensuring that the integrity of the data is maintained is a mandate that cannot be overlooked, as discussed further in this chapter.

Foundational to defining big data and information systems are contemplating how the first three industrial revolutions impacted modern society. Each industrial revolution basically changed the world, from the steam engine to the age of science and production to the ascent of technology. With the advent of the fourth industrial revolution (FIR, and referenced in the literature as 4I or Industry 4.0), change in the healthcare industry is occurring at an exponential rate. Although blurred boundaries between the physical, biological, and digital worlds exist, the FIR fuses a myriad of intricate advances being produced by data and technology.

Based upon historical and current impacts, big data is defined as large data sets that are available for computational analysis in order to reveal patterns, trends, and related associations in human behavior and interactions. Information systems are defined as mixtures of hardware, software, and networks interconnected for creation, collection, and distribution of data that support decisions within an organization (Bourgeois & Bourgeois, 2014; Gandomi & Haider, 2015; Laudon & Laudon, 2012; Valacich & Schneider, 2010).

As interprofessional project improvement teams form and are involved in change, data will continue to be analyzed to understand the causative factors that limit efficient operations. Through technology, the evolution from power to value becomes a reality. Opportunities necessary to change existing management styles and historical patterns of operation toward an environment embracing dedication to innovation and discovery emerge.

Expanded innovative systems and discoverable technologies will advance artificial intelligence, recording and data sharing, computational technologies, virtual reality, biotechnology, robotics, and personalized patient experiences. As the centrality of a global economy is expanded, big data will become the exchange of a digital landscape (Argarwal et al., 2010; Comstock, 2018; Schwab, 2017). Big data and information systems value focused on successful improvement will become commonplace as managers and teams are challenged to meet the healthcare demands of a global society.

Big Data and Information Systems as a Facilitator for Improvement

Electronic networks 24/7 provide access across points of care and offer numerous advantages for improvement. Improving outcomes and remaining competitive will be enhanced if teams understand informatics, computers, and the value of big data (Kelly, 2012). Knowledge is being familiar with the environment through experience and association that provides understanding for reasoning and decisions. Knowledge is the culmination of what is known that creates outcomes (Carper, 1978; Collins, 2021).

Information systems have created multiple opportunities for assisting healthcare systems and provider's response to patient needs as an advantage for big data. The multiple sources of big data, when understood and used efficiently, assist in identifying what is occurring without answering why. Big data is supported by small data as specific questions are addressed and creates new knowledge necessary to advance care (Beal, 2014; Henly, 2014; McCartney, 2015).

As facilitators for big data and information systems, the organizational mission statement and critical success factors (CSF) support improvement. Data-centrality is recognized as the nucleus for patient-centric care. As the project is planned, reviewing the organizational mission statement and linking the project focus to the mission can directly and indirectly prove beneficial in securing buy-in and support. Examples of the benefits from such links may include financial benefits, meeting quality service and patient and/or employee satisfaction objectives, or continuous opportunities that provide value for learning and growth.

CSFs must work effectively to ensure high performance within an organization. For example, CSFs are used to prioritize operational initiatives and assist leaders in choosing the most pressing and relevant activities and projects to initiate and support. Being cognizant of these factors and linking them to the project improvement processes will yield positive outcomes.

The Importance of Stakeholders, Partnerships, and Information Systems Using Data Big or Small as Improvement Projects Are Developed

Identifying and engaging stakeholders, developing lasting partnerships dedicated to improvement, and using available data (big or small) are critical to any improvement project's success. Information systems and current technology must be an integral part of data retrieval, sharing, and meaningful use to an organization. Stakeholders and partner participation reinforce the centrality and importance of big data when supported by state-of-the-art information systems.

An imperative for participation by stakeholders and ongoing partnerships is the commitment and value that the information systems and technology development provide in advancing project improvements within any organization. The demand for improvement endeavors that add value and invest in information systems will continuously be emphasized. Otherwise, gaps in clinical care will not be closed. End users must assist in communicating to stakeholders and partners the utility that supporting all improvement projects, implementation, and their sustainability will create.

As a student or expert project developer considers and plans improvement projects or redesigns those that may have previously failed, big data and small data, information systems, technology investment, and partnerships among project leaders and departments will create a competitive edge for any organization. The magnitude of this effect will depend on how well information systems and the use of technology are designed in relationship to other business and organizational metrics. As knowledge is generated and spread, and the information generated in terms of local project outcomes is interconnected with national and international information resources, variability among data (big or small) will be minimized. Information exchanges will therefore guide clinical and organizational decisions (Sicotte & Paré, 2010; Tang et al., 2018). Opportunities for avoiding and managing risk will be created and errors reduced. The content of information exchanges will be strengthened as informatics core competencies and skill sets are developed and utilized, as discussed in Chapter 9. Although initially viewed as a challenge, potentials for big data use, analysis, and sharing are a greater potential (Collins, 2021; Sivarajah et al., 2017).

Keys to Positive and Sustainable Project Outcomes: The Five Vs of Big Data

Data produces value and guides healthcare decisions. Big data offers healthcare managers opportunities to evaluate processes, quantify outcomes, and translate knowledge into improved decisions and performance (McAfee & Brynjolfsson, 2012). The evolution of big data and its significance for health care are demonstrated by the five Vs of big data (volume, velocity, variety, veracity, and value) (Brennan & Bakken, 2015; Broome, 2016; Laney, 2001).

Volume refers to the size of data that extends beyond use and management of the right tools used such as Microsoft Access or Oracle. Understanding why data is being analyzed exceeds the tool used. *Velocity* describes data rates generated and can be more valuable than volume. *Variety* focuses on numerous sources and data types. Examples include data from smartphones, social networks, electronic communication, and other digital information. *Veracity* is related to questioning if the integrity of data can inform decisions. In 2015, Brennan and Bakken stated multiple uncertainties could exist by the very nature of how data are collected and analyzed. Lastly, *value* refers to opportunities for healthcare organizations to be innovative as volumes of data are transformed into a cost–benefit analysis (Brennan & Bakken, 2015; Broome, 2016; Collins, 2021; Laney, 2001).

Unquestionably, big data is generated from substantial amounts of public data from multiple sources and measures. Examples include provider data, surveys, numerators, denominators, risk-adjusted rates and factors, and regulatory by-products that are linked to performance and reimbursement. Big data exist as information is synthesized and used to create knowledge, new measures of performance and reimbursement, policies, standards, and publicly reported data. Big data has and will continue to offer huge opportunities for healthcare organizations and enterprises. The ultimate prize for any enterprise is the knowledge and wisdom from big data that may be used to produce value (Collins, 2021).

Data Integrity, Accuracy, Relevance, and Use for Future Improvement Priorities

Health information systems and technology make it possible for all providers to engage in patient-centered care and to manage care through secure use and sharing of health information. Maintaining data integrity, security, and privacy is a shared responsibility. It is necessary for all care providers, including students, to receive the necessary education to support safe, secure, and trustworthy practice in the healthcare system. As changes in the care delivery system continue to multiply, it is imperative to consider all of the regulatory and technological changes and any changes that impact practice—including any data that are collected during projects and used to change practice. These considerations provide a blueprint for future improvement opportunities and priorities.

Meaningful project improvement requires a commitment to both data security and protection of human subjects. This understanding is steered by the sensitivity of the data and the consequences for data compromise. Despite precautions, cybercrime continues to rise (Conaty-Buck, 2017). As an improvement project or research begins and data are collected and stored, adhering to the mandates of the Health Insurance Portability and Accountability Act (HIPAA) is essential. This act outlines administrative, physical, and technical safeguards to ensure confidentiality, integrity, and availability of electronic protected health information (U.S. Department of Health and Human Services, 2014b).

Being mindful of data integrity, security, and human-subject protection must happen in parallel with measures to address ethical, legal, and security issues. Although these issues may be primary responsibilities of the organization as outlined in various organizational policies and procedures, the shared responsibility of users of that information cannot be dismissed. Numerous safeguards and processes may be established, but individual responsibility in adhering to and respecting them is the key to maintaining the integrity and protection of data and an individual's privacy.

Summary

- The footprint of data and processes related to information that systems provide are foundational to understanding the value of data in the healthcare market.
- Big data and its value in health care cannot be minimized.

- When data integrity is questioned, the five Vs of big data provide processes to solve issues for the achievement of stated goals and continuous improvement.
- Without information, knowledge development is diminished and organizational stability is in jeopardy.
- Data and human protection are essential to avoid ethical, legal, and security issues.

Reflection Questions and Learning Activities

1. How can the five Vs of big data be used for large data set analyses? Based on your response, develop key talking points that could be used during a discussion with the chief of information management.
2. What are the key ways that big and small data are collected and used by organizations that contribute to the outcome of an improvement initiative?
3. How may value be identified using data? Develop a brief white paper for your response.
4. What are three ways a clinical project may engage stakeholders and partners in achieving meaningful outcomes?
5. Why would improvement teams be concerned with the ethical, legal, and human protection of individuals when using and managing data?

References

Agarwal, R., Guodon, G., DesRoches, C., & Jha, A. K. (2010). Research commentary—The digital transformation of healthcare: Current status and the road ahead. *Journal of Management Information Systems, 21*(4), 796–809. https://doi.org/10.1287/isre.1100.0327

Beal, V. (2014). *Big data*. https://www.webopedia.com/TERM/B/big_data.html

Bourgeois, D., & Bourgeois, D. T. (2014). Chapter 1: What is an information system? In *Information Systems for Business and Beyond* (pp. 1–15). Saylor Academy.

Brennan, P. F., & Bakken, S. (2015). Nursing needs big data and big data needs nursing. *Journal of Nursing Scholarship, 47*(5), 477–484. https://doi.org/10.1111/jnu.12159

Broome, M. E. (2016). Big data, data science, and big contributions. *Nursing Outlook, 64*(2), 113–114. http://dx.doi.org/10.1016/j.outlook.2016.02.001

Carper, B. A. (1978). Fundamental ways of knowing in nursing. *Advances in Nursing Science, 1*(1), 13–24.

Collins, B. (2021). Big data: Understanding its value. In P. L. Thomas, J. L. Harris, & B. Collins, *Data-driven quality improvement and sustainability in healthcare: An interprofessional approach* (pp. 99–116). Springer Publishing.

Comstock, J. (2018). *Digital therapeutics alliance releases definition, best practices for burgeoning space.* https://www.dtxallince.org/wp-content/uploads/2018/09/DTA-Report_DTx-Industry-Foundations.pdf

Conaty-Buck, S. (2017). Cybersecurity and healthcare records. Tips for ensuring patient safety and privacy. *American Nurse Today, 12*(9), 62–65.

Donabedian, A. (1978). The quality of medical care. *Science, 4344*, 856–864. https://doi.org/10.1126/science.417400

Gallagher, T. (2012, October 8). The role of informatics in project management. *HIMSS Clinical Informatics Insights.* http://www.himss.org/News/NewsDetail.aspx?ItemNumber=3128

Gandomi, A., & Haider, M. (2015). Beyond the hype: Big data concepts, methods, and analytics. *International Journal of Information Management, 35*(2), 137–144. https://doi.org/10.1016/j.ijinfomgt.2014.10.007

Henly, S. J. (2014). Mother load and mining tools: Big data for science. *Nursing Research, 63*(3), 155.

Kelly, P. (2012). *Nursing leadership and management* (3rd ed.). Delmar.

Laney, D. (2001). *3D data management: Controlling data volume, velocity, and variety*. https://blogs
.gartner.com/doug-laney/files/2012/01/ad949-3D-Data-Management-Controlling-Data-Volume
-Velocity-and-Variety.pdf

Laudon, K. C., & Laudon, J. P. (2012). *Management information systems* (12th ed.). Prentice-Hall.

McAfee, A., & Brynjolfsson, E. (2012). Big data: The management revolution. *Harvard Business
Review*, *90*(10), 60–66.

McCartney, P. R. (2015). Big data science. *The American Journal of Maternal/Child Nursing*, *40*(2),
130.

Porter-O'Grady, T., & Malloch, K. (2015). *Quantum leadership: Building better partnerships for sustainable health*. Jones & Bartlett Learning.

Schwab, K. (2017). *The fourth industrial revolution*. Penguin Random House.

Sensmeier, J. (2015, April). Big data and the future of nursing knowledge. *Nursing Management*,
46(4), 22–27. https://doi.10.1097/01.NUMA.0000462365.53035.7d

Sicotte, C., & Paré, G. (2010). Success in health information exchange: Solving the implementation
puzzle. *Social Science & Medicine*, *8*(70), 1159–1165.

Sivarajah, U., Kamal, M. M., Irani, Z., & Weerakkody, V. (2017). Critical analysis of big data challenges and analytical methods. *Journal of Business Research*, *70*, 263–286.

Tang, T., Lim, M. E., Mansfield, E., McLachlan, A., & Quan, S. D. (2018). Clinician user involvement in the real world: Designing an electronic tool to improve interprofessional communication and collaboration in a hospital setting. *International Journal of Medical Informatics*, *110*,
90–97.

U.S. Department of Health and Human Services. (2014a). 42 CRF Part 495. *Federal Register*,
79(171).

U.S. Department of Health and Human Services. (2014b). *FY 2014 HHS agency financial report*.
https://www.hhs.gov/sites/default/files/afr/fy2014-agency-financial-report-final.pdf

Valacich, J., & Schneider, C. (2010). *Managing in the digital world* (4th ed.). Prentice-Hall.

Case Exemplars

Data and Information Systems: A Valuable Asset for Nursing Informatics Projects

Todd Harlan

As technology has evolved, so has information systems and nursing informatics. As a leader of an informatics program preparing master's and doctoral nursing students, an overarching theme is coaching students to strengthen their skill sets for success within the industry and organizations. As students matriculate nationally through informatics tracks, project plans and products must be developed that are based on need and data to address constantly changing care needs. Outcomes from the developed products will be evaluated both directly and indirectly, as patient care processes are improved and their sustainable value is realized economically.

Students engage in a series of purposeful activities during the process of selecting improvement projects. A needs assessment is central to understanding challenges in all organizations, whether at the micro-, meso-, or macro-level. The assessment findings require validation, and teams are often used to perform this task. Of note, more interprofessional team validation of findings has become commonplace with the advent of the EMR and big data sets of information publicly available, as it crosses all disciplines. The improvement project plan is then developed based on the assessment findings, industry standards, best available evidence, and stakeholder engagement. Students seek and attain approval before progressing with any project, including institutional review board (IRB) approvals. Throughout the process, venues are abundant for additional student knowledge attainment and synergy of stakeholders as the plan matures and informatics products are created and implemented.

According to McGonigle and Mastrian (2015), the time interval between conduct of research, project outcome dissemination, and clinical translation can be significant. Both patient and system outcomes may be affected adversely by such delays. The issue within many organizations is translating the data that are embedded within the EMR and trying to extrapolate that information for improved patient outcomes.

During their tenure as informatics program leaders, several students have collaboratively developed systems that support an infrastructure aimed at ensuring quality and safety. One example of a value-based collaborative project is a computerized provider order entry (CPOE) system. Such systems allow physicians to capture order information and access other materials that can improve the overall delivery of care and improve patient outcomes. The Healthcare Information Technology for Economic and Clinical Health (HITECH) provision of the American Recovery and Reinvestment Act provided the supporting rationale for the project. This act provides funding to assist with the development of a health information technology (IT) infrastructure that subsequently improves quality and healthcare safety (Radley et al., 2012). Among the provisions noted were incentive payments to physicians and healthcare facilities to support health IT, including CPOE implementation.

Whereas the CPOE example was specific to one discipline's actions, other projects have focused on issues that directly affect patient care and outcomes. Regardless of the IT project, students tend to identify that the task can be daunting and in some cases very difficult to implement. The constantly changing healthcare landscape, reimbursement issues, and accreditation mandates will require easily extractable data for project success. All student projects are vital to the overall knowledge gained within the theory portions of the informatics track. For the primary instructor, ensuring that students are attaining the stated learning objectives and are assigned to knowledgeable preceptors is essential for success.

Nursing informatics will continue to emerge as a dynamic and value-added asset as care delivery shifts to community settings. The development of integrated IT systems will only expand in the coordination of healthcare delivery. Nurses are in pivotal positions to address this call to action.

Reflection Questions

1. When assessing the process of an improvement project, what is a central requirement that is crucial to the success of the project? Describe this process, and discuss the advantages and disadvantages if it is not followed.
2. Discuss the premise of data research and dissemination, and explain how the time between these two phases can affect desired outcomes.
3. As discussed in the case study, CPOE and big data offer many advantages to physicians and other healthcare providers. Expand on these advantages; also discuss any disadvantages that may exist and become constraints to progress.

References

McGonigle, D., & Mastrian, K. (2015). *Nursing informatics and the foundation of knowledge* (3rd ed.). Jones & Bartlett Learning.

Radley, D., Wasserman, M., Olsho, L., Shoemaker, S., Spranca, M., & Bradshaw, B. (2012). Reduction in medication errors in hospitals due to adoption of computerized provider order entry systems. *Journal of the Medical Informatics Association*, 20(3), 470–476. https://doi.org/10.1136/2012-001241

Increasing Nurse Awareness When Administering Medications: The Creation of a Dashboard Warning System

Amy Campbell

Problem Statement

The Institute of Medicine (IOM) has identified medication errors as being a significant problem causing over 400,000 serious injuries and between 48,000 and 98,000 deaths yearly (IOM, 1999). Medication errors are defined by the Agency for Healthcare Research and Quality (AHRQ) as being any discrepancy in the medication dispensing process from pharmacy handling to the nurse administering the medication. A distracted nurse is at a higher risk for committing an error. In the complex healthcare environment where there are bells, warnings, and alerts everywhere, a central question remains: How can the nurse increase awareness before administering medications and avoid additional warning fatigue?

Knowledge Gap

How can a nurse be warned that they are at risk for committing an error without adding to the nurse's workload or indirectly causing more distraction?

Project Process and Evaluation Methods

A review of the literature on medication errors was completed to identify multiple causes and contributing factors in medication errors. Six main themes of errors were identified as the most common for affecting the nurse and increasing the risk for medication error: (1) working more than 40 hours a week, (2) large medication loads, (3) large patient loads, (4) large task loads, (5) interruptions, and (6) patient acuity. Quality improvement projects such as "quiet spaces," staffing changes, and modified scheduling were met with mild to moderate success in reducing errors, but old habits and rising healthcare costs mitigated the long-term success of these changes.

A workflow analysis of a medical–surgical/oncology floor found that nurses were often multitasking while working and were frequently interrupted during documentation and direct patient care by call-lights. The manager worked to maintain a maximum patient–nurse ratio of 1:6 and to schedule staff for no more than 3 days on before giving them 2 days off. A review of documentation revealed that data pertaining to the six identified factors were being gathered and stored in the hospital databases.

Stakeholders composed of the manager, quality improvement team, IT team, clinical analyst team, and leadership sponsor met with the doctor of nursing practice (DNP) student to review the problem, clearly define the scope of the project, and identify barriers and potential solutions to improve the project's success. Additional considerations related to the hospital's limited resources were also addressed. IRB and administration approval were obtained as part of the planning process.

A pre-post survey on patient safety was given to the nursing staff before the dashboard implementation and 30 days following. Data pertaining to the six risk factors were then harvested from the hospital databases for a 60-day period. The data were organized in order to match each patient's data risk factors (number of times the patient used the call-light, number of medications ordered for the patient, sepsis score, etc.) with the nurse who was providing care for that patient. The nurse's lack of situational awareness while administering medications was measured by the number of near-misses (NM) the nurse committed when scanning the wrong patient, wrong medication, or wrong dose or tried to administer a medication in the wrong time frame using a bar-code medication administration system (BCMA). The time frame for when the NM occurred and the nurse's current workload, patient acuity, and level of distraction in relation to the six risk factors were aligned.

An analysis of the historical data found that, even though not all six factors affected each nurse, at least one or two of the six influenced most nurses negatively. NM thresholds were then determined by the potential risk each factor had on each nurse. After speaking with the nursing staff and the manager, a dashboard design was created that allowed each nurse currently working to quickly visualize both their own NM risk level and that of peers using a stoplight color-coded system. The dashboard also identified which of the six factors were currently influencing each nurse's increased risk, allowing for the nurses to make personal modifications to their workflow and allowing for their peers to know how and when to offer assistance. The dashboard was placed within the same room as the automated medication dispensing system so that it would be easily visualized as nurses were getting ready to secure medications for their patient. During the 30-day implementation of the dashboard, NMs were reduced by 15.6%. The postimplementation survey suggested that the dashboard not only improved overall teamwork by 13%, with significant changes specifically noted in the area of respect for team, but also revealed a positive increase in 9 of the 12 patient safety culture areas measured, including a 37% increase in nursing-perceived overall patient safety and a 119% increase in frequency of error reporting. As an indirect result of improved teamwork, the average length of stay and discharge turnaround were both reduced. Results were presented to management, and two additional full-time employees were added to the unit to help reduce workload levels and NM risks.

Reflection Questions

1. What are the benefits of identifying causative factors for near-miss medication errors?
2. What role can members of an interprofessional project team play in developing a project to eliminate medication errors?

Reference

Institute of Medicine. (1999). *To err is human: Building a safer health system*. National Academies Press.

CHAPTER 12

Measuring the Value of Projects Within Organizations, Healthcare Systems, and Globally

Patricia L. Thomas
Michael Bleich

CHAPTER OBJECTIVES

1. Define value in project management.
2. Explore principles of project evaluation.
3. Identify team attributes, engaging experts, and project oversight responsibilities.
4. Describe communication requirements and dissemination strategies.

KEY TERMS

Communication
Dissemination
Evaluation plan

Evidence
Information management
Value

ROLES

Communicator
Decision-maker
Influencer
Information manager

Integrator
Leader
Risk anticipator

PROFESSIONAL VALUES

Altruism   Social justice
Integrity

CORE COMPETENCIES

Assessment   Evaluation
Coordination   Interpersonal influence
Critical thinking/appreciative inquiry   Leadership
Data analysis   Measurement
Data management   Risk reduction
Design   Systems thinking
Emotional intelligence

Introduction

When an organization undertakes a project, a major driver in decision-making is intention to align the work with the organization's mission and vision. Strategic alignment with the mission leverages constrained resources to be assigned to a proposed project as a priority. Allocation of resources typically requires shifting existing resources away from one project or program for use in the proposed project. This simple frame belies the essence of this chapter—that value must be attained and measured to ensure that the allocation of resources did, in fact, advance the organization's mission and vision and that the investment of resources yielded value to stakeholders.

Measuring value is difficult, both conceptually and practically. In recent years, significant efforts to establish consistent data definitions for reporting and transparency purposes have emerged that highlight key attributes of cost-effective, high-quality, low-cost care. Notably, the Institute for Healthcare Improvement's (IHI) Triple Aim, to provide quality care to populations served that is efficient, effective, and low cost, serves as a framework and driver for care improvement (IHI, 2021).

In 2012, the Centers for Medicare and Medicaid Services (CMS) introduced value-based purchasing, a program that provides incentive payments for the quality of care in hospitals, home health, and skilled nursing facilities. Centered on the Triple Aim, value-based programs move away from the quantity of care provided (volume) to the quality of care. Incentives also align to readmission rates and hospital-acquired conditions (CMS, 2017). The CMS hospital, home care, and skilled nursing facility comparison websites provide information on location-specific quality indicators and core measure benchmarks that define cost and quality parameters expected and achieved in organizations. The Hospital Quality Alliance, accreditors, regulators, and third-party payors have created and generated evidence and reporting mechanisms to influence organizational priorities for resource allocation to promote efforts that demonstrate value-added care delivery.

Recently, the COVID-19 pandemic has highlighted how investments in technology-based resources yielded high value and efficiency that enabled productivity and sustained operations when traditional care settings restricted access to traditional facilities for care. These provisions identified both regulatory modifications and care delivery setting modifications that expanded hospital care at home (or in the community) and modifications to existing practice settings to modify current practice settings or locations to meet care needs (CMS, 2020a, 2020b).

How Value Is Defined in Health Care

In recent years, U.S. healthcare spending represented nearly 18% of the gross domestic product (GDP), or $3.8 trillion, reflecting stabilization compared with predicted long-term spending trends; however, sustainability of the system remains a concern. In 2019, healthcare spending grew 4.6% (CMS, 2020c). Figures are not yet available to establish how the global COVID-19 pandemic and response will be reflected. The Institute of Medicine (IOM) stated, "The only sensible way to restrain costs is to enhance the value of the system, thus extracting more benefit from the dollars spent" (IOM, 2013, p. xi). With this context, improving productivity, efficiency, effectiveness, and coordination of care are the foci for value-added processes, projects, and programs. Although much has been written about quality improvement, project design, and measurement as vehicles to hardwire evidence-based practices in care delivery, variation in practice, variation in care delivery, and variation in outcomes remain. Now, coequal partner concepts, cost, and quality are cornerstones in healthcare debates, policy making, and care delivery decisions, whereas in the past, quality reigned as the principal goal. Irrespective of the project or program, measurement of financial impacts is a necessity and inclusion and transparency related to cost are key to the credibility of the team, project sponsor, and project manager.

Notable change in the *Future of Nursing 2020–2030* report highlight definitions and goals to explicate value in payment systems, recognition of scope of practice, and contributions of disciplines in primary and acute care services that heretofore were not visible from a health and wellness perspective (National Academies of Science, Engineering, and Medicine, 2021). Recognizing team-based care and intervention, value is defined and articulated, recognized in payment structures, revealed in care delivery design, and showcased with an emphasis on the influence and impact of social determinants of health to foundationally change how care is delivered and outcomes are reported.

The American Hospital Association (AHA, 2019) established screening tools to engage care teams in assessment of social needs. In this value initiative, the AHA created screening tools to facilitate conversations and engage patients and care team members in conversation about nonmedical needs that were creating barriers to health. The focus of the value initiative is to facilitate dialogue and drive value by learning from patients to lower cost and improve outcomes by addressing social needs (AHA, 2019).

Measurement

To generate value, measurement of information is needed, usually drawn from databases but often collected specifically for a project, based on anticipated and desired outcomes. The information collected must be informative, meaning that a predesigned plan for its use has been determined. If it informs, then it must also be relevant to the project and sensitive so that it measures real differences in the project's anticipated impact. Further, information must be unbiased and comprehensive to capture the scope and magnitude of the project, such that the integrity of the project's impact is real. Measuring the impact of a project also requires timely information. Additionally, how that information is stored and maintained must be considered so that impact can be measured throughout the project's duration and in sustainability. In project management, information must be performance targeted to the goals and objectives of the project, collected in a uniform manner, and, importantly, cost-effective and possible to obtain. These attributes, as per Austin (1979), have been a foundation for project management and quality improvement changes over time.

The next challenge is how to capture value. Although the cost or expense of a service can define value, the healthcare industry has, at its foundation, people and the experiences they have while interacting with providers and health systems at the core. The perceptions of care held by all stakeholders, patients, family members, employees, and care-providing professional disciplines, as well as the organization's governing board, are guided by their unique and shared interests. Value is expressed by first knowing the stakeholders' interests. In the case of a project that influences organizational efficiencies, this may be measured in time saved, simplifying a complex task, replacing a way of working that is distasteful with one that is opposite, supplanting one method for another, and so on. There may be dimensions of cost-effectiveness, job autonomy, and other factors. The project manager must be clear about the stakeholders' needs and wants to form a baseline for comparison of outcomes. Similarly, if the project impacts patient care, then the patient's perceptions must be considered. Will the project create ease of access to care? Or will it provide for symptom management, influence quality of life, diminish pain or discomfort, or reduce the advancement of disease to a higher stage of chronicity? The project leader must be clear about the aim of the project and establish this from a value perspective. As stated earlier, measuring value is complex and requires considerable forethought and design (Fitzgerald, 2004; Koomans & Hilders, 2017). This is an often-missed step in healthcare project improvement initiatives.

If it is not already apparent, the project manager will play multiple roles in the measurement of project value. Measuring the value and impact of any project must be considered during design and before the onset of the project activities. The project manager must understand the genesis of the project, especially when a project is delegated as an opportunity for visibility and growth of the project manager. What were the organizational dynamics that led to the project? What are the strategic and operational impacts desired from the project? Who are the affected stakeholders? What, in the creation of change, is going to be lost and gained as a result of the project? The role of leadership comes into play by venturing into the unknown. The role of a manager is executed by guiding the project through a defined process. However, additional roles germane to this chapter are also relevant: The project manager must be strategic and must function as a planner, the communicator (which includes being a sleuth in order to understand people, processes, and structures that influence the project), a data analyst, and even a database administrator. Value, then, based on stakeholder expectations, may be expressed in terms of time saved, cost, convenience, access, simplicity of use, and more.

Project Evaluation

A common and accepted definition of project evaluation is, "The systematic collection of information about the activities, characteristics, and outcomes of program, services, policy, or processes, in order to make judgments about the program/process, improve effectiveness, and/or inform decisions about future development" (Bowen, 2012, p. 6; International Labour Organization, 2018). With this context, program evaluation informs management decisions where evaluation research generates knowledge that may be applicable to other settings. Value and valuing are central to evaluation. Scriven (1991) defined *evaluation* as "the process of determining the merit, worth, or value of something, or the product of that process" (p. 139), emphasizing that descriptive data are not considered evaluation. Evaluation is often used to improve and demonstrate the merit of programs or activities (summative evaluation) or to improve or refine a program (formative evaluation). In the design or development of a program, developmental evaluation is used. Where knowledge is limited, evaluation may be used to generate new knowledge (Bowen, 2012; Centers for Disease Control and Prevention [CDC], n.d.).

Steps in Program Evaluation

Although activities of program evaluation are presented sequentially, it is often an iterative process that is completed through different orders. Typically, a program evaluation includes:

1. Considering the evaluation purpose
2. Identifying stakeholders
3. Assessing evaluation expertise
4. Gathering relevant evidence
5. Building consensus (Bowen, 2012; CDC, n.d.)

Aligning Metrics with Project Aims

Projects vary in terms of the magnitude and scope of the change, the stakeholders involved, and the degree of linearity or complexity associated with the approach taken to manage the project. **Table 12-1** provides a useful framework for examining a project's level of complexity (Berger, 2005).

An example of a simple project might be the introduction of a product that is available at the point of care to encourage hand hygiene. The aim of the project has a defined location (bedside), a defined target audience (bedside caregivers), and a targeted aim (nosocomial infection reduction or prevention). As simple as this might seem, the project leader must consider what to measure. Should we measure handwashing compliance using the product? Should we measure changes in nosocomial infection rates? Will we measure the impact of the product in real time or retrospectively? Is there an existing database from which to draw information? Does one need to be created? Will we sample for outcomes or include the entire population? When is the best time to collect the data to represent the results with integrity and to reduce risk? Who will collect the data, and how will data collection be coordinated? From this example, there are many clues to indicate that the complexities of measuring value are endless.

Table 12-1 Project Characteristics as a Precursor to Metric Selection

Simple Project	Mid-Range Project	Complex Project
Stakeholders are limited to a select few, often with readily aligned values and needs.	Stakeholders are modest in number and cross boundaries within an organizational setting where values and needs are similar.	Stakeholders are large in number or are of varying disciplines with often disparate values and needs.
The project is primarily linear with clearly defined outcomes targeted at individuals and groups.	The project is both linear and nonlinear in that the outcomes extend to influence behaviors that are less defined and that focus at the group level of attainment.	The project is primarily nonlinear with less defined structure, and the outcomes cannot be clearly defined and are aimed at social change.
The project manager retains the ability to oversee and control each aspect of project activities.	The project manager works with a team to oversee and provide general direction while the project unfolds and morphs to meet unanticipated needs.	The project manager does not exist in one individual but rather extends to intersecting groups, all of whom share a common aim, and multiple strategies emerge to shape the direction of the project.
Metrics are simple to retrieve from existing data and can be readily observed or collected; feedback loops are easy to define and are often from a single source.	Metrics are retrieved from multiple data sources and may require development beyond what is available, with feedback loops required from multiple sources.	Metrics are retrieved from large databases and public opinion and must capture the multiple interests within divergent populations and stakeholders.
Metrics are focused on project completion and simple outcomes.	Metrics are focused on organizational impact and more complex outcomes, beyond project completion to project impact.	Metrics are focused on social change with complex social outcomes.
The value to measure is tied to a few defined concepts within a narrow range.	The value to measure is tied to multiple concepts within a broad organizational range.	The value to measure is tied to social concepts that cross organizational boundaries.

Case Study Application

A project manager has been appointed based on a community desire to be more heart healthy. The hospital responded favorably to this community request, which emanated from several organizations, including the YMCA, the statewide affiliate of the AHA, and civic leaders whose concern was a healthy workforce. A cardiovascular nurse leader was selected by the hospital CEO to lead the hospital's efforts to make a huge impact on cardiovascular health. The project aims included assuring that exercise was available to all age groups year-round, having one or more citizens trained in CPR reside on every city block, and placing a defibrillator device in all public buildings with an occupancy of 75 or more people. Note that, fortunately, the project aims were all measurable, which is not always the case.

The nurse leader charged with this project had a number of complex design challenges to think through, beginning with a willing spirit and strong personal values that the project was a good thing. Using Table 12-1 as a reference, the nurse determined that there were components of the project that could be subdivided and that crossed over all project levels from simple to complex. The leader recognized that the project had dimensions that addressed social justice and that there was an altruistic component to it. Evidence about cardiovascular disease supported the project and could be used for ideas about measuring the project's impact. Evidence that did not already exist also needed to be gathered. The following questions needed to be answered: How many establishments exist that accommodate 75 or more people? How many have automatic external defibrillators? Further, how many city blocks exist, and where do the city limits end? Does the charter really mean city blocks, or should suburbs be included? What are the ramifications if they are not included? What is the anticipated risk of limiting the project to the city? How does one define *exercise*? What are socially acceptable norms relating to exercise given weather conditions and public safety issues? How will the communities of interest value and accept the risk associated with exercise or the lack thereof?

Only when these and similar questions were answered could an effective metric design and information management plan emerge. Systems thinking was needed by the nurse leader to understand the interrelated components of the project and to recognize which parts of the project had linear, systematic, and predictable components to them versus other aspects of the project that targeted larger social and policy issues. In a brainstorming session around metrics, the following suggestions emerged:

- We could collect data on satisfaction with CPR training.
- We could count the number of individuals who exercise on a regular basis.
- We could look at the number of heart-related procedures that are performed at the local hospital and see if those go down.
- We could look at claims databases to check for cardiac risk factors.
- We could mandate that vending machines have their food choices altered to include healthy alternatives and count the changes.
- We could count the number of people who attend a health fair and have their blood pressure taken.
- We could restrict public smoking because of its link to heart disease and monitor heart disease occurrences.
- We could count the number of new exercise programs that are held in public places, including long-term-care facilities.

If you were going to use this list, how useful would it be to you? Which data are tied to simple, mid-range, and complex social change? How accessible is the information suggested? Is it performance targeted? Are they new or existing data? How do the data tie to the project objectives set forth? How do the metrics suggested integrate with the project? What would you change?

Principles of Project Evaluation Methods

Project evaluation is an effort to measure the impact of project-based change. The value proposition to be measured is derived from the stakeholders themselves, which often are diverse. One stakeholder (e.g., a shareholder) may have a singular interest in profit. Another stakeholder (e.g., a patient) may have an interest in access, cost, and quality. Regulators may want adherence to a defined set of standards. Many projects evolve from quality improvement initiatives, where metrics are a close "cousin" to project management metrics. In fact, the principles of developing metrics for quality improvement serve as a substantive guide for project evaluation (Berger, 2005; Bowen, 2012; Hamilton et al., 2020; Lloyd, 2004; McLees et al., 2015).

In order to adequately meet the needs of the stakeholders, the project manager (note that this is not a formal title but rather a temporary job assignment, such as in the case study) bears responsibility for measuring the impact of project objectives or aims. These objectives should be readily aligned with the organization's mission and purpose if the level of change is targeted within an institutional setting. However, some projects extend to multiple settings and are therefore more complex for determining a single value proposition. Insurance companies may have a desire to provide different health education, for instance, than what is desired by a provider–patient relationship. These differences must be accounted for in complex changes.

Some researchers describe project evaluation methods as being closely aligned with the field of program evaluation. As defined by Fink (1993), program evaluation is a diligent investigation of a program's characteristics and merits. Its purpose is to provide information on the effectiveness of projects so as to optimize the outcomes, efficiency, and quality of health care. Evaluations can analyze a program's structure, activities, and organization and examine its political and social environment. They can also appraise the achievements of a project's goals and objectives and the extent of its impact and costs.

Fink (1993) differentiated project and program evaluation from other types of research in that its major task is to judge a program's merits. She defined a meritorious program/project as one that has "worthy goals, achieves its standards of effectiveness, provides benefits to its participants, fully informs its participants of potential risks of participation, and does no harm" (1993, p. 2). Developing value metrics in an organizational context, then, can relate to measuring program objectives and activities, program outcomes, and program impact.

The methods used to capture data include both quantitative and qualitative strategies. As used here, quantitative methods include approaches that measure impact through mechanisms such as data retrieval from existing administrative and national databases; economic cost-effectiveness determination; surveys measuring perceptions; and targeted research instruments that measure patient, family, and societal outcomes that align with the project objectives and aims. Examples of quantitative data include selecting metrics from the following:

- Clinical/epidemiologic databases, such as those contained in disease registries or through epidemiologic surveys (Johantgen, 2005; Thomas et al., 2020)
- Administrative claims data at the organization or state level (Johantgen, 2005; Thomas et al., 2020)
- Sociodemographic data, such as that available through census reports and state-level vital statistics records (Thomas et al., 2020)
- Patient satisfaction data, such as that available through proprietary databases at the institutional level (Hayes, 2008; Thomas et al., 2020)
- National Data on Nursing Quality Indicators (NDNQI) data, applied at the institutional level (Montalvo, 2007; Trossman, 2006)
- Marketing data that specify lifestyle and other useful population practices (Thomas et al., 2020)

Similarly, qualitative data provide rich context for project impact. These data are available through the following:

- Focus groups with project-oriented aims
- Appreciative inquiry/storytelling methods aligned with stakeholder groups (Hung et al., 2018; Whitney & Trosten-Bloom, 2003)
- Internet and social networking approaches to capture context

Recently, engaging in data analytics and data mining has become a cornerstone of project evaluation. Given the expanded use of technology and multiple technological interfaces with individuals and groups, evaluation of projects through the analysis of processes integrated in electronic health records, self-reported assessments, health apps, and telehealth care visits has expanded. Recognition of the goal-directed touchpoints in health care, as well as interest in data mining and analysis, is growing (Erdogan & Tarhan, 2018; Thomas et al., 2020).

Information Dissemination: Roles and Responsibilities for Communication

The project manager has the ultimate responsibility to ensure that the impact of project implementation is reflected in useful ways to stakeholder groups. As early data are collected, the dissemination of information is critical to the stabilization of the project. Those engaged in the change need and want feedback on how the project is progressing. Although the full impact of change may be unknown in the early stages of data collection, it does provide motivation toward meeting project aims and objectives. Chapter 13 gives greater detail on the dissemination process.

Face-to-face communication is helpful, but when it comes to data presentation, it simply is not enough. The accountable project manager displays data using charts, survey tools, graphs, and other means to fully reflect the impact of the project during its implementation and at the conclusion of the intervention and continues to monitor postintervention effectiveness and restabilization. Today, electronic support of data presentation and analysis underscores the need to be transparent in all facets of program accountability.

Rarely do projects turn out exactly as planned. If the right metrics are selected, namely those that show sensitivity to the project aims and objectives, and if the data are reliably collected and displayed, then variation will occur from the plan. This does not mean failure of the project but, rather, presents an opportunity for the project leader and stakeholder groups to "torture the data," as John Ruskin was quoted as saying, such that meaning emerges from the data (Ruskin, 2010). In other words, data themselves do not signify the success or failure of a project. Only collective meaning and an eye toward improvement derive a project's success (Thomas et al., 2020). Too often, project managers feel the obligation to measure that which appears to denote success rather than capture what is successful—or not—about a project.

The presentation of feedback through quantitative and qualitative data presents the opportunity for the project leader to anticipate risk, integrate findings with lived reality, communicate a sense of purpose to the stakeholders, and design plans for improving the project past its due date and into the fabric of the work of the organization.

Especially in the case of projects that lead to system change, the use of statistical process control charts helps to determine the impact of the change and resets the new and improved standard, such that variation can be identified as that which is created by the system change itself (known as common cause variation) or as a major aberrancy that rests outside of the system change (special cause variation) (Deming, 1986). These techniques, used in quality improvement, are critical to help determine whether a changed system is performing in a desirable manner and quickly draw attention to special causes that are not related to the change itself. Although outside of the scope of this chapter, statistical process control tools should be within the realm of project managers to aid in decision-making and direction setting (Carey & Lloyd, 2001; Thomas et al., 2020).

Lastly, it is important to portray the effects of change to stakeholder groups. A final report, a summary email, a closure event to mark achievements, or the presence of run charts with notes attached to denote accomplishments are all mechanisms that can be employed to tell the story of the value that the project brought to the organization, its stakeholders, and others who evaluate the organization, such as external regulators, public constituency groups, and so on. Today, nurse leaders are not present often enough in the boardroom to discuss change, but a well-educated project leader, with the right tools for communication and data presentation, should be present at the venue to advance patient care and to inform others of the contributions of nursing and other healthcare professionals.

Tools of the Trade

In project management, inexpensive statistical process control software is readily available. Some basic procedures can be performed with an Excel spreadsheet. When these tools are used, the process changes that have occurred can be monitored for common cause and special cause variation, as described previously. The control chart that emanates from statistical process control powerfully documents change and variability (Best Excel Tutorial, 2021; Kelley, 1999).

Similarly, graphic presentation of data is useful, particularly when it can be modeled in a dashboard style of presentation. A dashboard presentation compares and contrasts metrics into a single document, such that patient outcomes, staff performance, economic data, and risk data, for example, can be studied as a set, aiding decision-making by displaying that one variable (e.g., cost savings) is not working against other variables (e.g., patient satisfaction). This is another important tool for decision-making and evaluation (Health IT Analytics, 2021; Nelson, 1995).

Summary

- Value is about knowing the specific stakeholder wants and needs related to the project. These can vary widely but often include access to service, cost-effective delivery of service, and satisfaction with the project's outcomes.
- Measuring value depends on the art and science of selecting metrics. Metrics must be informative, relevant, unbiased and comprehensive, action oriented, performance targeted, and cost-effective.
- Projects vary in complexity, and the metrics will vary accordingly.
- Metrics can include both quantitative and qualitative data; the former provides information about specific points of achievement, whereas the latter provides context. They are complementary.
- Project leaders are accountable for a fair and honest representation of the project and should be prepared to reveal progress toward the aims, as well as unanticipated outcomes, both positive and negative.
- Project leaders should use decision science tools, such as those associated with statistical process control and dashboard mapping, to represent their work and to adapt projects as needed.
- Data should support the project from before the onset of the project through to project stabilization, until the work is sustained as part of the way work is done.

Reflection Questions

1. What is the importance of defining a clear end-point vision before implementing a project? What role should stakeholders play in articulating this vision?
2. What role do standards setting play in selecting metrics? Does the role of Donabedian's (2003) structure → process → outcome model have any relevance in choosing metrics?
3. How do the research principles of data validity and reliability tie into data collection in project management? Do data that do not have confirmed validity and reliability play any role in evaluation?
4. How does one determine the cost of data collection and management compared with its relative value in project evaluation?

Learning Activities

1. Take an existing project and determine whether or not clear outcomes for the project were stated early on. Examine who the stakeholders were/should have been to establish these outcomes. Did a data collection plan exist that would measure the impact of the project?
2. Develop measurable and obtainable metrics for a project. Include with these metrics an operational definition to focus on what the metric measures and how it ties to the project. Develop a sampling plan for data collection including whether the data will be collected in real time or on a retrospective basis. Determine who will collect and display the data and whether it comes from an existing database or must be collected as new data. Prepare a plan for using the data at various phases during and after the project. Anticipate how the data will affect decision-making and provide feedback to stakeholders.

3. Generate a project evaluation plan based on a proposed project. What information was readily available to support evaluation? What was missing? Were values considered as part of the overall data management plan, and were specific metrics identified related to value?

References

American Hospital Association. (2019). *Screening for social needs: Guiding care teams to engage patients.* https://www.aha.org/system/files/media/file/2019/09/screening-for-social-needs-tool-value-initiative-rev-9-26-2019.pdf

Austin, C. (1979). *Information systems for hospital administration.* Health Administration Press.

Berger, S. (2005). *The power of clinical and financial metrics: Achieving success in your hospital.* Health Administration Press.

Best Excel Tutorial. (2021). *Statistical process control chart.* https://best-excel-tutorial.com/56-charts/371-statistical-process-control-chart

Bowen, S. (2012). *A guide to evaluation in health research.* Canadian Institutes of Health Research. http://www.cihr-irsc.gc.ca/e/45336.html

Carey, R. G., & Lloyd, R. C. (2001). *Measuring quality improvement in healthcare: A guide to statistical process control applications.* ASQ Quality Press.

Centers for Disease Control and Prevention. (n.d.). *Building our understanding: Key concepts of evaluation. What is it and how do you do it?* https://www.cdc.gov/nccdphp/dch/programs/healthycommunitiesprogram/tools/pdf/eval_planning.pdf

Centers for Medicare and Medicaid Services. (2017). *What are the value-based programs?* https://www.cms.gov/Medicare/Quality-Initiatives-Patient-Assessment-Instruments /Value-Based-Programs /Value-Based-Programs.html

Centers for Medicare and Medicaid Services. (2020a). *CMS announces comprehensive strategy to enhance hospital capacity amid COVID-19 surge.* https://www.cms.gov/newsroom/press-releases /cms-announces-comprehensive-strategy-enhance-hospital-capacity-amid-covid-19-surge

Centers for Medicare and Medicaid Services. (2020b). *CMS Innovation Center models COVID-19 related adjustments.* https://www.cms.gov/files/document/covid-innovation-model-flexibilities .pdf

Centers for Medicare and Medicaid Services. (2020c). *Historical.* https://www.cms.gov/Research -Statistics-Data-and-Systems/Statistics-Trends-and-Reports/NationalHealthExpendData /NationalHealthAccountsHistorical

Deming, W. E. (1986). *Out of the crisis.* MIT Press.

Donabedian, A. (2003). *An introduction to quality assurance in health care.* Oxford University Press.

Erdogan, T. G., & Tarhan, A. (2018). A goal-driven evaluation method based on process mining for healthcare processes. *Applied Sciences, 8*(6), 894. https://doi.org/10.3390/app8060894

Fink, A. (1993). *Evaluation fundamentals: Guiding health programs, research, and policy.* Sage.

Fitzgerald, M. (2004, July 15). Don't stop thinking about the value. *CIO Magazine, 17*(19), 66.

Hamilton, S., Jennings, A., & Forster, A. (2020). Development and evaluation of a quality improvement framework for healthcare. *International Journal for Quality in Health Care, 32*(7), 456–463. https://doi.org/10.1093/intqhc/mzaa075

Hayes, B. E. (2008). *Measuring customer satisfaction: Survey design, use, and statistical analysis methods* (3rd ed.). ASQ Quality Press.

Health IT Analytics. (2021). *Using visual analytics, big data dashboards for healthcare insights.* https://healthitanalytics.com/features/using-visual-analytics-big-data-dashboards-for -healthcare-insights

Hung, L., Phinney, A., Chaudhury, H., Rodney, P., Tabamo, J., & Bohl, D. (2018). Appreciative inquiry: Bridging research and practice in a hospital setting. *International Journal of Qualitative Methods, 17*(1). https://doi.org/10.1177/1609406918769444

Institute for Healthcare Improvement. (2021). *Triple Aim for populations: Overview.* http://www .ihi.org/Topics/TripleAim/Pages/Overview.aspx

Institute of Medicine. (2013). *Variation in health care spending: Target decision making, not geography.* The National Academies Press.

International Labour Office. (2018). *Project evaluation. Development cooperation internal governance manual/International Labour Office, Partnerships and Field Support Department*. https://www.ilo .org/wcmsp5/groups/public/---dgreports/---exrel/documents/genericdocument/wcms _172679.pdf

Johantgen, M. (2005). Uses of existing administrative and national databases. In C. Waltz, O. L. Strickland, & E. R. Lenz (Eds.), *Measurement in nursing and health research* (pp. 326–338). Springer.

Kelley, D. L. (1999). *How to use control charts for healthcare*. ASQ Quality Press.

Koomans, M., & Hilders, C. (2017). Design-driven leadership for value innovation in healthcare. *Design Management Journal, 11*(1), 43–57. https://doi.org/10.1111/dmj.12031

Lloyd, R. (2004). *Quality health care: A guide to developing and using indicators*. Jones & Bartlett Publishers.

McLees, A., Nawaz, S., Thomas, C., & Young, A. (2015). Defining and assessing quality improvement outcomes: A framework for public health. *American Journal of Public Health, 105*(suppl 2), S167–S173. https://doi.org/10.2105/AJPH.2014.302533

Montalvo, I. (2007, September 30). The national database of nursing quality indicators (NDNQI). *The Online Journal of Issues in Nursing, 12*(3), Manuscript 2. https://doi.org/10.3912/OJIN .Vol12No03Man02

National Academies of Sciences, Engineering, and Medicine. (2021). *The future of nursing 2020– 2030: Charting a path to achieve health equity*. The National Academies Press. https://doi .org/10.17226/25982

Nelson, E. (1995). Report cards or instrument panels: Who needs what? *Journal of Quality Improvement, 21*(4), 155–166. https://doi.org/10.1016/s1070-3241(16)30136-5

Ruskin, J. (2010). *The complete works of John Ruskin: Stones of Venice, Volume III*. National Library Association.

Scriven, M. (1991). *Evaluation thesaurus* (4th ed.). Sage.

Thomas, P., Collins, B., & Harris, J. (2020). *Data-driven quality improvement and sustainability in health care: An interprofessional approach*. Springer Publishing Company.

Trossman, S. (2006). Show us the data! NDNQI helps nurses link their care to quality. *The American Nurse, 38*(6), 1, 6.

Whitney, D., & Trosten-Bloom, A. (2003). *The power of appreciative inquiry: A practical guide to positive change*. Berrett-Koehler Publishers. PMID: 17283912

Innovation, Diffusion, and Dissemination of Improvement Project Outcomes

James L. Harris
Catherine Dearman

CHAPTER OBJECTIVES

1. Define *innovation, diffusion*, and *dissemination* with the context of improvement project outcomes.
2. Demonstrate how the alignment of innovation, diffusion, and dissemination advance continuous improvement and add value within an organization.
3. Discuss different forums, techniques, and other considerations for disseminating project outcomes.
4. Identify the role of appreciative inquiry in presentations.
5. Discuss the value of presentation and information sharing.
6. Recognize potential pitfalls in dissemination.

KEY TERMS

Appreciative inquiry	Outcomes
Diffusion	Posters
Dissemination	Presentations
Improvement	Publications
Information	Value
Innovation	

ROLES

Diffusor of evidence and outcomes	Presenter
Disseminator	Team member
Innovator	

PROFESSIONAL VALUES

Inclusivity   Professionalism

CORE COMPETENCIES

Adaptability   Measurement
Communication   Professionalism
Leadership

Introduction

Innovation, diffusion, and information dissemination are predominant factors recognized for success within contemporary health care. Although each has different meanings, their interconnectedness is fundamental to new ideologies of discovery and sharing of information. For innovation to occur, healthcare systems must consider different strategies and reasoning, questioning the status quo. Compendiums of different ideas that are respected and shared provide a solid foundation for continuous improvement. Without innovation, the discovery of new evidence, as well as its diffusion and dissemination, is absent. Missed opportunities occur and progress is stationary. For purposes of this chapter, the following definitions of innovation, diffusion, and dissemination apply.

Innovation is a process of knowledge creation and a mindset of creatively assimilating information along a continuum as problems are defined, solutions are found, and differing alternatives are accepted from project team outcomes (Fagerberg et al., 2005; Innovation SIG, 2017). The discovery of new knowledge is random by nature. Being adaptive, imaginative, and consistent in investment accelerates innovation, efficiency, and capacity within any organization. Christensen et al. (2016) proposed that as individuals and teams innovate, they are attempting to achieve solutions and progress in various situations. Without a rigorous and deliberate process to manage and guide innovation, the benefits become unlikely. A designated and skilled project leader is an essential element for innovation as teams ideate, innovate, and capitalize on the success inherent in a well-developed project (Shaker, 2015).

Diffusion is defined as "the process in which innovation is communicated through certain channels over time among the members of a social system" (Rogers, 2003, p. 5).

Diffusion involves effective communication, and meaning is assigned to various events and situations. For information to be useful, it must be tested and questioned. Otherwise, information and new methods are not adopted and knowledge attainment is a lost opportunity. Accepting the status quo becomes the norm with the loss of new opportunities and knowledge. As improvement team outcomes are created, information will inform processes and create a relative advantage adaptable to healthcare situations. Practice approaches are adopted and a culture of adaptation and adoption of new knowledge occurs.

Dissemination is an action associated with sharing information and knowledge widely using a variety of methods and techniques. What begins as a successful outcome in one setting is adopted by others to guide operational improvement. Value is therefore attributed to the successes that follow.

Dissemination of the results of projects and creative work promotes the exchange of information and extends impact. It is essential to sustaining innovation and applying outcomes into various outlets. Dissemination of designs, processes, and outcomes allows others to understand the value of a project and determine how a similar project within a system is applicable. Without dissemination, potential consumers within and outside the primary organization or system are unaware of project outcomes, which may impact use and future outcomes.

Projects naturally lend themselves to replicability within a system by the same team or similar teams. Replication of projects can, and arguably should, occur in other parts of an organization or in other organizations. Replicating a project can yield distinct and positive results that provide new opportunities to integrate findings. As a result, improved sustainability occurs and improvements are evidenced in quality and safety outcomes. Sustainability and replicability are inextricably linked to projects and outcomes. Dissemination is not to promote replication of the project itself; rather, dissemination provides a sample or a plan of how any innovation can be completed and applied.

Dissemination takes many forms and to some extent depends on the venue in which a project occurred. Nurse educators and those in the academic setting typically focus on the publication of articles in journals or papers and posters for verbal presentation. Clinicians and nurse executives, in contrast, share innovative work at a practice-based level. Healthcare systems attempting Magnet status must demonstrate participation in quality improvement projects and provide evidence of processes and results that are disseminated and sustained throughout a system. Larger healthcare systems use projects and other creative and innovative work to advance team members on a career ladder. Dissemination becomes an integral part of all of those processes.

The impact of a practice project or innovation is not limited to one or more healthcare systems or even one form of dissemination. Some innovations are best shared through social media, or blogs, in "lay" literature such as magazines.

Aligning Innovation, Diffusion, and Dissemination: The Value for Continuous Improvement

The alignment of innovation, diffusion, and dissemination, which are associated with improvement projects, requires a nonlinear progression of actions. Otherwise, the impact and value of continuous improvement project outcomes within a healthcare system is diminished (Rosing et al., 2011).

Inclusion of different perspectives offers opportunities for systems to align innovative projects to the mission and goals of a system or other organizations. The inclusion provides an avenue to explore different processes and individual ideas available that traditionally may have not challenged methods and patterns of care delivery. Clavelle et al. (2016) proposed the belief that the value of individual and team ideas provides an impetus to innovate and disseminate knowledge.

Consider how to use design thinking as a strategy for aligning innovation, diffusion, and dissemination to improve care. Historically used in business and engineering for developing services and products, design thinking is applicable to healthcare settings as the complexities levied by social, political, and financial pressures are confronted. Through a process of divergent and convergent thinking, the four phases of design thinking (discovery, define, develop, and delivery) provide a framework for aligning innovation, diffusion, and dissemination.

Discovery offers a healthcare system or any organization the opportunity to identify information regarding a population. *Define* provides an understanding of the identified population's issues that were discovered. *Develop* is a collaborative process whereby solutions are identified and tested. *Delivery* involves testing and analysis of solutions (Brooks-Carthon et al., 2021; Design Council, n.d.; Hasso et al., 2009). Each of the phases provides advantages necessary when one considers the alignment of innovative ideas and solutions, diffusion within any healthcare system, and dissemination.

As implementation science has advanced and been recognized as valuable to a healthcare setting, innovative inquiry for population health and future care advancement are being aligned through diffusion and dissemination of thought and acquired knowledge (Brown et al., 2017). This recognition supports the goals of the *Future of Nursing 2020–2030 Report* and embraces the need to reexamine strategies and actions used to advance health care within a global society (National Academies of Engineering, Science, and Medicine, 2021; Weberg & Davidson, 2019). Measuring innovation, its diffusion, and its dissemination will be an informant for change and future innovation. Void of innovation, diffusion, and dissemination, information and new knowledge are lost that would inform future constellations of healthcare systems (Davidson et al., 2017).

Forums and Techniques: Considerations for Disseminating Improvement Project Outcomes

The imperative to innovate, diffuse knowledge in healthcare systems, and share improvement project outcomes is a constant reminder of professional responsibility. Multiple forums, techniques, and considerations exist to achieve this goal. Examples include publications, presentations, social and informal forums, and the impact of appreciative inquiry. Although the examples provide valuable information for project outcomes, there are certain consequences associated with dissemination that must be considered. Different forums and techniques, followed by consequences of dissemination and the value of appreciative inquiry, will be discussed further in the chapter.

Most formal and many informal presentations involve the use of audio, audiovisual, or supportive technology, such as Microsoft's PowerPoint program, flip charts, storyboards, videos, and posters. The literature is replete with models and strategies to structure such presentations. Acronyms provide an easy method to remember the components a speaker needs to consider and address during preparation of a presentation. APPLE, which designates audience, presentation, purpose, language, and engagement, provides a simple framework that is amenable to any presentation, whether one will address a group of students or peers during an international meeting.

Consideration of the audience is critical to an effective presentation. Structuring a presentation that effectively represents the project and is predicated on the type of audience enhances the potential for a positive experience for each individual or group involved. Effective presentations reach out to and engage the audience as active participants in the experience.

The audience aspect of the APPLE model represents the intended audience or the actual one. The intended audience is the group one intends to reach, whereas the actual audience includes individuals who are exposed to the presentation. In any given venue, one may prepare a presentation for a group of individuals, but the attendees may not share the same views as evidenced by unexpected ways. The presenter needs to be prepared to address the audience (intended or actual) effectively and manage the interaction in order to achieve a successful presentation outcome.

The presentation itself may be oral or written and may or may not include visual aids. Most presentations are planned, but others may be formatted as spontaneous for sharing information and data. For example, a faculty member may be walking across campus when approached by a student or group of students who pose a question. The resulting dialogue could be termed a presentation of data, although little about the data is considered formal.

Personal preference and presentation style, as well as the venue itself, guides whether the presentation is formal or informal. A research conference venue that requires statistical methods and data outcomes to be presented in a formal style may be required. A conference designed to showcase teaching strategies or unit-specific interventions highlights various teaching strategies and engender dialogue may be the objective. Most presentations include a question-and-answer session, which allows the audience to fully engage with the content and the presenter. Successful interactions in the question-and-answer sessions can extend and expand the impact of the presentation. As one prepares to present, consider potential questions that may be raised by the audience and prepare to respond in a cogent manner.

In many cases, an abstract of the presentation is provided to the audience. With some instances, a completed manuscript is required with a verbal presentation. The abstract or paper is included in a "proceedings" document for the conference, which is recognized as a publication, doubling the benefit to the presenter in many organizations.

Poster presentations are another forum that provides a one-on-one opportunity to share the outcomes of the project and answer questions with an audience. A poster template is provided later in this chapter to guide content and placement.

The purpose of any paper or poster presentation has two primary aspects: explicit and implicit. The explicit purpose is the stated reason; the implicit purpose is what the presenter ultimately desires to accomplish. For example, one may state as a primary purpose to share the processes and outcomes of a project or innovation. The implicit purpose may be to further the presenter's career through sharing scholarly activity. The presenter's implicit purpose will be to shape the presentation to some extent and create outcomes that are consistent with and combined with an audience and an individual's presentation style.

The purpose of any presentation is to guide the development of the actual information to be presented and, combined with personal preference in style, drive the manner in which information is presented. For example, a researcher may wish to share outcomes formally that describe the internal processes and the outcomes. Sharing the outcomes of a project in a less formal style may identify the overall purpose of a presentation if an audience is encouraged to interact with the information and the presenter.

The language component of any presentation is another consideration where the tone by presenters includes diction and formality, voice and tense, objectivity versus self-reference, and scientific/professional versus lay terminology or street language. The evidence or the information being conveyed impacts the language used throughout a presentation. The audience must be considered as well. The astute presenter observes an audience's reaction and adjusts the presentation accordingly. The language may be supported by data, facts, opinions, direct observations, references to the work of others, and hearsay, among other forms. Language and tone flexibility will significantly enhance the presentation, similar to body language impacts to a one-on-one interaction.

Presenters are responsible for tailoring the language to the audience. Failure will negatively impact the entirety of the presentation. For example, if one prepares for a small, intimate gathering and encounters a large, boisterous audience, the language and style of presentation may need to be adjusted.

Engaging an audience requires maintaining eye contact, projecting a positive facial expression, and asking questions that elicit responses, either verbal or nonverbal. Other methods of engaging the audience include ensuring that objectives match content, ensuring that the abstract or description provided to a potential audience is congruent with the actual presentation, and maintaining a less formal style. Engagement, similar to beauty, can frequently be in the eye of the beholder. Individuals adopt a minimalistic personal style; others are effusive and ebullient. One's personal style may affect engagement in presentations offered in a different tone.

Remembering APPLE will facilitate the speaker's ability to structure an effective presentation. Other considerations for presentations include honoring time constraints imposed by the conference to facilitate smooth operation. Extending over time impacts both audiences and other speakers.

Presentations may also occur at a group event or a panel discussion. In those cases, the time frame is for the entire group, not for each individual speaker. Participating as a part of a group or a panel means a far more restrictive environment, resulting in less opportunity for individual members of the group to tailor personal presentations.

Visual and/or auditory aids are typically included along with the oral components of the presentation. Many speakers embed short videos or short computer interactions that make their point effectively and efficiently. If including these adjunctive methods, the speaker must be aware of the software and hardware interfaces available at the conference. Embedding a critical auditory or visual aid that is not effective in the venue can have a significant negative impact on the presentation. Presenters must always be aware that equipment may fail, be incompatible with the venue, be cumbersome, or be lost in transit; it is therefore critical to have a backup.

Additionally, entering the room allocated to the presentation in advance offers an opportunity. For example, the size of the room typically reflects the number of anticipated attendees, which may impact handouts, visual aids, or presentation style. A large room may have "inappropriately" placed barriers that inhibit viewing. Viewing a few slides from the presentation before beginning can assist the presenter to determine font size and color, the need for speakers to support audiovisual efforts, and a multitude of other considerations. In the case of presentations, it is generally better to be safe than sorry.

Role of Appreciative Inquiry in Presentations

Appreciative inquiry also must be considered as innovative project outcomes are diffused and disseminated. Appreciative inquiry is the coevolutionary search for the best in people, their organizations, and the relevant world around them. Appreciative inquiry gives life to a living system; presentations using appreciative inquiry provide an opportunity to share the hidden aspects of a system or a project that are not obvious to the audience. Appreciative inquiry includes the art and practice of asking questions that strengthen a system's capacity to comprehend, anticipate, and heighten the positive potential of a project or innovation (Cooperrider & Whitney, 2010).

Traditionally, a project is not communicated until it is completed, and an innovation is not considered complete until outcomes are communicated. In appreciative inquiry, communication of outcomes occurs throughout the entire process of innovation, thereby creating transparency and an evidence-based culture (Marchionni & Richer, 2007). The approach to be used to communicate outcomes requires forethought, flexibility, willingness to capitalize on the differing presentation strengths of team members, and the ability to view the innovation process entirely.

The personal style of the presenter is critical to an effective presentation. The component of personal style addresses the unique strengths and characteristics that blend well with different people and situations at different times. Identifying and capitalizing on one's strengths and matching them to the characteristics of the intended audience increase the opportunity to make a truly successful presentation. When presenting early findings, matching one's personal style with the intended audience is especially critical. Early findings are more tenuous and can be ambiguous. Even skilled presenters can be challenged if the audience is not receptive to the data. Presentation of information about an innovation is considered successful if the information is remembered favorably and implemented or applied to new situations.

Personal style includes personal appearance, ease of interacting in different settings, vocal qualities (including volume, tone, pitch, and intonation), and personal power. Habitual and deliberate use of gestures, ease of making eye contact, ability to listen, ability to communicate interest and enthusiasm about the topic, and willingness to accept criticism can either add to or detract from a presentation. Being aware of one's personal style is essential to making effective presentations (Rutledge et al., 2007).

Ensuring the sustainability of an innovation requires understanding the various factors that influence its dissemination. Appreciative inquiry provides the context for disseminating results that directly contribute to sustaining innovations within systems by making the implicit connections more explicit. In other words, sustainability rests on presentations making essential hidden connections more obvious for all to see. The result is transparency for the team, the system, and the audience (Havens et al., 2006).

Value of Publications and Information Sharing

Publications in academic circles are more valuable than other types of data sharing, such as posters, books, and book chapters. In this context, the word *publication* typically refers to an in-print or online paper that appears in a peer-reviewed journal.

"Peer-reviewed" indicates a level of quality review that exceeds that performed in non-peer-reviewed or any other type of publication. Other terms indicating a peer review are *refereed* (as in "contested and emerging victorious") and *juried* (as in "from a jury of one's peers"). Academicians, especially those in competitive systems, consider only peer-reviewed publications when making tenure and promotion decisions. Although online publications are becoming more mainstream, print journals remain at the top of the academic pecking order.

Tappen (2011) provided the following advice for would-be authors seeking publication of their work in peer-reviewed journals: endure criticism, maintain staying power, and tolerate revision. Seldom is one's paper accepted without revisions. Other advice regarding peer-reviewed publications includes choosing the journal wisely (i.e., read the articles in the journal, look at the purpose and types of articles typically published, and tailor the submission to those elements). Additionally, authors should read and follow the journal's requirements; compile the literature review properly; organize the paper appropriately with headings and other elements; proofread, proofread, proofread; format the manuscript correctly and double-check it; be willing and able to change the manuscript based on reviewers' comments; and refuse to concede defeat. Persistence and perseverance frequently win the day.

Books and book chapters are valuable learning and sharing tools, especially for those professionals early in their career or for health systems. Books and book chapters contain more of the surrounding details than can be shared in a poster or podium presentation and, therefore, are extremely useful for teaching others and for developing a strong writing style.

Posters are useful as mechanisms to share a lot of information quickly. A poster typically consists of a problem statement, findings, data elements, and outcomes. The poster presenter must consider how to provide these elements in a visually pleasing manner that is easy to read and understand (**Figure 13-1**). Poster sessions are frequently held during a conference at lunch or during breaks to allow larger exposure of presentations than can be accommodated with paper presentations. Poster presentations are far more informal and occur many times in a one-on-one fashion as interested audience members approach and read about the study. Handouts are especially helpful for poster presenters because they allow viewers to take the presentation with them.

Professional publications, presentations, books and book chapters, and posters all share some commonalities in terms of preparation, such as tailoring the submission to the audience, being aware of the sponsor's requirements and ensuring that they are followed, and being tolerant of suggestions to improve. The final element is perhaps the most difficult to accept, especially when people consider themselves to be "experts" on the topic.

Lay literature can be a valuable teaching tool for the general public. Academicians, however, would not presume to count a submission to a women's magazine or a newspaper as evidence of deserving tenure or promotion. However, publications that reach a wider population can be quite impactful, especially when the goal is to share "need-to-know" health information or to propose lifestyle changes. Many practitioners will find publication in lay journals to be as challenging as publication in peer-reviewed journals. Not only is the venue different, but also the purpose and the manner in which the information is produced are vastly different. The same

Figure 13-1 Sample Poster Format. Landscape Format Is Desired for Display

advice applies when submitting a manuscript to this type of publication: know the reputation and readership, follow directions, proofread, and take criticism well.

Social networking, such as via blogs, wikis, email, and face-to-face sharing, can be very valuable for disseminating a project. Many individuals can be reached through social media rather than through more traditional methods. In social networking, the message is more personal and more reflective of opinion based on evidence rather than limited to the evidence itself. In all social networking, presenters must be keenly aware of the audience, group dynamics, and spread of information.

Written reports can be a very valuable means of sharing information within a system, especially if one seeks to sustain the project or innovation. This type of publication requires the author to make a more businesslike and more streamlined presentation. A business case must be made and arguments formulated to achieve sustainability. Written reports are frequently shared with internal and external audiences such as external regulators. Above all, the author of such a report should avoid verbosity and adhere to the system's guidelines.

Press releases for television, radio, and newspaper can be another valuable tool for sharing information in a more informal fashion with a more selective audience. However, if you are being interviewed in these venues rather than writing the script yourself, be aware that you may be misquoted or "bumped" if a bigger story occurs. To avoid being misquoted, make an attempt to get review privileges before publication; you may encounter resistance from the media outlet because timing is critical, but such a review can save you from heartache.

Potential Pitfalls in Dissemination

It is critical to be aware of two major pitfalls that can occur with any sharing of information: redundant publication and self-plagiarism. Sometimes an innovation is innovative only for one's own system and is widely accepted outside that system. Becoming an expert on the information contained in the broader literature will prevent this error.

Self-plagiarism occurs when the researcher shares the same information with more than one publication or in more than one presentation. Typically, when one is invited to present or publish, the conference or the journal becomes the owner of the information shared. Subsequent publication or presentation of the data, even if you are the researcher who discovered the findings, is problematic. Focused presentations and publications that present one finding or a very limited amount of information can prevent this faux pas and can result in multiple publications and presentations, all different, from a single study, project, or innovation.

Projects typically involve teams of contributors rather than a single researcher. Dissemination opportunities expand exponentially with the number of people involved in the project development. Sharing a common understanding of how dissemination will occur and keeping the entire team apprised of all developments is critical to limit overexposure and reduce the potential for jeopardizing the data.

Because dissemination requires an ongoing exchange of information between and among project staff, specific planning for dissemination and audiences must be addressed at the inception of project development. Several factors and conditions affecting dissemination, adoption of a project's outcome, and the sustainability of the project must be included in all presentations: the advantages that the innovation has brought to the organization, the compatibility of the innovation with the organization, the complexity of the innovation, the ability to track and observe the elements of the innovation, the inherent risks to the project, the expected reversibility and ability to revise each individual element and the project as a whole, and the leadership and support of the organization. All of these elements are based on effective communication within the organization and an assessment of the agency's readiness to change.

Summary

- Diffusion and dissemination of innovative projects are parts of the natural progression of any endeavor.
- Innovation involves knowledge creation as learning occurs along a continuum that requires adaptation because of its random order.
- As innovations are shared, a critical mass of data are created that can be used to create value within healthcare systems.
- Various stimuli and information provide innovators to sustain a spirit of inquiry.
- Diffusion occurs through the communication and sharing of innovations.
- Relative advantage is an output of diffusion and dissemination of information.
- As others are engaged in improvement processes, innovative outcomes are adopted.

- Measuring the value of innovation is a required competency for leaders across numerous domains.
- Project diffusion and dissemination offer healthcare systems and audiences new knowledge and create an exchange of information.
- A number of forums are available for dissemination of information, including journal publications, book chapters, and poster and podium presentations.
- Multiple presentation methods and models are available; however, the APPLE model is widely used by individuals to prepare presentations.
- Presentations using appreciative inquiry provide opportunities to share aspects of a system or project that may not be obvious to the audience.
- Careful consideration should be given to where one publishes and presents findings, who maintains the copyright, and which pitfalls of dissemination may be encountered.

Reflection Questions

1. What strategies may be used to ensure innovation is supported and used to the relative advantage in any system?
2. Compare and contrast innovation, diffusion, and dissemination. Identify ways each are valued within healthcare systems.
3. Consider presentations you have attended in the past. What aspects engaged you? What aspects distracted you? How would you have changed the presentation had you been at the podium?
4. Which personal characteristics can impact a presentation or poster?
5. What strategies can be employed during and after a presentation to enhance the positives and decrease the negatives?
6. What actions do presenters need to take following a presentation to prepare for the next opportunity?

References

Brooks-Carthon, J. M., Brom, H., Kim, V., Hedgelan, T., Ponietowicz, E., & Cacchione, P. (2021). How innovation and design thinking can improve care. *American Journal Nurse, 16*(6), 30–33.

Brown, C. H., Curran, G., Palinkas, L. A., Aarons, G. A., Wells, K. B., & Cruden, G. (2017). An overview of research and evaluation designs for dissemination and implementation. *Annual Review of Public Health, 38,* 1–22. https://doi.org/10.1146/annurev-publhealth-031816-044215

Christensen, C. M., Hall, T., Dillon, K., & Duncan, D. S. (2016). *Competing against luck: The story of innovation and customer choice.* HarperCollins Publishers.

Clavelle, J. T., Porter-O'Grady, T. P., Weston, M. J., & Verran, J. V. (2016). Evolution structural empowerment: Moving from shared to professional governance. *Journal of Nursing Administration, 46*(6), 308–312. https://doi.org/10.1097/nna.0000000000000350

Cooperrider, D., & Whitney, D. (2010). A positive revolution in change: Appreciative inquiry. *AI Commons.* http://appreciativeinquiry.case.edu/intro/whatisai.cfm

Davidson, S., Weberg, D., Porter-O'Grady, T., & Malloch, K. (2017). *Leadership for evidence-based innovation in nursing and health professions.* Jones & Bartlett Learning.

Design Council. (n.d.). *What is the framework for innovation? Design Council's evolved Double Diamond.* https://design-council.org.uk/news-opinion/what-framework-innovation-Design-councils-evolved-double-diamond

Fagerberg, J., Mowrey, D. C., & Nelson, R. (2005). *The Oxford handbook of innovation.* Oxford University Press.

Hasso, P., Meinel, C., & Weinberg, U. (2009). *Design thinking.* Springer.

Havens, D. S., Wood, S. O., & Leeman, J. (2006). Improving nursing practice and patient care: Building capacity with appreciative inquiry. *Journal of Nursing Administration*, *36*(10), 463–470. https://doi.org/10.1097/00005110-200610000-00007

Innovation SIG. (2017). *Definition of innovation* (Unpublished document). The University of Iowa.

Marchionni, C., & Richer, M. C. (2007). Using appreciative inquiry to promote evidence-based practice in nursing: The glass is more than half full. *Nursing Leadership*, *20*(3), 86–97. https://doi.org/10.12927/cjnl.2007.19291

National Academies of Sciences, Engineering, and Medicine. (2021). *The future of nursing 2020–2030*. The National Academies Press. https://doi.org/10.17226/25982

Rogers, E. M. (2003). *Diffusion of innovations* (5th ed.). Free Press, A Division of Simon & Schuster, Inc.

Rosing, K., Frese, M., & Bausch, A. (2011). Explaining the heterogeneity of leadership-innovation relationship: Ambidextrous leadership. *The Leadership Quarterly*, *22*(5), 956–974. https://doi.org/10.1016/j.leaqua.2011.07.014

Rutledge, P. A., Bajaj, G., & Mucciolo, T. (2007). *Special edition: Using Microsoft Office PowerPoint 2007*. Que.

Shaker, K. (2015). Framing innovation. *PM Network*, *29*(7), 22–23.

Tappen, R. M. (2011). *Advanced nursing research: From theory to practice*. Jones & Bartlett Learning.

Weberg, D., & Davidson, S. (2019). *Leadership for evidence-based innovation in nursing and health professions*. Jones & Bartlett Learning.

Case Exemplar

Presentations Supplemented with PowerPoint Tips and Examples

Catherine Dearman

PowerPoint is an instructional design tool for presentations that is commonly used, especially in business and academic settings. Because PowerPoint presentations are extensions of the traditional presentation, the typical rules for presenting evidence apply. The information that follows provides novice presenters with essential information related to PowerPoint presentations.

A PowerPoint presentation is an adjunct to the verbal presentation, and as such it needs to supplement—not replace—the presenter's oral discussion. Most instructional design specialists indicate that there should be a maximum of one slide for each minute scheduled for the presentation. This basic setup includes the introductory slide, the reference slide, and the "Questions?" slide.

The basic rule of thumb for slide makeup is to include seven lines of text with seven words on each line (at most), for a total of 49 words per slide. At its best, the PowerPoint slide serves as a guide, prompting the presenter to mention salient points. The slides are not expected to contain every word that a presenter needs to say.

Inclusion of pictures on PowerPoint slides can be great, especially if they link to the topic at hand. For example, if the presentation is addressing community work groups building a playground, then including before, during, and after pictures would give a complete image to the audience and would replace words.

Most audiences typically prefer lighter backgrounds with darker text. Colors should complement, not detract from, the presentation.

Slide layouts sometimes intrude on the words the presenter wanted to show on the slides. Previewing the slides carefully before finalizing the layout will facilitate clarity and attractiveness.

Slide transitions, animation, and sound are all effective attention-getting devices. Use them cautiously, however. Not every slide needs a transition for each word. Flashing words are distracting to some viewers.

Before a presentation where visual aids (including PowerPoint slides) are used, the presenter is well advised to assess the environment of the presentation. Go into the room and look around. How many chairs are there? How large is the space? Is it square or rectangular? Are there impediments to full view of the screen, such as poles and projectors? Following this inspection, load the presentation onto the computer and display it. Go to the back of the room and see if the slides are clear or if adjustments in font or other elements are needed. Sometimes a color scheme for a slide looks great on a personal computer but does not communicate as well in a large group.

If the presentation is a result of funding, the funding agency typically prefers to be mentioned in some way. Some funders actually publish the statement they want used with every publication and/or presentation. Be sure to include these statements if they exist.

Index

Note: Page numbers followed by *f* or *t* indicate material in figures or tables, respectively.